CW00557374

# Vascular and Endovascular Consensus Update —Pathways of Care

BIBA Publishing, BIBA Medical Limited, 526 Fulham Road, Fulham, London, SW6 5NR.
www.bibamedical.com
First published in 2017 by BIBA Publishing.
ISBN: 978-0-9570419-6-7

©Roger M Greenhalgh, 2017

The right of Roger M Greenhalgh to be identified as editor of this work has been asserted by BIBA Publishing in accordance with sections 77 and 78 of the Copyright, Designs and Patents Act 1988.

British Library Cataloguing-in-Publication Data: A catalogue record for this book is available from the British Library.

All rights reserved. No part of this publication may be reproduced, stored in or introduced into a retrieval system, or transmitted, in any form, or by any means [electronic, mechanical, photocopying, recording, or otherwise] without prior written permission of the Publishers. This publication may not be lent, resold, hired out or otherwise be disposed of by way of trade in any form of binding or cover other than which it is published without prior consent of the Publishers. Any person who does any unauthorised act in relation to this publication may be liable to criminal prosecution and civil claims for damages.

Permissions may be sought from the Publishers at the shown address.

The use in this publication of trade names, trademarks, service marks, and similar terms, even if they are not identified as such, is not to be taken as an expression of opinion as to whether or not they are subject proprietary rights.

The author(s) have attempted to trace the copyright holders of all material reproduced in this publication.

### Limit of Liability/Disclaimer Warranty

The Publishers and author(s) make no representation or warranties with respect to the accuracy or completeness of the contents of this publication and specifically disclaim any warranties, including without limitation warranties of fitness of particular purpose. No warranty may be created or extended by sales of promotional materials. The advice and strategies contained herein may not be suitable for every situation. The publication is sold with the understanding that the Publishers are not rendering legal, accounting or other professional services. If professional assistance is required, the service of a competent professional person should be sought. No responsibility is assumed by the Publishers or author(s) for any loss of profit or any other commercial damages, injury and/or damage to persons or property as a matter of products liability, negligence or otherwise, or from the use or operation of any methods, products, instructions or ideas contained in the materials herein. The fact that an organisation or website is referred to in this publication as a citation and/or potential source of further information does not mean that the Publishers nor the author(s) endorse the information of the organisation or website may provide or recommendations it may make. Further, readers should be aware that the internet websites listed in this Work may have changed or disappeared in the period between when this publication was written and when it was read. Because of the rapid changes in medicine and medical sciences, independent verification should be made, especially in regards to drug usage and whether it complies with legislation and current standards of practice.

Head of Publishing: Marcio Brito; Managing editor: Dawn Elizabeth Powell. Subediting team: David Brennan, Susan Couch, Angela Gonzalez, Katherine Hignett, Urmila Kerslake and Amanda Nieves

Typeset by Naomi Amorra

Printed in the UK by Henry Ling Printers.

Published by BIBA Publishing, 2017

# Acute stroke consensus update—Pathways of care

# Thoracic aortic consensus update—Pathways of care

## Juxtarenal consensus update—Pathways of care

### Intervention methods & outcomes

## Radiation dose awareness in aortic interventions

# Abdominal aortic aneurysm consensus update— Pathways of care

# Peripheral arterial consensus update—Pathways of care

# Acute and critical ischaemia consensus update

# Drug-coated balloon consensus update

## Stent use consensus update

### Popliteal aneurysm and angiosome concept

### Below the knee

### Diabetic foot consensus update

# Venous consensus update—Pathways of care

## Investigations of superficial and deep venous anatomy

## Pelvic vein congestion and reflux

## Varicose vein management

## Leg ulceration

# Contributors

## A

**Agrusa CJ, MD**
New York-Presbyterian
Weill Cornell Medicine
New York, USA

**Aho P, MD, PhD**
Department of Vascular Surgery
Helsinki University Hospital
University of Helsinki
Helsinki, Finland

**Allan RB, B Hlth Sc, DMU**
Department of Vascular Surgery
Flinders Medical Centre and Flinders
University
Bedford Park, Australia

**Ameli-Renani S, MBBS, FRCR**
Department of Radiology
St George's Hospital
Blackshaw Road
London, UK

**Ancetti S, MD**
Vascular Surgery
Department of Experimental, Diagnostic
and Specialty Medicine
Policlinico Sant'Orsola Malpighi
University of Bologna
Bologna, Italy

**Ante M**
Department of Vascular and Endovascular
Surgery
University Hospital Heidelberg
Heidelberg, Germany

**Auricchio F, PhD**
Department of Civil Engineering and
Architecture
University of Pavia
Pavia, Italy

## B

**Bachhuber S, MD**
Department of Anaesthesiology
Kaiser Sunnyside Medical Center
Clackmans, USA

**Baderkahn H, MD**
Department of Surgical Sciences
Section of Vascular Surgery
Uppsala University
Uppsala, Sweden

**Batchelder AJ, MBChB (Hons), BSc,
MMedSci (Med Ed), MRCS, MAcadMEd**
University Hospitals of Leicester NHS Trust
Department of Vascular Surgery
Leicester Royal Infirmary
Infirmary Square
Leicester, UK

**Bicknell CD, BM, MD, FRCS**
Imperial College London
London, UK

**Bischoff MS, MD**
Department of Vascular and Endovascular
Surgery
University Hospital Heidelberg
Heidelberg, Germany

**Björck MD, PhD**
Department of Surgical Sciences
Uppsala University
Uppsala, Sweden

**Böckler D, Prof Dr MHBA**
Department of Vascular and Endovascular
Surgery
University Hospital Heidelberg
Heidelberg, Germany

**Boersen JT, MSc**
Department of Vascular Surgery
St Antonius Hospital
Nieuwegein, The Netherlands

**Bremer C, MD, PhD, Professor Radiology**
Westphalian Centre for Radiology
Münster, Germany

**Brinster CJ, MD**
Ochsner Clinic Foundation
New Orleans, USA

**Bruce S, Med Phys**
Department of Medical Physics
Uppsala University Hospital
Uppsala, Sweden

**Budtz-Lilly J, MD**
Department of Vascular Surgery
Århus University Hospital,
Århus , Denmark

## C

**Cafasso DE, DO, MPH**
New York-Presbyterian
Weill Cornell Medicine
New York, USA

**Cannavale A, MD**
Interventional Radiology Unit
Department of Radiology
Queen Elizabeth University Hospital
NHS Greater Glasgow and Clyde
Glasgow, UK

**Cervin A, MD**
Department of Surgical Sciences
Uppsala University
Uppsala, Sweden

**Cipollari S, MD**
Department of Cardiothoracic Surgery
Falk Cardiovascular Center
Stanford University School of Medicine
Stanford, USA

**Cleveland TJ, B Med Sci BM BS FRCS FRCR**
Sheffield Vascular Institute
Sheffield Teaching Hospitals
Northern General Hospital
Sheffield, UK

**Conti M, PhD**
Department of Civil Engineering and Architecture
University of Pavia
Pavia, Italy

**Criado FJ, MD**
MedStar Union Memorial Hospital
Baltimore, USA

## D

**D'Abate F, MSc, Clinical vascular scientist**
St George's Healthcare NHS Trust London
London, UK

**Dake M, MD**
Department of Cardiothoracic Surgery
Falk Cardiovascular Center
Stanford University School of Medicine
Stanford, USA

**De A Sandri G, MD**
Division of Vascular and Endovascular Surgery
Mayo Clinic
Rochester, USA

**De Beaufort HWL, MD**
Thoracic Aortic Research Centre
Policlinico San Donato IRCCS
Milan, Italy

**Debus ES, Prof, MD, FEBS, FEBVS**
Professor and chair
German Aortic Centre
Department for Vascular Medicine - University Heart Centre Hamburg
University Clinics of Hamburg-Eppendorf
Hamburg, Germany

**Despa OR, MD**
Angioclinic Vein Centers
Berlin, Germany

**De Vries JPPM, MD PhD**
Head of Department of Vascular Surgery
St Antonius Hospital
Nieuwegein, The Netherlands

**Diderrich A, RN**
Division of Vascular and Endovascular
Surgery
Mayo Clinic
Rochester, USA

**Djavani-Gidund K, MD, PhD**
Department of Surgical Sciences
Uppsala University
Uppsala, Sweden

**Donas KP, Assistant Professor**
St Franziskus Hospital
Münster, Germany

**Donayre C, MD**
Chief, Division Vascular Surgery
Irvine Medical Center, University of
California
Orange, USA

**Donselaar EJ, MD**
Division of Vascular Surgery
Rijnstate Hospital
Arnhem, The Netherlands

**Dwivedi K, B Med Sci BM BS**
Sheffield Vascular Institute
Sheffield Teaching Hospitals
Northern General Hospital
Sheffield, UK

# E

**El-Chamali S, MD**
Angioclinic Vein Centers
Berlin, Germany

**El-Sayed T, MRCS**
Academic Department of Vascular Surgery
Guy's and St Thomas' NHS Foundation
Trust
Cardiovascular Division, King's College
London
St Thomas' Hospital
London, UK

**England A, BSc(Hons), MSc, PhD**
University of Salford
Salford, UK

**Ersryd S, MD**
Department of Surgical Sciences
Uppsala University
Uppsala, Sweden

# F

**Faggioli G, MD, PhD, Prof**
Vascular Surgery
Department of Experimental, Diagnostic
and Specialty Medicine
Policlinico Sant'Orsola Malpighi
University of Bologna
Bologna, Italy

**Fanelli F, MD, EBIR**
Vascular and Interventional Radiology Unit
Department of Radiological Sciences
"SAPIENZA" – University of Rome
Rome, Italy

# G

**Gaines P, MB, ChB, FRCP, FRCR**
Sheffield Hallam University
Sheffield, UK

**Gallitto E, MD, PhD**
Vascular Surgery
Department of Experimental, Diagnostic
and Specialty Medicine
Policlinico Sant'Orsola Malpighi
University of Bologna
Bologna, Italy

**Gargiulo M, MD, PhD, Prof**
Vascular Surgery
Department of Experimental, Diagnostic
and Specialty Medicine
Policlinico Sant'Orsola Malpighi
University of Bologna
Bologna, Italy

**Gazzetti M, MD, PhD**
Villa Stuart Medical Center
Rome, Italy

**Geisbüsch P, MD, PhD**
Department of Vascular and Endovascular
Surgery
University Hospital Heidelberg
Heidelberg, Germany

**Giannoukas A, MD, MSc, PhD, FEBVS**
Department of Vascular Surgery
University Hospital of Larissa
Faculty of Medicine
School of Health Sciences
University of Thessaly
Larissa, Greece

**Gibbs R, MD FRCS**
Imperial College London
London, UK

**Girsocz E, MD, MSc**
Vascular Surgery and Kidney Transplant
Department
Nouvel Hopital Civil
Strasbourg, France

**Goodyear SJ MD, FRCS**
The Vascular Unit
Worcestershire Royal Hospital
Worcester, UK

**Gosslau Y, MD**
Department of Vascular Surgery
Klinikum Augsburg
Augsburg, Germany

**Grant SW, MBChB (Hons), MRCS, PhD**
Institute of Cardiovascular Sciences
University of Manchester
Manchester, UK

**Griffiths O, MBBS, MRCS**
Department of Vascular Surgery and
Wound Healing
Ysbyty Gwynedd
Bangor, UK

**Grover G, BSc, MBBS, MRCS**
Imperial College London
London, UK

# H

**Holewijn S, MSc, PhD**
Division of Vascular Surgery
Rijnstate Hospital Arnhem
Arnhem, The Netherlands

**Hoter J, RN**
Division of Vascular and Endovascular
Surgery
Mayo Clinic
Rochester, USA

**Hunckler J, M Eng**
Division of Surgery and Interventional
Science
University College London
London, UK

# J

**Jaffer U, BSc (Hons), MSc (Surgery), MSc
(Ulrasound), PhD, PGCE, FRCS**
Department of Vascular Surgery
Imperial College NHS Healthcare Trust
London, UK

**Jakob R, MD**
Department of Vascular Surgery
Klinikum Augsburg
Augsburg, Germany

**Jangland L, Med Phys**
Department of Medical Physics
Uppsala University Hospital
Uppsala, Sweden

## K

**Kanapathy M, MD, MRCS, MSc**
Division of Surgery and Interventional
Science, University College London
Department of Plastic Surgery, Royal Free
Hospital
London, UK

**Khoynezhad A, MD, PhD, FACS**
Director, Aortic Surgery
Cedas-Sinai Medical Center
Los Angeles, USA

**Kölbel T, MD, Prof**
German Aortic Centre
Department for Vascular Medicine -
University Heart Centre Hamburg
University Clinics of Hamburg-Eppendorf
Hamburg, Germany

**Kopchok G, BS**
Project Scientist
Division Vascular Surgery
Irvine Medical Center, University of
California,
Orange, USA

## L

**Laine M, MD**
Department of Vascular Surgery
Helsinki University Hospital
University of Helsinki
Helsinki, Finland

**Li MM, MBBS, BSc**
Imperial Vascular Unit
Division of Surgery and Cancer
Imperial College
London, UK

**Litchenberg M, MD**
Professor of Angiology
Klinikum Arnsberg
Arnsberg, Germany

## M

**Macedo T, MD, Professor**
Department of Radiology
Mayo Clinic
Rochester, USA

**Maili L, MD**
Department of Radiology
St George's Hospital
Blackshaw Road
London, UK

**Majoie CBLM, MD, PhD, Professor**
Department of Radiology
Neurovascular Interventional Center
Academic Medical Center
Amsterdam, The Netherlands

**Mani K, MD, PhD, FEBVS**
Department of Surgical Sciences
Section of Vascular Surgery
Uppsala University
Uppsala, Sweden

**Marrocco-Trischitta, MM**
Thoracic Aortic Research Centre
Policlinico San Donato IRCCS
Milan, Italy

**Martin-Gonzalez T, MD, PhD**
Royal Free Hospital
London, UK

**Mascoli C, MD**
Vascular Surgery
Department of Experimental, Diagnostic
and Specialty Medicine
Policlinico Sant'Orsola Malpighi
University of Bologna
Bologna, Italy

**Mastracci TM, MD**
Royal Free Hospital
London, UK

**Maurel B, MD, PhD**
University Hospital of Nantes
Hospital Nord Laennec
Nantes, France

**McCollum CN, MBChB, MD, FRCS**
Professor of Surgery
Academic Surgery Unit
University of Manchester
Manchester, UK

**McKeever S, DO**
University of Arkansas for Medical Sciences
Little Rock, USA

**McWilliams R, FRCR, EBIR**
Department of Radiology
Royal Liverpool University Hospital NHS Trust
Liverpool, UK

**Milner R, MD, FACS, Professor of Surgery**
Pritzer School of Medicine
University of Chicago
Chicago, USA

**Modarai B, PhD, FRCS**
Academic Department of Vascular Surgery
Guy's and St Thomas' NHS Foundation Trust
Cardiovascular Division, King's College London
St Thomas' Hospital
London, UK

**Moll FL, MD, PhD**
Department of Vascular Surgery
University Medical Center Utrecht
Utrecht, The Netherlands

**Morgan RA, MRCP, FRCR, EBIR**
Department of Radiology
St George's Hospital
Blackshaw Road
London, UK

**Morganti S, PhD**
Department of Civil Engineering and Architecture
University of Pavia
Pavia, Italy

**Mosahebi A, MBBS, FRCS, PhD, MBA**
Division of Surgery and Interventional Science, University College London
Department of Plastic Surgery, Royal Free Hospital
London, UK

## N

**Nauta FJH, MD, PhD**
Thoracic Aortic Research Centre
Policlinico San Donato IRCCS
Milan, Italy

**Nicolaides A, MS, FRCS, PhD (Hon)**
Emeritus professor of vascular surgery
Imperial College London, UK
Honorary professor of surgery
University of Nicosia Medical School
Nicosia, Cyprus

**Nicotera P, MD**
Service of International Radiology
Ospedale Regionale di Lugano
Lugano, Switzerland

**Normahani P, MBBS, BSc (Hons), MSc, MRCS (Eng)**
Department of Vascular Surgery
Imperial College NHS Healthcare Trust
London, UK

**Noronen K, MD, PhD**
Department of Vascular Surgery
Helsinki University Hospital
Helsinki Finland

**Nyamekye IK MD, FRCS**
The Vascular Unit
Worcestershire Royal Hospital
Worcester, UK

## O

**Oderich GS, MD, professor**
Division of Vascular and Endovascular Surgery
Mayo Clinic
Rochester, USA

# P

**Patel AS, PhD, MRCS**
Academic Department of Vascular Surgery
Guy's and St Thomas' NHS Foundation
Trust
Cardiovascular Division, King's College
London
St Thomas' Hospital
London, UK

**Pavlidis, MD, MSc, EBIR**
Department of Radiology
St George's Hospital
Blackshaw Road
London, UK

**Pini R, MD**
Vascular Surgery
Department of Experimental, Diagnostic
and Specialty Medicine
Policlinico Sant'Orsola Malpighi
University of Bologna
Bologna, Italy

**Powell-Chandler A, MBChB, MRCS**
Department of Vascular Surgery and
Wound Healing
Ysbyty Gwynedd
Bangor, UK

# R

**Ragg JC, MD**
Angioclinic Vein Centers
Berlin, Germany

**Reijnen MPJ, MD, PhD**
Division of Vascular Surgery
Rijnstate Hospital Arnhem
Arnhem, The Netherlands

**Ribeiro MS, MD, PhD**
Division of Vascular and Endovascular
Surgery
Mayo Clinic
Rochester, USA

**Richards T, MD, FRCS**
Division of Surgery and Interventional
Science
University College London
London, UK

**Riding DM, MSc, MEd, MBChB, MRCSEd**
Clinical Research Fellow
Academic Surgery Unit
University of Manchester
Manchester, UK

**Riga CV, MBBS, BSc, MD, FRCS**
Imperial Vascular Unit
Division of Surgery and Cancer
Imperial College
London, UK

**Romarowski RM, MSc**
Department of Civil Engineering and
Architecture
University of Pavia
Pavia, Italy

# S

**Santoni M, MD**
Vascular and Interventional Radiology Unit
Department of Radiological Sciences
"SAPIENZA" – University of Rome
Rome, Italy

**Sardanelli F, MD, PhD**
Department of Radiology
Policlinico San Donato IRCCS, University of
Milan
Milan, Italy

**Schneider DB, MD**
New York-Presbyterian
Weill Cornell Medicine
New York, USA

**Schnitzler L**
Chair for experimental physics, Biophysics
Working Group
University of Augsburg
Augsburg, Germany

**Secchi F, MD, PhD**
Department of Radiology
Policlinico San Donato IRCCS
Milan, Italy

**Settembre N, MD**
Department of Vascular Surgery
Helsinki University Hospital
Helsinki, Finland

**Skrypnik D**
Department of Vascular and Endovascular
Surgery
University Hospital Heidelberg
Heidelberg, Germany

**Smeds M, MD**
University of Arkansas for Medical Sciences
Little Rock, USA

**Smith A, PhD**
Academic Department of Vascular Surgery
Guy's and St Thomas' NHS Foundation
Trust
Cardiovascular Division, King's College
London
St Thomas' Hospital
London, UK

**Spanos K, MD, MSc, PhD**
Department of Vascular Surgery
University Hospital of Larissa
Faculty of Medicine
School of Health Sciences
University of Thessaly
Larissa, Greece

**Spark JI, MBChB, MD, FRCS (Eng), FRCS
(Gen Surg), PGCert Med US, FRACS
(Vasc)**
Department of Vascular Surgery
Flinders Medical Centre and Flinders
University
Bedford Park, South Australia

**Standfield NJ, MD, FRCS**
Department of Vascular Surgery
Imperial College NHS Healthcare Trust
London, UK

**Stella A, MD, PhD, Prof**
Vascular Surgery
Department of Experimental, Diagnostic
and Specialty Medicine
Policlinico Sant'Orsola Malpighi
University of Bologna
Bologna, Italy

**Stoyanova K, MD**
Angioclinic Vein Centers
Berlin, Germany

**Sullivan T, MD, FACS, FSVS, FACC**
Chairman of Vascular and Endovascular
Surgery
Minneapolis Heart Institute at Abbott
Northwest Hospital
Minneapolis, USA

# T

**Tepe G, MD**
Professor of Radiology
RoMed Clinic Rosenheim
Rosenheim, Germany

**Thaveau F, MD, PhD**
Vascular Surgery and Kidney Transplant
Department
Nouvel Hopital Civil
Strasbourg, France

**Torsello GB, University Professor**
Münster University Hospital
St. Franziskus Hospital
Münster, Germany

**Torsello GF, MD, BA**
Westphalian Centre for Radiology
Münster, Germany

**Treurniet K, MD, PhD student**
Department of Radiology
Neurovascular Interventional Center
Academic Medical Center
Amsterdam, The Netherlands

**Trimarchi S, MD, PhD**
Thoracic Aortic Research Centre
Policlinico San Donato IRCCS, University of Milan
Milan, Italy

**Trojan M, MD**
Department of Vascular and Endovascular Surgery
University Hospital Heidelberg
Heidelberg, Germany

**Tsilimparis N, MD, PhD**
German Aortic Centre
Department for Vascular Medicine - University Heart Centre Hamburg
University Clinics of Hamburg-Eppendorf
Hamburg, Germany

# V

**Van Bakel, TMJ, MD**
Thoracic Aortic Research Centre
Policlinico San Donato IRCCS
Milan, Italy

**Van den Berg, MD, PhD**
Centro Vascolare Ticino
Service of International Radiology
Ospedale Regionale di Lugano
Lugano, Switzerland
Universitätsinstitut für Diagnostische, Interventionelle und Pädiatrische Radiologie
Inselspital
Bern, Switzerland

**Van den Ham, LH, MD**
Division of Vascular Surgery
Rijnstate Hospital
Arnhem, The Netherlands

**Van Herwaarden, JA, MD, PhD**
Department of Vascular Surgery
University Medical Center Utrecht
Utrecht, The Netherlands

**Van Wijcj I**
Division of Vascular Surgery
Rijnstate Hospital Arnhem
Arnhem, The Netherlands

**Venermo M, MD, PhD**
Department of Vascular Surgery
Helsinki University Hospital
University of Helsinki
Helsinki, Finland

**Vikatmaa L, MD, PhD**
Department of Anaesthesiology, Intensive Care and Pain Medicine
Helsinki University Hospital
University of Helsinki
Helsinki, Finland

# W

**Wagstaff A MBChB**
The Vascular Unit
Worcestershire Royal Hospital
Worcester, UK

**Wanhainen A, MD PhD**
Department of Surgical Sciences
Section of Vascular Surgery
Uppsala University
Uppsala, Sweden

**White RA, MD, FACS**
Medical director/professor of surgery
Vascular Surgery
Long Beach Memorial Heart & Vascular Institute
Long Beach, USA

**Wigham JR, RN**
Division of Vascular and Endovascular Surgery
Mayo Clinic
Rochester, USA

**Williams DT, BSc, MSc, MD, FRCS**
Department of Vascular Surgery and Wound Healing
Ysbyty Gwynedd
Bangor, Wales, UK
School of Medical Sciences
Bangor University
Bangor, UK

**Wisely NA, MBChb, FRCA**
Department of Anaesthesia
University Hospital South Manchester
Manchester, UK

# Z

**Zeller T, MD, PhD**
Universitäts-Herzzentrum Freiburg – Bad
Krozingen
Bad Krozingen, Germany

**Zerwes Z, MD**
Department of Vascular Surgery
Klinikum Augsburg
Augsburg, Germany

# INTRODUCTION

This year we have **consensus** in the three-yearly cycle of controversies, challenges, consensus: **controversies** that enable a world-class faculty and an expert audience to **challenge** the available evidence to reach a **consensus** after discussion.

These introductory comments are made at a time when the Charing Cross Symposium is designed and all the speakers are in place. Selected speakers have written chapters for this book to give a flavour of some key education that will occur in April 2017 at CX 2017. However, the whole story is not told in the book and there will be new information on the day. This companion book has absolutely up to date comments written and finalised within two months of the event. Especially of interest are the references of the chapters such that the book is an excellent source of current knowledge.

In this **consensus** year, we have chosen to focus upon **pathways of care:**
- **WHETHER** to intervene and the benefit from it
- **WHEN** to intervene and at what threshold?
- **INTERVENTION METHOD** and evidence
- **FOLLOW-UP** and outcomes of intervention.

The authors have been asked to orientate their comments to the pathways. This is never more important than in the **Acute Stroke Consensus** section. This is because it is now clear that stroke from thoracic endovascular procedures has become a matter of interest since CX 2016. The endovascular surgeon performing procedures involving the ascending aorta, the arch, the great vessels off the arch or the subclavian artery, as well debranching procedures involving zone 2, are aware of the risk of stroke. Therefore, embolic filters have been employed in the attempt to reduce stroke risk in the thoracic endovascular aortic repair. The filters are catching all types of pathologies including materials from the stent graft as well as thrombus and pieces of atherosclerosis from the artery wall, but cannot stop air embolism!

Dissecting aortic aneurysms is another area where **pathways of care** have become crucial. Therefore, the re-look at the very definition of types A and B, the relevance of acute, subacute and chronic as clinical entities as well as methods of intervention come into focus. This caused us to ask authors to consider **whether** to intervene, if so, **when** to intervene and finally **method of intervention** and then **follow-up** of the method. It seems incumbent upon the operator to know if the operation is essential or not and **whether** to intervene has to be considered at all times. In some cases, there is a threshold of intervention and this has to be considered and re-considered taking into account all of the evidence of the moment. Once having decided to intervene, **when** to intervene becomes relevant. Results will tell us by the evidence of the data available the preferred **method of intervention** and as **long-term follow-up** as possible, desirable to establish the best method of treatment. For dissecting aneurysm, the big question seems to be that, if the type B dissection is in the chronic phase, should one intervene and if so, when, by what criteria and with what outcome expectation.

Radiation dose awareness in aortic interventions was a highlight of CX 2016 and the increase in this subject is marked.

**Whether, when** and **method of intervention** and **follow-up** is plain to see in the section of abdominal aortic aneurysm consensus update. On the day, we are lucky to expect to hear new data from the podium for the first time on aortic matters. During the section on screening, we shall hear for the first time the Screening in Women for Abdominal aNeurysms (SWAN) trial. In addition, we shall hear the EVAR 2 (Endovascular repair of AAA in patients physically ineligible for open repair—very long-term follow-up) and the three-year results of the IMPROVE trial.

Peripheral arterial consensus update Pathways of care concern the best method of intervention for the increase of blood flow in the lower limb. There remains interest in the approach of **"leaving nothing behind"** or **"leaving something in"**. Leaving nothing behind would include percutaneous transluminal angioplasty with or without drug-coated balloon. It would also include atherectomy and any procedure that clears the blockage without leaving behind any non-absorbable material. The alternative is the use of a stent or a stent graft. Finally, there is the consideration of the place of bypass surgery.

Surgeons have come to recognise that the endovascular-first approach is swamping the scene. This will certainly be discussed at CX 2017. We shall see many first podium presentations in peripheral arterial disease, especially in terms of drug-coated balloon. The question is just how far the drug-coated balloon can go in the lower limb to correct disease without the use of a stent. It can fairly confidently be claimed already that drug-coated balloon is superior to angioplasty alone. Whether it will go on to become the treatment of choice for total occlusions, very long lesions or in-stent restenosis will be a matter of great interest. The CX audience will seek to understand when a stent should be used. In addition, if a stent is used, the type of stent can make a difference. Factors that will be discussed and appear in this book are swirling flow, flexibility of the stent and the radial strength of a stent.

Diabetic foot care is highlighted in the book and the diabetologists understand the need to work in an interdisciplinary group and this is favoured in this book and at the Charing Cross Symposium. Equally, the diabetologists are calling for early revascularisation. This is one of the reasons why endovascular procedures are given the first opportunity. Whether the endovascular procedure is durable or whether surgery should follow is a matter for discussion.

The endovenous revolution is with us and pathways of care apply here also. At the centre of the discussion is the need for availability of deep and superficial state-of-the-art duplex scanning. It will be seen that condition of the deep veins and the pelvic veins is becoming of great importance in predicting the long-term results of every venous procedure. Once, superficial venous interventions took place without consideration of the deep system. Rapidly those times are passing as it is realised that the condition of the deep venous system has much to do with the outcome and the durability of procedures for the superficial veins.

I am personally extremely grateful to the Faculty of Charing Cross who provided chapters for the book and to the BIBA Publishing team that has been able to create such an excellent book in time for the Symposium.

Roger Greenhalgh

# Acute stroke consensus update—Pathways of care

# HERMES collaboration and care structures for acute ischaemic stroke

K Treurniet and CBLM Majoie

## Introduction

Intra-arterial treatment quickly became the new standard approach for managing ischaemic stroke after seven studies—published in 2015 and in 2016—proved the benefit of the treatment compared with usual care. However, uncertainties remain about the benefit of endovascular thrombectomy in patient groups that were under-represented in these individual trials. These include patients who presented to treatment late, were elderly, were not eligible for intravenous alteplase and who had mild deficits. The trials were: MR CLEAN (Multicentre randomized clinical trial of endovascular treatment for acute ischaemic stroke in the Netherlands); ESCAPE (Endovascular treatment for small core and anterior circulation proximal occlusion with emphasis on minimising CT to recanalization times); SWIFT-PRIME (Solitaire with the intention for thrombectomy as primary endovascular treatment); REVASCAT (Randomized trial of revascularization with Solitaire FR device *vs.* best medical therapy in the treatment of acute stroke due to anterior circulation large vessel occlusion presenting within eight hours of symptom onset); EXTEND IA (Extending the time for thrombolysis in emergency neurological deficits—intra-arterial); PISTE (Pragmatic ischaemic stroke thrombectomy evaluation); and THRACE (Mechanical thrombectomy after intravenous alteplase *versus* alteplase alone after stroke). The investigators of these studies have pooled the data of their individual patients to address these questions within the HERMES group. This chapter covers the results published in two major papers from the HERMES group—the first concerning extended subgroup analyses, and the second concerning the effect of time on patient outcome.

## A meta-analysis of the five randomised trials

A total of 1,287 patients included in MR CLEAN, SWIFT-PRIME, ESCAPE, EXTEND-IA and REVASCAT were analysed in a meta-analysis.[1] The intervention arm contained 634 patients and the control arm 653. Baseline variables were largely balanced, except for a lower rate of IV alteplase administration in the intervention arm (p=0.04). Patients treated with endovascular treatment had a reduced chance of disability at 90 days (adjusted common odds ratio [acOR] of 2.49; 95% confidence interval [CI] 1.76-3.53, determined with mixed effect ordinal logistic regression). This resulted in an overall number needed to treat of

2.6 for one patient to have reduced disability of at least one point on the modified Rankin Scale (mRS). No heterogeneity of treatment effect was observed across the prespecified variables. These included age, sex, National Institutes of Health Stroke Scale (NIHSS) scores, site of intracranial occlusion (ICA-T, M1 or M2), administration of tissue plasminogen activator (tPA), Alberta Stroke programme early CT score (ASPECTS), time from onset to randomisation and presence of tandem cervical carotid occlusion. Across all groups the direction of the acORs favoured treatment, but there was not a significant difference for patients younger than 50 years, patients with low ASPECTS or NIHSS scores and patients with an M2 segment occlusion. It is important to note that there were probably not enough of these patients to provide sufficient power to assess treatment effect. Interestingly, for patients older than 80 years and patients randomised after five hours from symptom onset, significant positive treatment effect was observed.

In conclusion, based on current data, endovascular treatment reduces disability for patients with anterior circulation large vessel occlusions. The treatment is effective across a wide range of subgroups. However, future studies are needed to address whether there is clinically significant treatment effect in patients younger than 50 years, with M2 occlusions or low ASPECTS and NIHSS scores.

## Effect of time to treatment on outcomes

Among the same patients included in the aforementioned meta-analysis, the effect of time to intra-arterial treatment was assessed in another meta-analysis.[2] The effect of treatment declined with longer times from symptom onset: acOR for lower disability scores of 2.79 (95% CI 1.96–3.98) at three hours, 1.98 (95% CI 1.30-3.00) at six hours, and1.57 (95% CI 0.86-2.88) at eight hours. The time for which the lower bound of the 95% CI first crossed the 1.0 and was no longer statistically significant was at a symptom onset-to-expected arterial puncture time of seven hours and 18 minutes. However, except for time intervals starting at the emergency department arrival, no significant treatment effect modification was observed. Among the group of patients in whom substantial reperfusion was achieved, every nine-minute delay in symptom onset to substantial endovascular reperfusion time resulted in one of every 100 patients treated to have a worse disability outcome. This effect was larger when the time interval from emergency department admission to reperfusion was considered. Then, every four-minute delay resulted in a worse outcome for every one in 100 treated patients. Rates of functional independence declined in a similar manner for subgroups based on age, stroke severity, clot location, ASPECTS, patient arrival (direct vs. transfer) and time from onset to tPA start. Interestingly, a steeper decline in rates of good functional outcome was observed for patients receiving tPA compared to tPA ineligible patients.

Based on these data, the authors recommend the following work-flow benchmarks: 50 minutes for brain imaging-to-arterial puncture time, 75 minutes for emergency department door-to-arterial puncture time, and 110 minutes for emergency department door-to-reperfusion time.

## Summary

- Intra-arterial treatment has quickly become the new standard treatment worldwide of acute ischaemic stroke in patients with proximal intracranial occlusions of the anterior circulation after the publication of seven clinical trials in 2015 and in 2016, proving the benefit over usual care only.

- Intra-arterial treatment is effective across a wide range of subgroups.

- The treatment effect declined with longer times from symptom onset.

## References

1. Goyal M, Menon BK, van Zwam WH, *et al*. Endovascular thrombectomy after large-vessel ischaemic stroke: a meta-analysis of individual patient data from five randomised trials. *Lancet* 2016; **387:** 1723–31.
2. Saver JL, Goyal M, van der Lugt A, *et al*. Time to treatment with endovascular thrombectomy and outcomes from ischemic stroke: A meta-analysis. *JAMA* 2016; **316:** 1279–88.

# Use of embolic filters to reduce the stroke risk in thoracic endovascular aortic repair

G Grover and R Gibbs

## Introduction

Population-based studies have shown a meteoric increase in admissions for thoracic aortic disease. This trend will continue because of the increasing recognition of thoracic aortic conditions and access to imaging. The combination of better understanding of thoracic aortic disease and equipment access[1,2] has also enabled an ageing population, which is increasingly prone to these conditions, to be treated. Thoracic endovascular aortic repair (TEVAR) has been adopted ahead of surgical repair as the standard method of treatment for a range of aortic pathologies because the need for thoracotomy and aortic cross-clamping are avoided, morbidity is reduced and hospital stay is significantly decreased.

The brain is extremely sensitive to both hypoperfusion and embolic complications, and stroke remains one of the most devastating complications of both open and endovascular treatment of descending and aortic arch pathologies. There is a 3% to 8%[3] risk of stroke with TEVAR and stroke is associated with early mortality of affected patients. Cerebral embolisation during aortic arch instrumentation has been shown to be one of the primary causes of perioperative stroke during TEVAR.[3] Passage of wires and catheters, and manipulation of device delivery systems, means embolic risk is inevitable. Greater degrees of athermanous burden in the arch and more proximal landing zones of the stents increase this risk.

## Silent cerebral infarction—not so "silent"

Asymptomatic or silent cerebral infarction is a brain injury that can be detected incidentally by diffusion-weighted magnetic resonance (MR) imaging. This technology has allowed the burden of "silent" microembolisation to be visualised, which has led to the concept that full-blown clinical strokes probably represent the tip of the iceberg of the cerebral insult. Studies have shown that silent cerebral infarction is a predictor of future development of clinically overt stroke and can increase it by two to four fold.[4] It can also increase the risk of dementia, depression and cognitive deficits demonstrated by neuropsychometric testing.[5] The American Heart Association consensus document has recognised these lesions as clinically significant infarcts.[6]

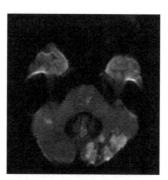

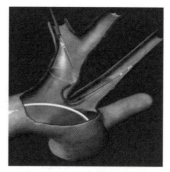

**Figure 1:** Silent cerebral infarction. Postoperative MR imaging patient with TEVAR and no clinical stroke.

**Figure 2:** Sentinel cerebral protection system (Claret Medical).

In addition to the risk of overt stroke, neuroimaging studies have demonstrated a significant rate of silent cerebral infarction associated with TEVAR. Kalhert *et al*[7] reported a 63% rate of cerebral injury on postoperative MR imaging in a cohort of patients undergoing TEVAR. Our own unit data of 52 consecutive TEVAR cases showed a 68% silent cerebral infarction rate, with an associated persistent early neurocognitive decline on neuropsychometric testing. Figure 1 shows an MR imaging displaying brain injury incurred by a patient who underwent TEVAR with no overt signs of stroke.

From an endovascular embolic perspective, intraoperative transcranial Doppler monitoring of the middle cerebral arteries has established two main risk periods: stiff wire placement and stent deployment.[8] We have observed maximum embolic high intensity transient signals in these procedural phases. What is yet to be determined is the nature of the emboli, so far assumed to be solid athermanous particles arising from a diseased arch. However, they could also be a gaseous release caused by the deployment of the stent. Studies have begun to look into flushing and prepping of these stents with carbon dioxide to reduce a potential embolic gaseous effect.[9] Our unit is furthering this research with emboli differentiation software to classify gas and solid emboli, which could help identify preventive mechanisms. Whether gas or solid, it has been established that cerebral insult is inevitable in TEVAR, and strategies to protect the brain and mitigate this risk are, therefore, necessary.

## Cerebral embolic protection

In a similar way to carotid filters being used in carotid artery stenting, cerebral embolic protection devices are currently used as adjuncts in other endovascular procedures, such as transcatheter aortic valve implantation (TAVI), to reduce the risk of cerebral injury. The Sentinel cerebral protection device (Claret Medical) is a dual filter embolic capture device, inserted via percutaneous access (6Fr radial or brachial) at the origin of the brachiocephalic and left common carotid arteries, designed to protect the brain throughout the procedure. The filters have 140μm pores and are retrievable, allowing for histopathological analysis of captured embolic debris. This device should protect all territories of the brain apart from the left posterior circulation as the left vertebral is not protected

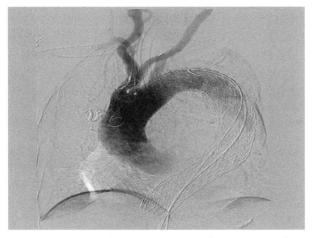

**Figure 3:** Embolic protection filters deployed at origin of innominate and left carotid.

The use of cerebral protection devices with TAVI has shown encouraging results. Recent randomised controlled trials using the Sentinel device have shown a significant decrease in number and volume of new silent cerebral infarction lesions.[10–12] Embolic debris was captured in more than 75% of cases. A meta-analysis of cerebral protection device use in TAVI has concluded a potential benefit in the embolic protection groups with a lower (although non-significant) risk of overt stroke and all-cause mortality, reduction in MR imaging markers of cerebral infarction and an early neurological benefit.[13]

A pilot trial, conducted in our unit, has applied this mechanism of cerebral embolic protection to TEVAR and we have demonstrated the safety and feasibility of the Sentinel dual filter protection system in 10 patients. Figure 3 shows the device *in-situ*. With the current device design, to ensure deployment and retrieval of the filters, the cerebral protection device would be suitable for TEVAR deployed distal to the left common carotid in landing zones 2, 3 and 4.

The early results have been encouraging. There has been a marked reduction in number and surface area of cerebral infarction compared to our retrospective unprotected cohort of TEVAR procedures. Additionally, there has not yet been any early neurocognitive decline during psychometric testing. Thoracic aortic disease monitoring has been performed and recorded in all cases, including analysis of the deployment of the protection filters. Embolic material was captured in all filters retrieved, with histopathological analysis demonstrating a mixture of arterial wall and acute thrombus in all cases and even

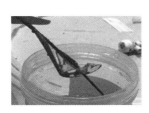 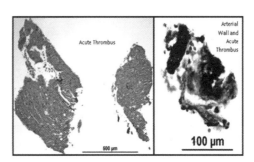

**Figure 4:** Retrieved proximal filter and histopathology.

polarisable foreign material captured in some filters, which could represent stent fibres. The mean number of particles retrieved was 473 (Figure 4).

## Conclusion

The aortic arch and thoracic aorta remains a hostile environment for both open and endovascular treatment and stroke is still the principle risk. As the use of TEVAR increases and becomes available to a wider and variable cohort of patients, measures to mitigate the neurological risk will be required.

## Summary

- Technical advances and gained expertise have resulted in increased and more complicated thoracic endovascular procedures.

- Stroke still remains a significant risk and periprocedural cerebral embolisation is a principal risk factor.

- Silent cerebral infarction identified on MR imaging is clinically significant and associated with detrimental neurological and cognitive decline.

- We have demonstrated the safety and feasibility of cerebral embolic protection in TEVAR, but larger scale studies may be required to justify the routine use of cerebral protection in patients undergoing the procedure.

## References

1. Allman RS, Anjum A, Powell JT. Incidence of Descending Aortic Pathology and Evaluation of the Impact of Thoracic Endovascular Aortic Repair: A Population-based study in England and Wales from 1999 to 2010. *E J VascEndovascSurg* 2013; **45** (2): 154–59
2. Chaikof EL, Mutrie C, Kasirajan K, Milner R. Endovascular repair for diverse pathologies of the thoracic aorta: an initial decade of experience. *J Am CollSurg* 2009; 208: 802–16.
3. Gutsche JT, Cheung AT, McGarvey ML *et al*. Risk factors for perioperative stroke after thoracic endovascular aortic repair. *Ann Thorac Surg*. 2007; **84** (4):1195–200.
4. Kobayashi S, Okada K, Koide H *et al*. Subcortical silent brain infarction as a risk factor for clinical stroke. *Stroke* 1997; **28**: 1932–39.
5. Vermeer SE, Prins ND, Den Heijer T *et al*. Silent brain infarcts and the risk of dementia and cognitive decline .*N Engl J Med* 2003; **348**: 1215–22.
6. Sacco RL, Kasner SE, Broderick JP *et al*. An Updated Definition of Stroke for the 21st Century. *Stroke* 2013; **44**: 2064–89.
7. Kahlert P, Eggebrecht H, Janosi RA et al.Silent Cerebral Ischemia After ThoracicEndovascular Aortic Repair: A Neuroimaging Study. *Ann ThoracSurg* 2014; **98**: 53–58.
8. Bismuth J, Garami Z, Anaya-Ayala JE et al.Transcranial Doppler findings during thoracic endovascular aortic repair. *J Vasc Surg*. 2011; **54**: 364–69.
9. Kölbel T, Rohlffs F, Wipper S *et al*. Carbon Dioxide Flushing Technique to Prevent Cerebral Arterial Air Embolism and Stroke During TEVAR. *J EndovasTher* 2016; **23** (2) 393–95.
10. Van Mieghem NM, van Gils L, Ahmad H *et al*. Filter-based cerebral embolic protection with transcatheteraortic valve implantation: the randomised MISTRAL-C trial. *EuroIntervention* 2016; **12**: 499–507.
11. Haussig S, Mangner N, Dwyer NG, Lukas Lehmkuhl. Effect of a cerebral protection device on brain lesions following transcatheter aortic valve implantation in patients with severe aortic stenosis. The CLEAN-TAVI randomized clinical trial. *JAMA* 2016; **316**: 592–601.
12. Kapadia SR, Kodali S, Makkar R *et al*. Cerebral embolic protection during transcatheter aortic valve Replacement SENTINEL trial. *J Am CollCardiol* 2016. Epub
13. Giustino G, Mehran R, Veltkamp R *et al*. Neurological Outcomes With Embolic Protection Devices in Patients Undergoing Transcatheter Aortic Valve Replacement. *J Am CollCardiol* 2016 24; **9** (20): 2124–33.

# Thoracic aortic consensus update—Pathways of care

# The potential for flow dynamics to inform stent sizing for thoracic aortic disease

HWL de Beaufort, TMJ van Bakel, M Conti, FJH Nauta, S Morganti, RM Romarowski, F Secchi, F Sardanelli, MM Marrocco-Trischitta, JA van Herwaarden, FL Moll, F Auricchio and S Trimarchi

## Introduction

Thoracic endovascular aortic repair (TEVAR) is well-established as a first-line treatment for aortic aneurysm, penetrating ulcer, dissection, intramural haematoma, trauma and coarctation. In each patient, the aortic wall will behave differently upon being manipulated by endovascular devices. Knowing the mechanical properties of a device and understanding how an individual's aorta will respond to its presence can clarify the occurrence of complications, and it may also explain some of the longer term effects of aortic stiffening induced by stent graft placement.[1] Studies on flow dynamics can increase knowledge on stent graft behaviour, aortic behaviour and the interaction between the two. In this chapter, we elaborate how the application of this knowledge can be helpful during crucial stages of preoperative planning, such as selection of stent graft type, size, and landing zones.

## Stiffness of the aorta and of endovascular devices

Aortic stiffness, which depends mainly on elastin and collagen content in the tunica media, varies along the aorta and increases with age.[2] Aortic valve morphology,[3] aortic arch geometry,[4] volume and direction of flow,[5] blood viscosity,[6] and surrounding tissues[7] determine, together with aortic stiffness, how the aorta will deform during the cardiac cycle. It is no surprise that aortic distensibility will vary between individuals.[2,8] The interaction between native aorta and aortic stent grafts is not fully understood and may depend on stent graft design, which has different mechanical properties according to the stent material, graft material, and other features such as longitudinal bars or fixation hooks.[9,10] Stent graft deployment has been shown to artificially induce aortic stiffening, which appears to be determined by stent graft length more than by any differences in stent graft design.[11-13] The long-term effects of this increased stiffness are unknown and need to be investigated to understand which patients will suffer severe adverse cardiovascular remodelling when using long stent grafts.[1]

## Consequences of compliance mismatch and incorrect sizing

Since endovascular devices are stiff and inert in comparison to the dynamic environment of the thoracic aorta, optimal sizing is crucial to ensure sufficient conformability. Poor stent graft conformability is associated with deployment-related complications such as bird-beaking,[14] and may also have an effect on cerebral microembolisation.[15] Postoperatively, poor conformability may be a cause of stent graft migration and type I or III endoleak.[16] Repeated excessive stresses caused by excessive oversizing can lead to stent graft fracture or collapse.[17] Compliance mismatch between stented and non-stented aorta in longitudinal[13] and radial direction[18] leads to increased wall stress in the aorta adjacent to the stent graft.[19] The relation between wall stress, wall degeneration and (retrograde) dissection has been established,[20] and the risk of excessive oversizing in patients treated for dissection is widely recognised.[21]

## Relation of flow dynamics to complications after TEVAR

ECG-gated computed tomography (CT) angiography allows measurement of time-resolved aortic geometry. Transesophageal Doppler-ultrasound and ECG-gated magnetic resonance (MR) angiography allow measurement of time-resolved aortic flow. These images can be post-processed using computational analysis to simulate intraluminal pressure, friction of flow on the endothelial surface (wall shear stress), as well as time-resolved flow in three dimensions (4D phase contrast magnetic resonance imaging). Computational fluid dynamics simulations can be performed to calculate blood flow and intraluminal pressure, structural analysis can be used to calculate intramural wall stresses. Previously, intraluminal pressure and wall stress measurements could only be obtained invasively or in *ex vivo* settings.

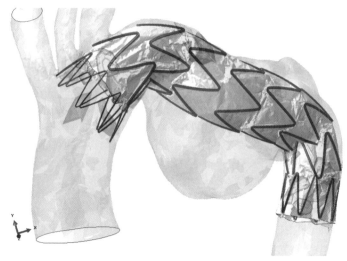

**Figure 1:** Visualisation of results from computational analysis in which the stress between the aortic wall and a stent graft was calculated.

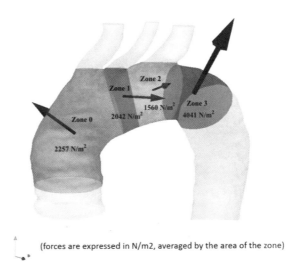

(forces are expressed in N/m2, averaged by the area of the zone)

**Figure 2:** Magnitude and orientation of drag forces in the different proximal landing zones of a patient's aortic arch (type II).

Using flow and pressure information gathered or simulated from dynamic imaging and computational modelling, many of the stresses, strains and forces that are at play in the aorta can be quantified (Figure 1). For example, the magnitude and direction of displacement forces acting on a stent graft can be calculated for any region of interest (Figure 2). The magnitude of displacement forces depends mostly on intraluminal pressure; flow-related forces determine a small part of the total displacement force.[22] The magnitude of the displacement force is much higher in the thoracic aorta compared to the abdominal aorta, and the direction is upward compared to downward orientation along with blood flow, respectively.[23] Increased blood pressure, stent graft length, and angulation lead to increased displacement forces, and are, therefore, risk factors for stent graft migration and endoleak.[23,24] The amount of oversizing, condition of the aortic wall and length of proximal sealing zone also have an effect on stent graft stability.[25] Consequently, stent graft manufacturers recommend increasing proximal sealing zone length in patients with high degrees of aortic arch angulation. Excessive oversizing does not have a significant impact on contact stability, but leads to disadvantageous stress distributions and stent graft collapse.[26] Increased stent graft angulation, as well as protrusion of the stent graft into the aortic arch—"bird-beaking"—leads to a transmural pressure load difference across the stent graft, which increases the risk of stent graft collapse.[27]

Flow-related stresses—such as wall shear stress and its derivatives oscillatory shear index, relative residence time, and platelet activation potential—describe the friction and changes in direction of blood flow. Some of these parameters are related to thrombogenic activity[28] and may possibly be used to predict thrombus-related complications after TEVAR[29] and false lumen thrombosis in cases of aortic dissection.[30]

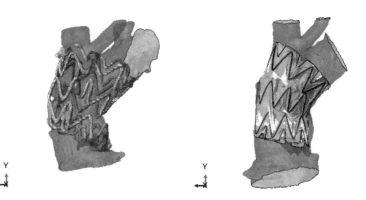

**Figure 3:** Patient-specific stent graft deployment in thoracic aortic pseudoaneurysm, comparison with postoperative situation (left) and simulation of stent graft deployment (right). (From Auricchio *et al*[31])

## The potential for flow dynamics to inform stent sizing

Dynamic imaging may help to optimise preoperative assessment for TEVAR planning. It is important to consider not only the circumferential, but also the axial pulsatile aortic deformations. This will allow more accurate choice of stent graft diameter and length. Subsequently, anatomical and physiological clues can be used to estimate flow dynamic parameters for that individual patient. An old patient, with a high pulse pressure and an angulated proximal aortic neck with a large diameter will probably experience high displacement forces, which may lead to an increased risk of type I endoleak. To reduce this risk and ensure stent graft stability, it may be judicial to choose a slightly longer sealing zone than the minimum recommended sealing zone length to ensure stent graft stability. However, a longer stent graft will also increase displacement force magnitude, so a balance needs to be found. In a young trauma patient with little angulation and high aortic distensibility, a high rate of oversizing may be adopted (both longitudinally and circumferentially) to reduce the risk of endoleak, but the risks of infolding and long-term complications due to increased aortic stiffness need to be taken into account too. In the future, stent graft deployment may be simulated preoperatively (Figure 3).[31] Calculation of flow dynamic forces may then be done in routine clinical practice to make a patient-specific risk prediction for stent graft related complications as endoleak, collapse and cardiac disease.[32]

## Conclusion

There are differences in the mechanical properties of commercially available stent grafts, but all are stiff in comparison to the dynamic environment of the native thoracic aorta. Complications after TEVAR may be caused by a compliance mismatch between the endovascular device and the native aorta. The relation between flow dynamic parameters and these complications has been shown in many different ways. It is, therefore, important to take these flow dynamic parameters into account during preoperative planning to choose the most suitable stent graft type, length, diameter and landing zone for the individual patient.

## Summary

- There are significant differences in aortic distensibility between individuals.

- Endovascular devices are generally stiffer and more inert than the native aorta, which leads to a compliance mismatch that can cause complications.

- Dynamic imaging and computational modelling provide information on flow, pressure and stresses in the aorta, which can be used to calculate displacement forces, wall shear stress, transmural pressure load, and other flow dynamic and structural parameters.

- There is increasing evidence for the association between flow dynamic parameters and the occurrence of complications.

- Anatomical and physiological factors that are associated with these flow dynamic parameters can be used to estimate the risk of complications.

- In the future, patient-specific risk estimation may be more accurate thanks to routine calculation of flow dynamic factors.

- Stent graft size may be adapted according to which complication is estimated to be most likely to occur.

# References

1. Nauta FJ, Kamman AV, Ibrahim EH, et al. Assessment of cardiovascular remodelling following endovascular aortic repair through imaging and computation: the CORE prospective observational cohort study protocol. BMJ Open 2016; 6 (11): e012270.
2. Roccabianca S, Figueroa CA, Tellides G, et al. Quantification of regional differences in aortic stiffness in the aging human. J Mech Behav Biomed Mater 2014; 29: 618–34.
3. Garcia J, Barker AJ, Murphy I, et al. Four-dimensional flow magnetic resonance imaging-based characterization of aortic morphometry and haemodynamics: impact of age, aortic diameter, and valve morphology. Eur Heart J Cardiovasc Imaging 2016; 17 (8): 877–84.
4. Marrocco-Trischitta MM, de Beaufort HW, Secchi F, et al. A geometrical reappraisal of proximal landing zones for thoracic endovascular aortic repair according to aortic arch types. J Vasc Surg 2017; (in press)
5. Andersson M, Lantz J, Ebbers T, et al. Quantitative assessment of turbulence and flow eccentricity in an aortic coarctation: Impact of virtual interventions. Cardiovasc Eng Technol 2015; 6 (3): 281–93.
6. Cecchi E, Giglioli C, Valente S, et al. Role of hemodynamic shear stress in cardiovascular disease. Atherosclerosis 2011; 214 (2): 249–56.
7. Liu Y, Dang C, Garcia M, et al. Surrounding tissues affect the passive mechanics of the vessel wall: theory and experiment. Am J Physiol Heart Circ Physiol 2007; 293 (6): H3290–300.
8. de Beaufort HW, Nauta FJ, Conti M, et al. Extensibility and distensibility of the thoracic aorta in patients with aneurysm. Eur J Vasc Endovasc Surg 2017; 53(2): 199–205
9. Kleinstreuer C, Li Z, Basciano CA, et al. Computational mechanics of Nitinol stent grafts. J Biomech 2008; 41 (11): 2370–78.
10. Morris L, Stefanov F, Hynes N, et al. An experimental evaluation of device/arterial wall compliance mismatch for four stent-graft devices and a multi-layer flow modulator device for the treatment of abdominal aortic aneurysms. Eur J Vasc Endovasc Surg 2016; 51 (1): 44–55.
11. Moulakakis KG, Kadoglou NP, Antonopoulos CN, et al. Changes in arterial stiffness and n-terminal pro-brain natriuretic peptide levels after endovascular repair of descending thoracic aorta. Ann Vasc Surg 2017; 38: 220–26.
12. Nauta FJ, de Beaufort HW, Conti M, et al. Impact of thoracic endovascular aortic repair on radial strain in an ex-vivo porcine model. Eur J Cardiothorac Surg 2017; (in press).
13. Nauta FJ, Conti M, Marconi S, et al. An experimental investigation of the impact of thoracic endovascular aortic repair on longitudinal strain. Eur J Cardiothorac Surg 2016; 50 (5): 955–61.
14. van Bogerijen GH, Auricchio F, Conti M, et al. Aortic hemodynamics after thoracic endovascular aortic repair, with particular attention to the bird-beak configuration. J Endovasc Ther 2014; 21 (6): 791–802.

15. Bismuth J, Garami Z, Anaya-Ayala JE, *et al.* Transcranial Doppler findings during thoracic endovascular aortic repair. *J Vasc Surg* 2011; **54** (2): 364–9.
16. van Prehn J, Bartels LW, Mestres G, *et al.* Dynamic aortic changes in patients with thoracic aortic aneurysms evaluated with electrocardiography-triggered computed tomographic angiography before and after thoracic endovascular aneurysm repair: preliminary results. *Ann Vasc Surg* 2009; **23** (3): 291–97.
17. Lin KK, Kratzberg JA and Raghavan ML. Role of aortic stent graft oversizing and barb characteristics on folding. *J Vasc Surg* 2012; **55** (5): 1401–09.
18. Nauta FJ, de Beaufort HW, Conti M, *et al.* Impact of thoracic endovascular aortic repair on radial strain in an ex vivo porcine model. *Eur J Cardiothorac Surg* 2017. Epub.
19. Raaz U, Zollner AM, Schellinger IN, *et al.* Segmental aortic stiffening contributes to experimental abdominal aortic aneurysm development. *Circulation* 2015; **131** (20): 1783–95.
20. Humphrey JD, Schwartz MA, Tellides G, *et al.* Role of mechanotransduction in vascular biology: focus on thoracic aortic aneurysms and dissections. Circ Res 2015; **116** (8): 1448–61.
21. Canaud L, Ozdemir BA, Patterson BO, *et al.* Retrograde aortic dissection after thoracic endovascular aortic repair. *Ann Surg* 2014; **260** (2): 389–95.
22. Cheng SW, Lam ES, Fung GS, *et al.* A computational fluid dynamic study of stent graft remodeling after endovascular repair of thoracic aortic dissections. *J Vasc Surg* 2008; **48 (2):** 303–9; discusion 9–10.
23. Figueroa CA, Taylor CA, Chiou AJ, *et al.* Magnitude and direction of pulsatile displacement forces acting on thoracic aortic endografts. *J Endovasc Ther* 2009; **16** (3): 350–58.
24. Wang X and Li X. Fluid-structure interaction based study on the physiological factors affecting the behaviors of stented and non-stented thoracic aortic aneurysms. J Biomech 2011; **44** (12): 2177–84.
25. Altnji HE, Bou-Said B and Walter-Le Berre H. Numerical simulation of the migration phenomena and type 1a endoleak of thoracic aneurysm endograft. *Comput Methods Biomech Biomed Engin* 2013; 16 Suppl 1 36–38.
26. Altnji HE, Bou-Said B and Walter-Le Berre H. Morphological and stent design risk factors to prevent migration phenomena for a thoracic aneurysm: a numerical analysis. *Med Eng Phys* 2015; **37** (1): 23–33.
27. Pasta S, Cho JS, Dur O, *et al.* Computer modeling for the prediction of thoracic aortic stent graft collapse. *J Vasc Surg* 2013; **57** (5): 1353–61.
28. Morbiducci U, Kok AM, Kwak BR, *et al.* Atherosclerosis at arterial bifurcations: evidence for the role of haemodynamics and geometry. Thromb Haemost 2016; **115** (3): 484–92.
29. Nauta FJ, Lau KD, Arthurs CJ, *et al.* Computational fluid dynamics and thrombus formation following thoracic endovascular aortic repair. *Ann Thorac Surg* 2017. Epub.
30. Cheng Z, Riga C, Chan J, *et al.* Initial findings and potential applicability of computational simulation of the aorta in acute type B dissection. *J Vasc Surg* 2013; **57** (2 Suppl): 35S–43S.
31. Auricchio F, Conti M, Marconi S, *et al.* Patient-specific aortic endografting simulation: from diagnosis to prediction. *Comput Biol Med* 2013; **43** (4): 386–94.
32. Brown AG, Shi Y, Marzo A, *et al.* Accuracy vs. computational time: translating aortic simulations to the clinic. *J Biomech* 2012; **45** (3): 516–23.

**Ascending aortic aneurysm:
Intervention method & outcomes**

# Ascending aortic aneurysm remodelling for various pathologies

## RA White, A Khoynezhad, GE Kopchok and CE Donayre

## Introduction

The success of endovascular stent graft repair of descending thoracic aorta has led to the application of these devices for the management of thoracic aortic diseases in other locations, such as aortic arch and the ascending aorta. Off-label use of descending thoracic stent grafts in the ascending aorta has been described since 2000 from outside of the USA,[1] while Ihnken and colleagues from Stanford reported the first off-label use in the USA in 2004.[2] There is also a series of case reports that (mostly) involve high-risk patients with high-risk features or pseudoaneurysms of the ascending aorta undergoing endovascular repair.[3–11]

The purpose of this chapter is to investigate the outcome of selected patients with ascending aortic pathologies including type A aortic dissection, retrograde type A aortic dissection, intramural haematoma, penetrating ulcer, or pseudoaneurysm with isolated diseases affecting the aorta between the sinotubular junction and the innominate artery orifice (with no involvement of aortic valve and the aortic root). These patients underwent thoracic endovascular aortic repair (TEVAR) with the Valiant stent graft (Medtronic) device as part of a physician-sponsored investigational device exemption approved by the US Food and Drug Administration (FDA).

This was a prospective trial of the Valiant device to determine the feasibility of successful implantation, as indicated by exclusion of the thoracic lesion and graft patency at implant, time of discharge, and one, six, and 12 months following implantation, and to determine the proportion of patients who die or experience adverse events during and after the implantation. The study protocol was approved by the Institutional Review Boards (IRBs) at Harbor-UCLA Medical Center and LA Biomed Research Institute in Torrance, USA, and Cedars-Sinai Medical Center in Los Angeles, USA, and was registered at ClinicalTrials.gov (identifier: NCT02201589) with RA White and A Khoynezhad as joint principal investigators.

Suitable candidates for inclusion included adult patients who signed a consent approved by the FDA and IRB and who agreed to follow-up. To be considered a candidate for endovascular repair, the patient must have had a type A thoracic aortic dissection, a retrograde type A thoracic aortic dissection, an intramural haematoma, a penetrating ulcer, or a pseudoaneurysm of the ascending thoracic aorta affecting the area between the sinus of Valsalva and the innominate artery orifice with no involvement of the aortic valve. The patient must also have at least 1cm of suitable landing zones both proximally and distally to the dissection, with an ascending aorta between 28mm and 44mm in diameter, and must be high-risk surgical candidate with an American Society of Anesthesiologists (ASA) score of IV.

We have recently reviewed our entire series of patient evaluated for entry in the study and those treated as part of the this study.[12] The cases presented in the following discussion are observations we have made from serial imaging of patients with frequently encountered pathologies.

## Regression of ascending aortic pathologies

### False/pseudoaneurysm

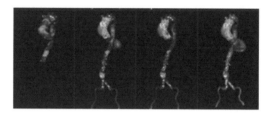

**Figures 1:** These images, obtained sequentially over two years, demonstrate that the device remains securely positioned as the lesion regresses in an 84-year-old male who developed a 65cm pseudoaneurysm in the ascending aorta several months after undergoing complicated coronary angiography interrogating patency of his coronary bypasses. Two thoracic endografts (92mm total/80mm covered length with proximal free flow and 52mm total/40mm covered proximal device). The second device was added to the greater curve of the aorta requiring more length than anticipated from preoperative images.

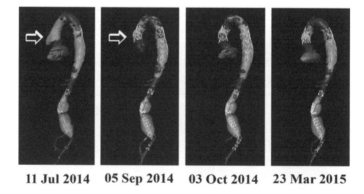

11 Jul 2014    05 Sep 2014    03 Oct 2014    23 Mar 2015

**Figures 2:** Exclusion of an aortic pseudoaneurysm suspected on surveillance computed tomography (CT) scans to be a needle puncture site in an ascending aortic Dacron graft. Two years' observation shows firm fixation of the ascending endograft with resolution of the pseudoaneurysm.

## Intramural haematoma

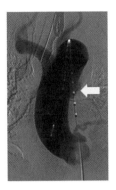 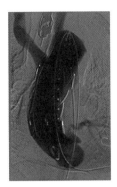

**Figures 3:** Entry site of an intramural haematoma in the ascending aorta with image following device deployment showing accurate deployment and exclusion of the lesion.

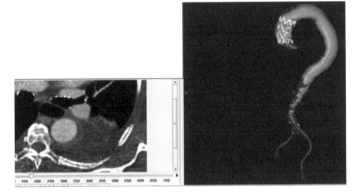

**Figures 4:** Seven-week follow-up CT of patient in Figure 3 showing stability of the ascending graft with exclusion of the ascending entry site (right figure), but with progression of the intramural haematoma in the descending thoracic aorta with suspected contained rupture (left image).

## Ascending dissection

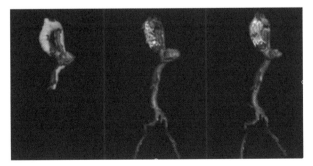

**Figures 5:** Sequential CT scans demonstrating an ascending dissection (left image, white colour showing the false lumen beginning approximately 1.5cm above the aortic valve) and follow-up CT scans at one and 30 days (centre and right images) with resolution of the ascending dissection and distal perfusion maintained by a stable remaining descending dissection.

## Conclusion

Valiant thoracic endografts provide durable treatment of non-aneurysmal lesions in the ascending thoracic aorta (penetrating ulcers, pseudoaneurysms, intramural haematomas, and ascending dissections). Secure fixation without migration in non-aneurysmal ascending aorta provided adequate (1cm) fixation length

Intramural haematoma, like ascending dissection, requires comprehensive surveillance and treatment to control and prevent distal complications.

## Summary

- Ascending aortic endografts successfully exclude penetrating ulcers, pseudoaneurysms, intramural haematoma, and ascending dissections in non-aneurysmal, non-infected tubular shaped aortic segments.

- Healing of ascending aortic lesions is similar to findings in descending aortic lesions with similar characteristics.

- Treatment of ascending aortic aneurysms is limited with endografts—inadequate fixation lengths and severely torturous anatomy limit utility of short devices without branches or fenestrations.

## References

1. Dorros AM, Planton S, O'Hair D, Zayed M. Transseptal guidewire stabilization facilitates stent-graft deployment for persistent proximal ascending aortic dissection. *Journal of Endovascular Therapy*. 2000; **7**(6): 506: 12.
2. IhnKen K. Successful treatment of a Stanford type A dissection by percutaneous placement of a covered stent graft in the ascending aorta. *J Thorac Cardiocasc Surg* 2004; **127**: 1808–10.
3. Chan YC, Cheng SW. Endovascular management of Stanford type A (ascending) aortic dissection. *Asian Cardiovasc Thorac Ann* 2009; **17**: 566–67.
4. Heye S, Daenens K, Maleux G, Nevelsteen A. Stent-graft repair of a mycotic ascending aorta pseudoaneurysm. *J Vasc Interv Radiol* 2006; **17**: 1821–5.
5. Hope TA, Markl M, Wigstrom L, *et al.* Comparison of flow patterns in ascending aortic aneurysms and volunteers using four-dimensional magnetic resonance velocity mapping. *J Magn Reson Imaging* 2007; **26**: 1471–79.
6. Kolvenbach RR, Karmeli R, Pinter LS *et al.* Endovascular management of ascending aortic pathology. *J Vasc Sur* 2011; **53**: 1431–37.
7. Senay S, Alhan C, Toraman F, Karabulut,H, Dagdelen S, Cagil H. Endovascular stent-graft treatment of type A dissection: Case report and review of literature. *Eur J Vasc Endovasc Surg* 2007; **34**: 457–60.
8. Szeto WY, Moser WG, Desai ND *et al.* Transapical deployment of endovascular thoracic aortic stent graft for an ascending aortic pseudoaneurysm. *Ann Thorac Surg* 2010; **89**: 616–18.
9. Zhang H, Li M, Jin W, Wang Z. Endoluminal and surgical treatment for the management of Stanford Type A aortic dissection. *Eur J Cardiothorac Surg* 2004; **89**: 616–18.
10. Zimpfer D, Czerny M, Kettenbach J *et al.* Treatment of acute type A dissection by percutaneous endovascular stent graft placement. *Ann Thorac Surg* 2006; **82**: 747–49.
11. Lin PH, Kougias P, Huynh TT, *et al.* Endovascular repair of ascending aortic pseudoaneurysm: Technical considerations of a common carotid artery approach using the Zenith aortic cuff endograft. *J Endovasc Ther* 2007; **14**: 794–98.
12. Khoynezhad A, Donayre CE, Walot I, *et al.* Feasibility of endovascular repair of ascending aortic pathologies as part of an FDA-approved physician-sponsored investigational device exemption. *J Vasc Surg* 2016; **63**: 1483–95.

# Arch aneurysm: When to intervene, intervention method & outcomes from follow-up

# Carotid-axillary bypass may be a better surgical option for revascularisation of the left subclavian artery in zone 2 TEVAR

FJ Criado

## Introduction

Endograft coverage of the left subclavian artery is often performed during thoracic endovascular aortic repair (TEVAR) of proximal descending and aortic arch pathologies. Consequently, debranching of the left subclavian artery frequently becomes necessary in such a setting, most commonly involving a left carotid-subclavian bypass.[1,2] The technique was first described by Lyons and Galbraith in 1957,[3] and was popularised by Diethrich *et al* who reported their large experience in a well-known article published 10 years later.[4] In the ensuing decades, carotid-subclavian bypass became the overwhelming favourite of surgeons performing left subclavian artery revascularisation for management of arterial occlusive disease and, more recently, in the context of a TEVAR procedure when over-stenting this vessel. The reported good results would seem to justify such preference,[5] but concern about possible technical complexity and potential complications, such as phrenic nerve and thoracic duct injury,[6] has been voiced consistently over the years. Our own early experience substantiated these reservations, prompting adoption of an alternative operative solution with use of the carotid-axillary bypass,[7] an operation first reported by Shumacker in 1973.[8] It has proved equivalent to the carotid-subclavian technique in terms of efficacy and durability, with the additional appeal of distinct practical advantages—mainly because the axillary artery tends to be an easier vessel to expose and handle, and through the avoidance of complications resulting from damage to anatomical structures that are often in harm's way when exposing the left subclavian artery.

## Technical aspects

We have essentially used the same basic technique since first adopting carotid-axillary bypass in the mid-1980s.[7] Unlike the single-incision carotid-subclavian bypass, targeting the axillary artery as the recipient vessel necessitates two incisions: one in the neck inferiorly and parallel to the anterior border of the sternocleidomastoid

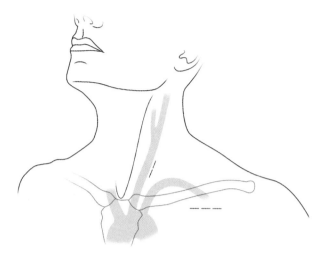

**Figure 1:** Cervical and infraclavicular incisions required for carotid-axillary bypass.

muscle; and an infraclavicular incision for surgical exposure of the axillary artery. (Figure 1).

The latter tends to be very familiar to most vascular surgeons because of prior experience with axillofemoral bypass. It involves splitting the fibres of the pectoralis major muscle, and division of the pectoralis minor which [I believe] facilitates exposure. A ringed PTFE vascular graft remains the preferred conduit, carefully tunnelled behind the internal jugular vein and under the clavicle. This operative step does carry a small risk of venous injury. However, we have not found it to be a major problem, as the haemorrhage—when it does occur—can be controlled with relative ease by applying firm pressure from above and below the clavicle for a few minutes.

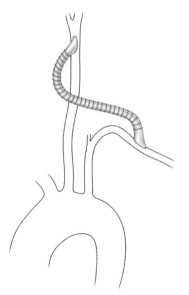

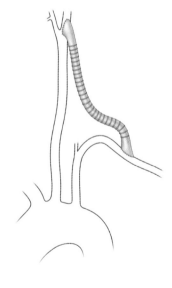

**Figure 2:** Illustration of completed left carotid-axillary bypass.

**Figure 3:** Technique for combined left carotid endarterectomy and carotid-axillary bypass.

Proximal and distal end-to-side anastomoses are constructed in routine manner (Figure 2). We do not use carotid shunting for this procedure.

At times, one may want to combine a carotid endarterectomy with the cervical bypass, in which case the vascular graft can be anastomosed to the carotid artery more distally, at the endarterectomy site (Figure 3).

The conduit length must be tailored with great care in order to achieve the desirable gently curving course without undue tension or redundancy (Figure 2).

Proximal ligation of the left subclavian artery, often performed during the carotid-subclavian bypass, cannot be a part of the carotid-axillary procedure because of inaccessibility. Some experts look upon this as a disadvantage, but I tend to view such limitation as advantageous because it eliminates the potential for a misplaced ligation distal to the left vertebral artery origin, which is now known to occur more frequently than previously suspected. If interruption of the left subclavian artery is deemed necessary, it is arguably best to use an endovascular (trans-brachial access) approach with precise **deployment of a vascular plug** device under angiographic guidance (Figure 4).

## Results

The carotid-axillary bypass has been shown to match the success and durability of the more popular carotid-subclavian operation,[7,9] being technically easier to perform and carrying little, if any, risk of lymphatic or nerve complications. The need to use two incisions is a small price to pay for such advantages.

## Conclusions

The carotid-axillary bypass emerges as a worthy alternative to the more popular carotid-subclavian operation and it ought to be considered more frequently than it is at present. In our hands (and that of others), it has proven technically simpler, and perhaps safer, through the avoidance of potential nerve and lymphatic

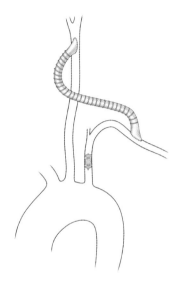

**Figure 4:** Vascular plug device delivered to occlude the proximal left subclavian artery (proximal to the origin of the vertebral artery).

complications. It deserves a place in the armamentarium of endovascular surgeons everywhere who perform left subclavian artery debranching in the context of zone 2 TEVAR.

## Summary

- Carotid-subclavian bypass is the acknowledged standard for left subclavian artery revascularisation, as it has been embraced by most surgeons performing these procedures.

- The carotid-axillary technique has been found to be an appealing and possibly superior technical option, offering an easier technical operation and avoidance of potential injury to the phrenic nerve and thoracic duct.

- Potential disadvantages of the carotid-subclavian bypass include the need for two incisions and the use of a longer graft conduit, but these have not been found to be detrimental in any way.

- The technical inability to perform proximal left subclavian ligation during carotid-axillary bypass is felt to constitute an actual advantage, as the potential for misplacing such ligature distal rather than proximal to the origin of the vertebral artery is eliminated altogether.

## References

1. Criado FJ, Barnatan MF, Rizk Y, *et al*. Technical strategies to expand stent-graft applicability in the aortic arch and proximal descending thoracic aorta. *J Endovasc Ther* 2002; **9** (suppl2): 1132–38.
2. Moulakakis KG, Mylonas SN, Markatis F, *et al*. A systematic review and meta-analysis of hybrid aortic arch replacement. *Ann Cardiothorac Surg* 2013; **2**: 247–60.
3. Lyons C, Galbraith G. Surgical treatment of atherosclerotic occlusion of the internal carotid artery. *Ann Surg* 1957;**146**: 487–94.
4. Diethrich EB, Garrett HE, Ameriso J, *et al*. Occlusive disease of the common carotid and subclavian arteries treated by carotid subclavian bypass: analysis of 125 cases. *Am J Surg* 1967; **114**: 800–08.
5. Woo EY, Carpenter JP, Jackson BM, *et al*. Left subclavian artery coverage during thoracic endovascular aortic repair: a single-center experience. *J Vasc Surg* 2008; **48**: 555–60.
6. Palchik E, Bakken AM, Wolford HY, *et al*. Subclavian artery revascularization: an outcome analysis based on mode of therapy and presenting symptoms. *Ann Vasc Surg* 2008; **22**: 70–8.
7. Criado FJ, Queral LA. Carotid-axillary bypass: a ten-year experience. *J Vasc Surg* 1995; **22**: 717–23.
8. Shumacker HB. Carotid-axillary bypass grafts for occlusion of the proximal subclavian artery. *Surg Gynecol Obstet* 1973; **136**: 447–48.
9. Archie JP. Axillary-to-carotid bypass grafting for symptomatic severe common carotid artery occlusive disease. *J Vasc Surg* 1999; **30**: 1106–12.

# Long-term feasibility data of thoracic single branched endograft in the aortic arch zones 0, 1, and 2

## MD Dake and S Cipollari

### Introduction

Open surgery currently remains the first choice for the treatment of pathologies involving the more proximal aortic arch (Ishimaru zones 0 and 1) in most cases,[1] given the durable long-term results. However, despite continuous improvements in graft design, advances in open surgical techniques and postoperative care, it still is a **complex and invasive procedure**, requiring a sternotomy, prolonged cardiopulmonary bypass, and deep hypothermic circulatory arrest, and is associated with high morbidity and mortality.[2] Furthermore, patients with multiple and severe comorbidities or absolute contraindications may not be eligible for surgical repair. Alternative approaches have, therefore, been developed with the goal of reducing the operative risks and enabling repair of aortic arch aneurysms in patients with contraindications to surgery. Hybrid techniques,[3] for example, involve a first stage surgical debranching procedure followed by stent graft placement. Although the introduction of hybrid repair has reduced to some extent the risks associated with the intervention, an entire endovascular approach would be more desirable.

Development of an endovascular device for the aortic arch has been delayed by the presence of several unique characteristics that make this anatomical location particularly challenging. First, its complex spatial geometry, consisting of curves and narrow three-dimensional angulations, complicate the achievement of an optimal endograft seal, thus predisposing to type I endoleaks. Additionally, higher haemodynamic forces compared to the descending aorta and their pulsatile nature subject stent grafts in this location to significant loading conditions that raise concern for the durability of devices. Finally, the presence of supra-aortic trunks branching off the aortic arch requires the development of stent graft designs able to maintain branch vessel perfusion.

Ideally, the optimal endovascular device would successfully address these challenges and facilitate a minimally invasive approach that can potentially achieve lower operative mortality and morbidity compared to open surgical repair and currently available hybrid techniques. It would also enable treatment of patients considered too high risk for surgery and be suitable for a wide range of anatomies and pathologies.

To date, no endovascular devices have been approved that satisfy these needs, but several strategies, each one with its own advantages and limitations, have been developed. These include parallel branch grafting (chimney technique),[4] homemade fenestrated stentgrafts,[5] *in-situ* fenestration[6] and branched devices.[7]

Branched endografts for aortic arch pathology were initially investigated in the form of homemade prototypical devices in 1999 and have subsequently been studied using both custom-made devices and different commercial designs, currently only available for investigational use.

The Gore TAG thoracic branch endoprothesis (TBE, Gore) is a novel, single branch stent graft designed and initially studied for the treatment of thoracic aortic aneurysms with an intended proximal landing in zone two. The applications of the device have then been expanded and it has been studied (with some modifications in terms of the size of the components) to target pathologies involving zones 0 and 1, based on promising preliminary results observed in the zone two study.[8]

## Device description

The Gore TBE is a modular system consisting of two key components intended for "off-the-shelf" use: a main aortic component (Figure 1) and a side branch stent graft (Figure 2). The system also includes an optional aortic extender cuff and an additional DrySeal side branch introducer sheath (Gore). The components are made of a nitinol-based stent frame with an expanded polytetrafluoroethylene graft. The main aortic component is 10–15cm long and features sealing cuffs on both ends and a proximal bare apex that aid in generating a circumferential seal. The key characteristic of the main aortic component is the integrated inner portal that allows insertion, seal and anchoring of the modular side branch component. The portal is oriented in a retrograde fashion, so that delivery of the side branch is performed through the same femoral artery access used for the main component. The distal edge of the portal (where the side branch component exits the main aortic component) is located 20mm to 40mm distal to the proximal bare apex of the main component. The side branch is a tapered nitinol-based expanded polytetrafluoroethylene stent graft with a covalently-bound heparin coating (CBAS heparin surface, Carmeda) which allows for long-term local inhibition of thrombosis. There are three distinct

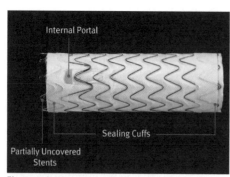

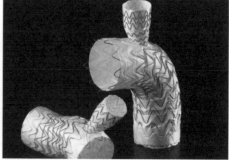

**Figure 1:** Aortic component of Gore thoracic branch endoprosthesis with side branch portal to accommodate branch component.

**Figure 2:** Assembled aortic and side branch components of Gore thoracic branch endoprosthesis. The device on the left is for use in zone one and two cases and the graft on the right with a longer segment between its proximal margin and the branch portal is for zone 0 anatomy with anchoring in the ascending aorta.

sections in the side branch component: the branch vessel segment, the tapered flex segment, and the internal portal segment. The leading 15mm branch vessel segment is designed to provide a circumferential seal in the branch vessel. The middle tapered segment is 20mm long and is designed for optimal flexibility, to accommodate arch movements. The trailing 25mm constitutes the internal portal segment, which provides a seal at the main aortic component portal and features three anchoring apices to prevent any slippage or migration. The optional aortic extender cuff is similar to the main aortic component without the portal and includes bare apices on the distal end. Each of the components is available in various sizes, with a variety of possible combinations that allow for treatment of a wide spectrum of anatomies.

## Procedure

Treatments with an intended landing in zones 0 or one require a first stage surgical revascularisation procedure of the left common carotid artery and/or the left subclavian artery. A variety of strategies can be used, depending on the segment treated and the specific anatomy of the patient, including left common carotid artery to left subclavian artery bypass, left subclavian artery and including left common carotid artery double transpositions, left common carotid artery transposition with left subclavian artery bypass, right common carotid artery to left common carotid artery bypass with left subclavian artery transposition, right common carotid artery to left subclavian artery bypass with reimplantation of the left common carotid artery. Suture ligation or coiling is required as well, in order to prevent retrograde type II branch endoleaks. Treatment in zone two can be completed without any adjunctive surgical procedure.

The device is delivered through a transfemoral route under general anaesthesia. First, guidewires are inserted into the aorta and the branch vessel. Through and through brachial to femoral guidewire access to facilitate the delivery of the side branch can be used depending on the individual arch anatomy and physician preference. The main aortic component is then introduced over both guidewires. A removable guidewire tube is provided to aid in passage of guidewire through the internal portal (Figure 3). The device is advanced into the proximal descending segment where care is taken to reduce any crossing of the guidewires by twisting

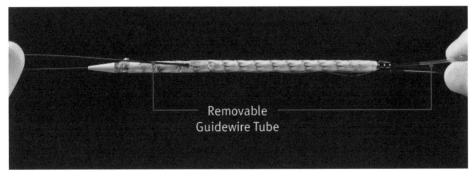

Removable
Guidewire Tube

**Figure 3:** Distal end of delivery system for aortic component with pre-cannulated loading tube within branch portal to facilitate guidewire passage through internal branch sleeve. The device is advanced in the aorta over the guidewire exiting the end hole and the second wire placed within the target branch artery.

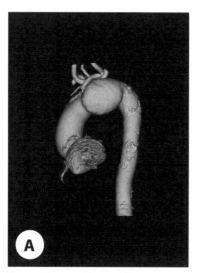

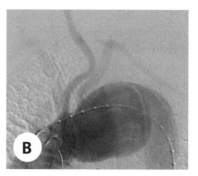

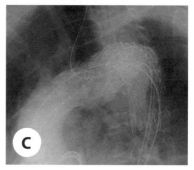

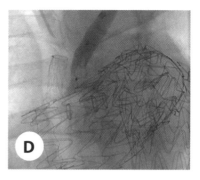

**Figure 4:** 76-year-old man with aortic arch aneurysm involving the left subclavian artery. (A) CT scan reconstruction of arch aneurysm and zone one landing zone between the innominate artery and the left common carotid artery origin; (B) Thoracic aortogram in left anterior oblique projection prior to TBE placement. (C) Post-deployment aortogram of the aortic component and side branch graft in left common carotid artery. A distal C-TAG extension into the proximal descending segment is evident. (D) Placement of Amplatzer vascular plug (Abbott) in the proximal left subclavian artery below left carotid to left subclavian surgical bypass graft is performed to prevent retrograde flow into the aneurysm via the left subclavian. The left common carotid side branch graft is well seen exiting from the portal of the aortic component of the TBE.

the delivery catheter to undo any wire wrap. Then, the device is positioned within the arch and deployed. After deployment of the aortic component, the delivery system is withdrawn. The DrySeal side branch introducer sheath and dilator are then advanced, over the branch guidewire, through the portal of the aortic component and into the branch artery. The dilator is removed, and the side branch component is advanced through the sheath to the side branch vessel. Once the device is properly positioned within the branch, the sheath is withdrawn into the aorta and the self-expanding branch stent graft is deployed.

## Advantages

The main benefit of using the Gore TBE for the treatment of zone 2 aneurysms is that it enables total endovascular repair, while maintaining perfusion of the left subclavian artery. As for its application to treat pathologies in zone 0, it allows for a relatively low risk hybrid repair, in conjunction with a revascularisation procedure of the left common carotid artery and left subclavian artery. Currently available alternative hybrid approaches in this setting would involve a surgical debranching of the innominate artery with a graft from the ascending aorta, a more invasive and complex procedure that requires a median sternotomy approach, with associated additional operative risks.

Several design features of the Gore TBE make it a suitable option for the treatment of pathologies of the aortic arch. The side branch features a flexible middle portion, allowing it to accommodate the arch movements relative to the branch vessels, one factor that raises concern for the durability of any branch stent graft. Additionally, the retrograde orientation of the side branch allows for an easier access from the femoral artery for deployment of both the main aortic component and the side branch graft. The easier deployment of the device and the side branch component compared to other solutions such as fenestrated endografts can help reduce extensive manipulations in the aortic arch, and in turn limit the risk of complications such as embolisation and retrograde dissection. Finally, being a modular device, a variety of configurations of the different components of the Gore TBE system are possible, enabling for treatment of a wide range of pathologies (e.g. the intended aortic diameter treatment range with the device is 16mm to 48mm).

## Limitations

Despite the availability of different sizes for the various components, there are still limitations in terms of the anatomies that can be targeted by this device. Specifically, the minimum required proximal landing zone ranges 16mm to 33.5mm, depending on the diameter of the aorta (and of the main aortic component used). In general, the larger the aortic diameter, the longer the distance from the portal segment to the proximal covered portion of the aortic component (proximal landing zone) and, hence, the longer the minimum spacing required between the side branch endograft and the adjacent proximal branch vessel (left common carotid artery or innominate arch). Additionally, the side branch stent graft is intended for placement in branch vessels 6mm to 18mm in diameter; therefore, patients with larger supra-aortic trunks may not be eligible for treatment with this device.

## Outcomes

Currently the device has been investigated in two studies that have evaluated the feasibility and early feasibility of the TBE for the treatment of aortic aneurysms in zones 2 and zone 0/1, respectively. Short-term results from the zone 2 trial have been recently published.[8] In total, 30 patients have been treated with the device: seven patients with a proximal landing zone in Ishimaru zone 0, one patient in zone one (Figure 4) and 22 patients in zone two. Details of the pathologies treated are listed in Chart 1.

The primary endpoints of successful access and deployment of the device and primary patency of the side branch stent graft (assessed by angiography at the conclusion of the procedure) were achieved in all patients (100%) (Figure 5). Additionally, primary patency of the side branch at one and six months has also

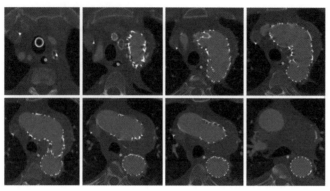

**Figure 5:** Axial CT images obtained prior to hospital discharge show the aortic and side branch grafts of the TBE. The aneurysm sac has thrombosed and there is no evidence of an endoleak. Contrast opacification of the innominate and left carotid arteries is evident as is the plug within the proximal left subclavian artery.

been evaluated, and only one case of side branch thrombosis with loss of patency at six months has been observed in the zone two study.

## Complications

Potential complications of the procedure include those associated with TEVAR: access site complications, endoleaks, retrograde aortic dissection, aortic rupture, paraplegia, stroke, stent fracture/kinking/migration. Additionally, complications involving the side branch component, such as occlusion, fracture or kinking, are possible as well.

Preliminary data from the feasibility studies have revealed no procedural or periprocedural (within 30 days) deaths. One death was reported in a patient with two aneurysms in the ascending and descending aorta. The patient was treated for the descending aneurysm and considered for subsequent ascending aortic surgery. The patient died four months after the TBE procedure. A post-mortem examination diagnosed a rupture of the ascending aortic aneurysm. It is unclear whether the death has been caused by the TBE device or a prior procedure during which a complication occurred when one of the two extender cuffs used was noted to invaginate during balloon aortoplasty.

| | Zone 2 | Zone 0/1 |
|---|---|---|
| Number of patients overall | | |
| | 31 | 9 |
| Number of patients per aneurysm type | | |
| Fusiform | 12 | 2 |
| Saccular | 19 | 7 |
| Max aneurysm diameter (mm) | | |
| Mean (std dev; range) | 54.8 (10.9; 39.7–77.0) | 63.8 (7.8; 54–75.5) |
| Total treatment length (cm) | | |
| Mean (std dev; range) | 17.3 (8.2; 10–32.7) | 19.6 (4.7; 15.0–26.5) |

**Chart:** Lesion characteristics.

Seven endoleaks have been observed in the zone 2 study, most of which resolved spontaneously at one month without treatment. Two type 2 endoleaks, however, were still present at six months without associated aneurysmal enlargement. There have been no endoleaks in the eight patients treated in Zone 0/1.

Of particular concern, as with any procedure involving the thoracic aorta, is the risk of neurological complications secondary to either embolisation or obstruction/occlusion of the side branch stent graft. In the first series of 30 patients, there has been only one case (in Zone 0) of a left middle cerebral artery stroke, probably due to embolisation from pre-existing extensive arch atheromatous disease. At one-month follow-up, the patient exhibits persistent right sided weakness and a Rankin score of 4. Two more patients suffered from procedure-related transient neurological impairment (right lower extremity paresis and right-sided hemiparesis) that resolved in one and two days, respectively, without intervention.

There have been no instances of spinal cord ischaemia. No aortic ruptures or retrograde dissection occurred.

## Conclusion

The Gore TBE is a single branch, modular stent-graft designed for use in the aortic arch which allows a novel approach for treating arch aneurysms while avoiding or reducing the use of adjunctive open surgical procedures. Preliminary data from two feasibility studies have shown promising short-term results and a low incidence of complications relative to surgical repair. Further trials with larger patient cohorts are anticipated. These will include the study of additional pathologies (e.g., dissection, trauma with involvement of zones 0, one, and two) and will help clarify the remaining questions regarding the long term durability of the device.

At the time of writing, the device is available only for investigational use for the treatment of aortic aneurysms.

### Summary

- The development of branched endografts for the aortic arch provides select patients with endovascular options to treat lesions extending into aortic zones 0, 1, and 2.

- Trials to study the use of branched endografts are now underway to treat arch pathologies, including dissection, trauma and aneurysm.

- Most branch endografts, including the Gore TBE device, include multiple components that are designed in modular configurations to provide branch perfusion.

- Initial results with the Gore TBE device in two feasibility studies have shown promising results with a low incidence of complications.

## References

1. Hiratzka LF, Bakris GL, Beckman JA, *et al.* 2010 ACCF/AHA/AATS/ACR/ASA/SCA/SCAI/SIR/STS/SVM guidelines for the diagnosis and management of patients with thoracic aortic disease: executive summary. A report of the American College of Cardiology Foundation/American Heart Association Task Force on Practice Guidelines, American Association for Thoracic Surgery, American College of

Radiology, American Stroke Association, Society of Cardiovascular Anesthesiologists, Society for Cardiovascular Angiography and Interventions, Society of Interventional Radiology, Society of Thoracic *Surgeons*, and Society for Vascular Medicine. Catheterization and cardiovascular interventions: J Soc Card Angio Interv 2010; **76:** E43–86.

2. Estrera AL, Miller CC, Lee TY, *et al.* Ascending and transverse aortic arch repair: the impact of retrograde cerebral perfusion. *Circulation* 2008; **118:** S160–66.

3. Cao P, De Rango P, Czerny M, *et al.* Systematic review of clinical outcomes in hybrid procedures for aortic arch dissections and other arch diseases. *J Thorac Cardiovasc Surg* 2012; **144:** 1286–300.

4. Criado FJ. A percutaneous technique for preservation of arch branch patency during thoracic endovascular aortic repair (TEVAR): retrograde catheterization and stenting. *J Endovasc Ther 2007*; **14:** 54–58.

5. Azuma T, Yokoi Y, Yamazaki K. The next generation of fenestrated endografts: results of a clinical trial to support an expanded indication for aortic arch aneurysm treatment. *Eur J Cardiotharc Surg* 2013; **44:** e156-63.

6. McWilliams RG, Fearn SJ, Harris PL, *et al.* Retrograde fenestration of endoluminal grafts from target vessels: feasibility, technique, and potential usage. *J Endovasc Ther* 2003; 10: 946–52.

7. Haulon S, Greenberg RK, Spear R, *et al.* Global experience with an inner branched arch endograft. *J Thorac Cardiovasc Surg* 2014; **148:** 1709–16.

8. Patel HJ, Dake MD, Bavaria JE, *et al.* Branched endovascular therapy of the distal aortic arch: Preliminary results of the feasibility multicenter trial of the Gore thoracic branch endoprosthesis. *Ann Thorac Surg* 2016; **102:** 1190–98.

# Dissecting aortic aneurysm & graft migration

# Debate: Types A and B terms are no longer satisfactory—for the motion

## D Böckler

## Introduction

Dissection of the aorta has been known since the 16th century, having been described by Fermelius in 1542 and by Vesalius in 1557. Later in 1769, Morgagni—and Maunoir in 1802—clearly described the anatomical and pathological changes in dissection aneurysms in detail. Laenned was the first who described the term dissecting aneurysm as "anevrysme disequant".[1] The disease remained somewhat obscure, with uncertainties about its pathogenesis, until Shennan in 1934 resolved much of this with a thorough review of the published literature. He concluded that cystic media necrosis was the underlying cause of dissection and also noted the rapidly fatal course of this aortic disease.[2]

Michael E DeBakey and his group were the first to classify aortic dissection into three types (Types I, II and III), based on their growing surgical experience and better understanding of anatomical and pathological patterns. Long-term studies from DeBakey, Cooley and Creech confirmed the validity of this classification with regard to application of appropriate surgical management and with regard to prognosis for survival.[3] Daily and colleagues attempted a simplified classification and in 1970, introduced the Stanford classification.[4] The European Society of Cardiology (ESC) published yet another (third) classification (classes 1–5) in 2014, but it did not find wide acceptance within the surgical community.[5]

The contemporary recognition and treatment management of aortic dissections was influenced and ushered in by two fundamental major developments. One was the creation of the International Registry of Acute Aortic Dissection (IRAD) and the other was the revolution of treatment by the introduction of endovascular stent graft placement into dissected aorta (Stanford type B).[6–8]

Fifty years after the introduction of the classification by Crawford, 37 years after the implementation of the Stanford classification and 18 years after the first report of a succesful endovascular treatment of aortic type B dissection, it is questionable whether the current definitions of type A and B dissections are still correct and/or useful. The following chapter will open the issue for discussion.

## Recent classifications

There are two anatomical classifications for aortic dissections existing contemporarily (Figure 1): the DeBakey classification and the Stanford classification. Presence of an intimal tear, location and extent of dissection flap are the characteristics for differentiation. Both classifications are still being used in daily practice to separate aortic dissections into those that need intervention, with either surgical or endovascular repair, and those that only require medical management.

The DeBakey classification divides dissections into:
- Type I: involves ascending and descending aorta (=Stanford A)
- Type II: involves ascending aorta only (=Stanford A)
- Type III: involves descending aorta only, commencing after the origin of the left subclavian artery (=Stanford B).

The Stanford classification from Daily *et al* divides dissections by the most proximal involvement:
- Type A affects ascending aorta and arch and accounts for about 60% of aortic dissections
- Type B begins beyond brachiocephalic vessels dissection distal to the left subclavian artery and accounts for about 40% of aortic dissections.

The redefinition by Daily and colleagues focused on the fundamental prognostic difference of whether or not the ascending aorta was involved, and the practical consequences deriving from this fact. In its natural evolution, without treatment, acute type A aortic dissection has been shown to have a mortality rate of about 1% per hour initially, with half of the patients expected to die the third day and almost 80% expected to die by the end of the second week. Death rates are lower but still significant in acute type B aortic dissection: 10% minimum at 30 days and ≥70% or more in the highest risk groups.[9]

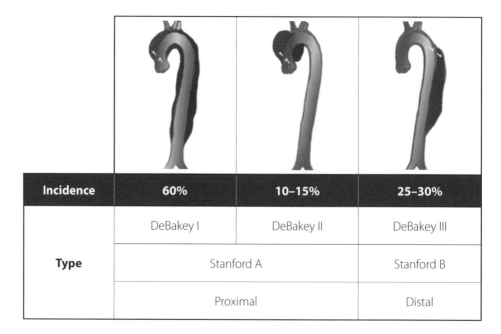

| Incidence | 60% | 10–15% | 25–30% |
|---|---|---|---|
| | DeBakey I | DeBakey II | DeBakey III |
| **Type** | Stanford A | | Stanford B |
| | Proximal | | Distal |

**Figure 1:** Classification of aortic dissection.

# Discussion

Outcome and management differ depending on localisation and extent of aortic dissection. Nevertheless, the management of aortic dissection, type A and B, acute and chronic, is considerably varied at present. Although substantial progress has been made over time, many important issues remain unclear or controversial; open surgical treatment of acute type B dissection is associated with suboptimal results because of continuing major morbidity, and it still has a 30-day operative mortality rate up to 25%.[10] On the other hand, clinical outcomes and mortality rates of best/optimal medical therapy for, e.g. uncomplicated acute type B aortic dissection, have improved considerably, with in-hospital mortality rates less than 10%.[11] Also, thoracic endovascular aortic repair (TEVAR) has added an entirely new dimension to the management of aortic dissection and is now emerging as a promising and probably preferable approach for patients who present with interventional imperatives and unstable situations. However, TEVAR for uncomplicated aortic dissection is not supported by currently available evidence. Nevertheless, there is a trend towards early TEVAR in selected uncomplicated acute type B dissection patients, a recommendation documented in the recently published guidelines of the European Society for Vascular Surgeons (ESVS).[12]

There are also preliminary reports and small series on successful endovascular treatment of type A dissection.[13–15] As development of endovascular technology proceeds ever closer to the aortic valve, endovascular repair for Type A aortic dissection deserves more attention and intensive investigation. A comprehensive literature search for studies reporting outcomes of endovascular repair in the ascending aorta was performed by Horton *et al.*[16] Hence, reconsideration of the long-standing dogma that type A needs immediate cardiothoracic repair in all cases is overdue.

The intention to classify complex diseases such as aortic dissection is important. However, aortic dissection is not a monomorphic entity but appears variable, individual and unpredictable in its natural course.

The armamentarium available to surgeons and interventionalists has been widened in the past decade by the introduction of endografting, branched and fenestrated stent graft design, false lumen management by candy plug and knickerbocker technique,[17] as well as the optimisation of best medical treatment and management modalities such as imaging.

Current definitions and terms of type A and B dissections were developed more than 40 years ago, by Daily in 1970, to simplify decision-making in clinical practice. But, with increasing evidence of the natural course, the variety of treatment options and the improving results of endovascular therapy since its first introduction in 1999 prohibits such a simplified approach. Individualisation of patient care, based on the most recent evidence available, is mandatory these days.

Applying Occam's razor has, on one hand, always been suitable in surgery. But from a forensic point of view, oversimplified approaches to complex disease (based on classification leading to guideline recommendations) can restrict the liberty of applying multimodal therapeutic options and may detain physicians from making life-saving treatment choices.[18] An example could be a patient with type A dissection being unfit for open but morphologically suitable for endovascular approaches being rejected because of the medicolegal concerns of the treating physician. There is a strong need for juridical coverage and safeguarding in these circumstances.

Regarding anatomical categorisation, type A is present when the entry site is in the ascending aorta, and type B is when it is distal to the left subclavian artery. Whereas the proximal thoracic aorta is almost always the site of the entry tear in Type B dissection, secondary or re-entry tears can occur either distally in the thoracic aorta or in the abdominal aorta or iliac arteries. Why and how all this occurs is somewhat mysterious and incompletely understood. Even retrograde haematoma or false lumen perfusion into the arch may occur, leading to different considerations for planning, judgment and therapeutic options. There is an overlap between type A and B kinds of transient pathologic morphologies and variants.

In a clinical setting, the beginning of a dissection can often be difficult to define: is it the aortic root, mid ascending aorta, distal ascending aorta or the distal aortic arch? Variants of intimal intussusception challenge interpretation and classification during imaging. How should one classify a patient showing a dissection flap starting in the aortic arch? What if supraortic branches are individually involved, as is observed in one third of patients with type A dissection? Local side branch involvement with natural fenestration or torn flap with branch stenosis remains uncomplicated, but dissection extending into branches or windsocking in the branch, causing stenosis or occlusion, are flow-limiting and cause malperfusion, which being misdiagnosed, may be fatal. Another variant of dissection is "limited intimal tear", also classified as class 3 by the ESC or type II by Svensson (Figure 2).[19]

The anatomical classification was useful for many years, informing everybody in the emergency room that type A has to be primarily referred to cardiac surgery, and type B should be primarily referred to vascular surgery. But it should not be the future. In the future, hopefully, we will not have to decide between cardiac and vascular surgery. The goal is to be treating patients together, in a hybrid room, taking care of the main entry tear, no matter where, but also malperfused organs

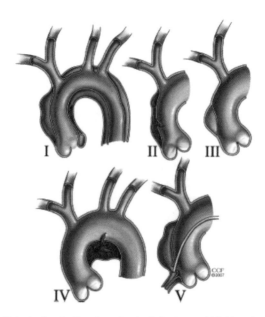

**Figure 2:** Variants of aortic dissections showing intimal tear with/without haematoma.[17]

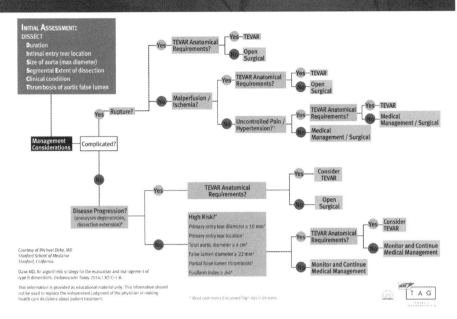

**A Physician Perspective When Treating Aortic Type B Dissections**

Courtesy of Michael Dake, MD
Stanford School of Medicine
Stanford, California

Dake MD. An algorithmic strategy for the evaluation and management of type B dissections. *Endovascular Today* 2014;13(11):1-8.

This information is provided as educational material only. This information should not be used to replace the independent judgment of the physician in making health care decisions about patient treatment.

* Most commonly discussed high-risk indicators.

**Figure 3:** DISSECT algorithm.

and blood pressure management. With treatment tools such as fusion imaging, intravascular ultrasound and transoesophageal echocardiogram in the hybrid operating room, the triage of cardiac or vascular surgery depending on the entry site is obsolete, and there is no longer a need to differentiate between types A and B.

Decision-making in daily practice becomes even more demanding with the clinical classification of acute, subacute and chronic: acute is defined as less than 14 days, subacute is between day 14 and six weeks, and everything after is defined as chronic. However, development of these criteria is an ongoing process. Different numbers of 15–90 days are found in the literature for subacute dissections demonstrating the necessity of a new classification. The terms of acute and subacute within, by convention-defined time windows, is not so useful anymore; there is need for a new classification. Michael Dake *et al* addressed this demand and developed an algorithm strategy for the evaluation and management of type B dissections not only based on the location of the main entry tear but initial assessment of duration, intimal entry tear location, maximal size of the aorta, segmental extent of the dissection, clinical condition and thrombosis of aortic false lumen (DISSECT; Figure 3).[20]

## Conclusion

In conclusion, therefore, too many and too strict classification systems followed by categorisation of individual patients should be stopped or at least become less rigid. Type A and Ttype B terms were helpful for decades, but are no longer relevant if we want to apply new knowledge, new tools, in an innovative, changing medical environment.

## Summary

- Therapy of dissections in 2017 became varied and multimodal, for both type A and B, best medical therapy, open repair, endovascular, false lumen treatment, etc.).

- Anatomical differentiation should not decide where the patient goes: type A to cardiac surgery and type B to vascular surgery or cardiology, etc.

- Treatment of dissection should be organised within interdisciplinary teams.

- Beside classic dissections, there are variants unable to be assigned within the Stanford classification.

- "White or black" (type A or B) excludes grey (variants) and limits adoption of therapeutic variety from a medicolegal perspective.

## References

1. Borst HG, Heinemann MK, Stone CD. Surgical treatment of aortic dissection. Churchill Livingstone Inc., 1996
2. T. Shennan: Dissecting Aneurysms. His Majesty's Stationery Office, London 1934. Medical Research Clinical Special Report Series No. 193
3. DeBakey ME, McCollum CH, Crawford ES, et al. Dissection and dissecting aneurysms of the aorta: twenty-year follow-up of 527 patients treated surgically. Surgery 1982; **92** (6):1118–34.
4. Daily PO, Trueblood HW, Stinson EB et al. Management of acute aortic dissections. Ann Thor Surg 1970; **10**: 237
5. Erbel R, Aboyans V, Boileau C, Bossone E et al. ESC Committee for Practice Guidelines. 2014 ESC Guidelines on the diagnosis and treatment of aortic diseases: Document covering acute and chronic aortic diseases of the thoracic and abdominal aorta of the adult. Eur Heart J 2014; **35** (41): 2873–26.
6. Hagan PG, Nienaber CA, Isselbacher EM et al. The International Registry of Acute Aortic Dissection (IRAD): new insights into an old disease. JAMA 2000; **283** (7): 897–903.
7. Nienaber CA, Fattori R, Lund G et al. Nonsurgical reconstruction of thoracic aortic dissection by stent-graft placement. N Engl J Med 1999; **340** (20):1539–45
8. Dake MD, Kato N, Mitchell RS et al. Endovascular stent graft placement for the treatment of acute aortic dissection. N Engl J Med 1999; **340 (20):** 1546–52.
9. Coady MA, Rizzo JA, Goldstein LJ, Elefteriades JA. Natural history, pathogenesis, and etiology of thoracic aortic aneurysms and dissections. Cardiol Clin 1999; **17** (4): 615–35
10. Criado F. Aortic Dissection. A 250-Year Perspective. Tex Heart Inst J 2011; **38** (6): 694–700.
11. Estrera AL, Miller CC, Goodrick J et al. Update on outcomes of acute type B aortic dissection. Ann Thorac Surg 2007; **83** (2): S842–45.
12. Riambau V, Böckler D, Brunkwall J, et al. Management of descending thoracic aorta diseases clinical practice guidelines of the European Society for Vascular Surgery (ESVS) Eur J Vasc Endovasc Surg 2017; **53:** 4–52
13. Zimpfer D,Czerny M, Kettenbach J et al. Treatment of acute type A dissection by percutaneous endovascular stent graft placement. Ann Thorac Surg 2006; **82** (2): 747e9.
14. Ye C, Chang G, Li S, et al. Endovascular stent graft treatment for Stanford type A aortic dissection. Eur J Vasc Endovasc Surg 2011; **42** (6): 787–94
15. Sobocinski J, O'Brien N, Maurel B et al. Endovascular approaches to acute aortic type A dissection: a CT-based feasibility study. Eur J Vasc Endovasc Surg 2011; **42** (4): 442–47.
16. Horton JD, Kölbel T, Haulon S et al. Endovascular Repair of Type A Aortic Dissection: Current Experience and Technical Considerations. Semin Thorac Cardiovasc Surg 2016; **28** (2): 312–17
17. Kölbel T, Lohrenz C, Kieback A, et al. Distal false lumen occlusion in aortic dissection with a homemade extra-large vascular plug: the candy-plug technique. J Endovasc Ther 2013; **20** (4): 484–89.
18. Berlin L. Medicolegal-Malpractice and Ethical Issues in Radiology. AJR Am J Roentgenol 2016; **206** (2): W41
19. Svensson LG, Labib SB, Eisenhauer AC, Butterly JR. Intimal tear without hematoma: an important variant of aortic dissection that can elude current imaging techniques. Circulation 1999; **99**: 1331–36
20. Dake M. An algorithm strategy for the evaluation and management of type B dissection. Endovascular Today 2014; **13** (11): 1–8

# Debate: Types A and B are no longer satisfactory— against the motion

K Spanos, AD Giannoukas, N Tsilimparis, ES Debus and T Kölbel

## Introduction

Aortic dissection is defined as the disruption of the media layer of the aorta with bleeding within and along its wall, resulting in separation of the aortic wall layers.[1] Two primary hypotheses of aortic dissection pathogenesis have been proposed: the first suggests that an intimal tear leads to blood flow into the media, thus separating the intima from the aortic wall; while the second suggests that it occurs after bleeding of the vasa vasorum situated in the media, resulting in a secondary intimal rupture.[2]

Population-based studies have suggested that the incidence of acute aortic dissection ranges from two to 3.5 cases per 10,0000 person/years.[3–7] Olsson and colleagues[7] noted that the incidence of aortic dissection appears to be increasing, independently of the ageing population, by 16 per 10,0000 men yearly. Aortic dissection more frequently affects men than it does women, and a male-to-female ratio of 5:1 has been reported.[8,9] The international registry of aortic dissection (IRAD) reported that the mean age at aortic dissection presentation was 63 years.[10] Regarding the prognosis of aortic dissection, 40% of patients die immediately, 1% die per hour thereafter, and between 5% and 20% die during or shortly after surgery.[9,11]

## Classification

Classification of aortic dissection is traditionally based on anatomic location and extent of the intimal flap and is critical for both treatment and prognostic purposes.

DeBakey and colleagues described the DeBakey system in 1965 and involved three types: type I arises in the ascending aorta and extends distal to the ascending aorta for a variable distance; type II is limited to the ascending aorta and terminates proximal to the origin of the innominate artery; and type III arises in the descending thoracic aorta, usually at or just distal to the left subclavian artery, below the left subclavian artery to the diaphragm (Figure 3A) or without distal boundary (3B).[12]

In 1970, a group of surgeons from Stanford University sought to simplify this classification system by reorganising it into two types. "Type A" denotes any involvement of the ascending aorta and "type B" indicates a dissection limited to the descending aorta.[13] Type Bs can be further classified as complicated and uncomplicated; approximately 25% of type Bs are complicated. Malperfusion is the most common complication, occurring in approximately 10% of patients and further complications are aortic rupture or impending rupture, peri-aortic haematoma, haemodynamic instability, spinal cord ischaemia, rapid aortic expansion and persisting hypertension.[14]

In 1994 von Segesser proposed the term "type non-A–non-B" for cases in which an intimal tear is localised beyond the ascending aorta.[15] However, there are also true "non-A–non-B" presentations that do not obviously fit with a definition of type As—instead they are limited to the aortic arch, or a retrograde dissection arising from the descending aorta extending into the arch and stops before the ascending aorta, resembling type B.[16] In the literature, ascending, arch, and descending aortic dissections have been reported to occur in 60–75%, 9–19%, and 30–35% of cases, respectively, showing that the arch is the least vulnerable location.[9,16–18]

The relative immunity of the aortic arch to intimal tears can be understood by looking at the pathophysiology and haemodynamic forces acting on the aorta. The heart is relatively fixed in position by the sternum and ribs anteriorly and by the vertebrae posteriorly. The ascending aorta and aortic arch are relatively mobile and are suspended by the arch vessels, similar to the pendulum of a clock, while the aorta is fixed just distal to the left subclavian artery by the previous ductus arteriosus botalli. A vulnerable point exists where the heart and ascending aorta connect, due to the junction of fixed and mobile structures. The mobile aortic arch and immobile descending aorta create an analogous situation. The vulnerability of these two locations to dissection and the tendency for distal rather than proximal propagation of dissections leads to a relatively low incidence of type non-A–non-B aortic dissection.[17,19]

Aortic dissection has been also clinically characterised as acute or chronic, based on the time of onset. A dissection is classified as acute within 14 days of onset and thereafter, it is defined as chronic. This classification has been based on the fact that 74% of overall mortality and most major adverse events occurred within 14 days from the symptoms onset.[4,6,9,11,20] A different temporal classification including a subacute phase has been proposed by recent studies.[21,22] The IRAD has identified four distinct time periods: hyperacute (symptom onset to 24 hours), acute (two to seven days), subacute (eight to 30 days), and chronic (>30 days). On the other hand, the VIRTUE registry,[22] a prospective multicentre clinical trial suggested a classification of acute (<15 days), subacute (15–92 days), and chronic (>92 days) dissection.

Recently, a working group on aortic dissection (the DEFINE Project) has developed a novel categorisation system that featured the specific anatomic and clinical manifestations of the disease process. This classification system is based on the mnemonic DISSECT (Duration of the disease—intimal tear location—size of the dissected aorta—segmental—extent of aortic involvement—clinical complications and thrombus within the aortic lumen), which is a more detailed classification system and intends to serve as a guide for critical analysis of contemporary therapeutic options and informed management decisions.[23] The authors suggested that this categorisation did not have the intention to dictate split-second emergent dispositions, but rather supplement the traditional Stanford classification schemes providing a framework that facilitates communication regarding the key aspects of aortic dissection.

## Treatment

### Type A aortic dissection

Type A generally requires immediate open surgical treatment including cardiopulmonary bypass and circulatory arrest. The aneurysmal ascending aorta and the proximal extent of the dissection is replaced using a supracoronary ascending repair, a hemiarch-repair or arch repair with or without a frozen elephant trunk. Replacement of the aortic valve depends on its involvement in the aortic dissection and valvular disease.[24,25]

The best surgical strategy for acute DeBakey type I aortic dissection is still controversial because of the inconsistent or even conflicting results of proximal aortic repair *vs.* extensive aortic repair on early and late prognostic outcomes. Extensive aortic repair refers to elephant trunk or frozen elephant trunk techniques. A recent meta-analysis including nine studies and 1,872 patients, indicated that proximal aortic arch dissection was associated with lower early mortality [risk ratio (RR) = 0.69, 95% confidence interval (CI) 0.54-0.90; p=0.005] but higher incidence of postoperative aortic events including reoperation of the distal aorta (relative risk [RR] = 3.14, 95% confidence interval [CI] 1.74-5.67; p<0.001).[24]

As far as it concerns age as a prognostic factor for type A treatment, a recent meta-analysis of elderly patients suggested that surgical repair remains the treatment of choice for type A, although it is associated with an increased risk of short-term mortality. Additionally, the main postoperative outcomes were comparable to younger patients and the mid-term survival rates were acceptable.[25]

Endovascular stent grafts have not yet been approved for aortic dissection involving the ascending aorta or aortic arch, while specific stent graft designs are currently being evaluated for clinical use. Despite the fact that in this first published series the graft was frequently used as a "rescue tool" outside its intended indication, treatment with the Zenith Ascend graft in this early experience appears to be safe and feasible for repair of ascending aorta pathologic processes in high-risk patients unsuitable for open repair.[26]

### Type B aortic dissection

Although best medical treatment is the traditional gold standard in uncomplicated type A,[1,20,] there is increasing evidence that thoracic endovascular aortic repair (TEVAR) is beneficial—at least in a selected subgroup of patients with certain risk factors.[27]

TEVAR, when feasible, is the first-line treatment for complicated acute type B. Compared with open surgery, TEVAR is associated with a survival benefit.[20] In a recent meta-analysis,[28] it was reported that endovascular repair provides a superior 30-day/in-hospital survival for acute complicated type B compared with surgical aortic reconstruction (7.3%; 95% CI, 5.3% to 9.6%. vs. 19.0%; 95% CI, 16.8% to 21.1%). Additionally, TEVAR seems to have a more favourable outcome regarding aortic remodelling and the aortic specific survival rate compared with medical therapy alone.[28] Despite TEVAR being associated with reasonably low early operative morbidity and mortality, there is the likelihood of aortic adverse events afterwards and all patients need to be followed with imaging after treatment.

Most chronic type B aortic dissections are managed medically unless complications develop. A tight control of systemic blood pressure is of utmost importance to limit false lumen aneurysmal dilation over time. Recurrence of symptoms or rupture, aneurysmal dilation (false lumen aneurysm of >5.5–6cm), a yearly false lumen growth (>5mm), or malperfusion should be considered signs of instability in the chronic phase and an indication for TEVAR or for open surgery if the patient has unsuitable anatomy for TEVAR. Early mortality in complicated chronic type B aortic dissection is lower with TEVAR compared with open surgery.[29]

In uncomplicated chronic type B aortic dissections, yearly clinical and imaging follow-up is recommended, irrespective of diameter and treatment applied (TEVAR/medical/open surgery).[20]

## Non-A-non-B aortic dissection; aortic arch dissection

Recent studies[16,30] suggest that there is a potential source of controversy regarding dissections with intimal flap extension into the aortic arch between the innominate and left subclavian arteries, and thus aortic dissection in this area is not adequately described with the widely-used Stanford classification. Urbanski et al[16] compared conservative with invasive treatment of aortic dissection involving the arch but sparing the ascending aorta (non-A–non-B aortic dissection) and showed that surgery seemed to offer improved clinical outcomes and, from a therapeutic point of view, non-A–non-B aortic dissection should be related to type A rather than type B. They concluded that conventional or endovascular surgery should be the preferred option in non-A–non-B aortic dissection, in which the dissection extends through the majority of the aortic arch, regardless of whether the tear is localised in the aortic arch or in the descending aorta. However, the small number of patients with non-A–non-B aortic dissection (2.8%; 8/281) and the lack of clear categorisation of type B into complicated and uncomplicated have been important limitations. Additionally, in another study, Valentine et al[30] highlighted the presence of uncertainty about whether acute type B aortic dissections involving the aortic arch (aortic dissection-arch) have an increased risk of retrograde extension into the ascending aorta or other dissection-related complications. They reported that aortic dissection of the arch was associated with a higher risk of cardiac and neurologic events, need for early intervention, and dissection-related death than aortic dissection of the descending aorta. However, in their conclusion, they suggested that medical management appeared, as the initial management strategy of aortic dissection involving the arch, to be safe and that surgeons should be aware of the increased risk of complications and the potential need for urgent interventions with these types of dissections.

On the other side of this controversy, there is convincing evidence that aortic dissection with arch extension does not limit the clinical value of the traditional Stanford classification. In IRAD study, Tsai et al[31] reported that aortic arch involvement in patients presenting with type B did not appear to increase the risk of either in-hospital or three year-follow-up mortality. In the context of IRAD study continuation, Nauta et al[32] recently suggested that arch extension was not an independent predictor of death at five years in patients with acute type

B. Thus, patients with an entry tear in the descending aorta and arch extension were associated with comparable outcomes to classic acute type B. The in-hospital mortality rate was similar for patients with (10.7%) and without (10.4%) retrograde arch extension (p= 0.96), and five-year survival was also similar (78.3% vs. 77.8%; p=0.27). Additionally, they highlighted that these patients require more diagnostic imaging tests, including echocardiography, angiography, and magnetic resonance imaging. This suggests that patients with type B and arch extension might typically require closer surveillance.

Additionally, there are authors who have suggested that because the prognosis of patients with arch extension in acute type B is virtually identical to that of others with type B, it is reasonable to extend the general management principles that are applied to classic acute type B even to patients with arch extension. Thus, there are supporters either of TEVAR with fenestrated and branched TEVAR techniques[33] or open surgery with arch replacement for the patients whose anatomy of target lesions is not manageable with TEVAR.[34]

## Conclusion

Although it has been almost half a century since the establishment of Stanford classification, there is still no evidence to dispute that this classification is satisfactory in clinical practice and decision-making. The main advantages of Stanford classification are its simplicity and coverage of most clinical situations. Although it does not include all thoracic aortic pathology such as non-A/non-B aortic dissection, and many factors like size and location of entry, extension etc. are not covered, this old classification is still primary choice as it guides the clinical treatment-algorithm in the acute situation. Thus, currently, recommendations for the management of aortic dissections are still based on the traditional classification systems such as that of Stanford. New classifications such as DISSECT may be helpful in scientific studies, but they are far too complex to be used in clinical practice, when acute decisions need to be made. In future, novel modifications or specifications may supplement the traditional Stanford classification.

## Summary

- Classification of aortic dissection is traditionally based on anatomic location and extent of the intimal flap and it remains critical for both treatment and prognostic purposes; Stanford classification (type A and B) is the most commonly used.

- In type non-A–non-B aortic dissection the intima tear is limited to the aortic arch or a retrograde dissection arising from the descending aorta extends into the arch and stops before the ascending aorta, resembling type B.

- The prognosis of patients with arch extension in acute type B is virtually identical to that of others with type B.

- Stanford classification system is simple and covers most of the clinical situations.

- There is still no evidence to support that Stanford classification (type A and B) is not satisfactory in clinical practice and decision making.

## References

1. Hiratzka LF, Bakris GL, Beckman JA, *et al*. 2010 American College of Cardiology Foundation/American Heart Association/American Association for Thoracic Surgery/ American College of Radiology/ American Stroke Association/ Society of Cardiovascular Anesthesiologists/ Society for Cardiovascular Angiography and Interventions/ Society of Interventional Radiology/ Society for Vascular Medicine for the diagnosis and management of patients with thoracic aortic disease. *Circulation* 2010; 6; **121** (13): e266–69.
2. Bonow RO, Mann DL, Zipes DP, *et al*. P. Braunwald's Heart Disease: A Textbook of Cardiovascular Medicine, Single Volume. 9th Edition. Amsterdam: Elsevier Health
3. Svensson LG, Labib SB, Eisenhauer AC, *et al*. Intimal tear without hematoma: an important variant of aortic dissection that can elude current imaging techniques. *Circulation* 1999; **99:** 1331–36.
4. Meszaros I, Morocz J, Szlavi J, *et al*. Epidemiology and clinicopathology of aortic dissection. *Chest* 2000; **117:** 1271–78.
5. Bickerstaff LK, Pairolero PC, Hollier LH, *et al*. Thoracic aortic aneurysms: a population-based study. *Surgery* 1982; **92:** 1103–08.
6. Clouse WD, Hallett JW, Jr, Schaff HV, *et al*. Acute aortic dissection: population-based incidence compared with degenerative aortic aneurysm rupture. *Mayo Clin Proc* 2004; **79:** 176–80.
7. Olsson C, Thelin S, Stahle E, *et al*. Thoracic aortic aneurysm and dissection: increasing prevalence and improved outcomes reported in a nationwide population-based study of more than 14,000 cases from 1987 to 2002. *Circulation* 2006; **114:** 2611–18.
8. Auer J, Berent R. Aortic dissection: Incidence, natural history, and impact of surgery. *J Clin Basic Cardiol* 2000; **3:** 151–54.
9. Hirst AE, Johns V, Dougenis D. Dissecting aneurysm of the aorta: A review of 505 cases. *Medicine* 1958; **37** (3): 217–19.
10. Hagan PG, Nienaber CA, Isselbacher EM, *et al*. The International Registry of Acute Aortic Dissection (IRAD): new insights into an old disease. *JAMA* 2000; **283:** 897–903.
11. Masuda Y, Yamada Z, Morooka N, *et al*. Prognosis of patients with medically treated aortic dissections. *Circulation* 1991; **84** (5 Suppl): 7–-13.
12. DeBakey ME, Henly WS, Cooley DA, *et al*. Surgical management of dissection aneurysms of the aorta. *J Thorac Cardiovasc Surg* 1965; **49:** 130–49.
13. Daily PO, Trueblood HW, Stinson EB, *et al*. Management of acute aortic dissections. *Ann Thorac Surg* 1970; **10** (3): 237–47.
14. Trimarchi S1, Eagle KA, Nienaber CA, *et al*. Importance of refractory pain and hypertension in acute type B aortic dissection: insights from the International Registry of Acute Aortic Dissection (IRAD). *Circulation* 2010; **122:** 1283–89.
15. von Segesser LK, Killer I, Ziswiler M, *et al*. Dissection of the descending thoracic aorta extending into the ascending aorta. *J Thorac Cardiovasc Surg* 1994; **108:** 755–61.

16. Urbanski PP, Wagner M. Acute non-A-non- B aortic dissection: surgical or conservative approach? *Eur J Cardiothorac Surg* 2016; **49** (4): 1249–54.

17. Lempel JK, Frazier AA, Jeudy J, *et al.* Aortic arch dissection: a controversy of classification. *Radiology* 2014; **271** (3): 848–-55.

18. Lansman SL, McCullough JN, Nguyen KH, *et al.* Subtypes of acute aortic dissection. *Ann Thorac Surg* 1999; **67** (6): 1975–78.

19. DeSanctis RW, Doroghazi RM, Austen WG, *et al.* Aortic dissection. *N Engl J Med* 1987; **317** (17): 1060–67.

20. Fattori R, Cao P, De Rango P, *et al.* Interdisciplinary expert consensus document on management of type B aortic dissection. *J Am Coll Cardiol* 2013; **61**: 1661–78.

21. Booher AM, Isselbacher EM, Nienaber CA, *et al.* The IRAD classification system for characterizing survival after aortic dissection. *Am J Med* 2013; **126**: 19-24.

22. VIRTUE Registry Investigators. Mid-term outcomes and aortic remodelling after thoracic endovascular repair for acute, subacute, and chronic aortic dissection: the VIRTUE Registry. *Eur J Vasc Endovasc Surg* 2014; **48**: 363–71.

23. Dake MD, Thompson M, van Sambeek M et al.; DEFINE Investigators. DISSECT: a new mnemonic-based approach to the categorization of aortic dissection. *Eur J Vasc Endovasc Surg* 2013; **46** (2):175-90.

24. Yan Y, Xu L, Zhang H *et al.* Proximal aortic repair *versus* extensive aortic repair in the treatment of acute type A aortic dissection: a meta-analysis. *Eur J Cardiothorac Surg* 2016; **49** (5): 1392-401.

25. Bruno VD, Chivasso P, Guida G *et al.* Surgical repair of Stanford type A aortic dissection in elderly patients: a contemporary systematic review and meta-analysis. *Ann Cardiothorac Surg* 2016; **5** (4): 257–64.

26. Tsilimparis N, Debus ES, Oderich GS *et al.* International experience with endovascular therapy of the ascending aorta with a dedicated endograft. *J Vasc Surg*. 2016; **63** (6): 1476–82.

27. Cooper M, Hicks C, Ratchford EV, Salameh MJ, Malas M. Diagnosis and treatment of uncomplicated type B aortic dissection. *Vasc Med* 2016; **21**(6): 547–52.

28. Moulakakis KG, Mylonas SN, Dalainas I, *et al.* Management of complicated and uncomplicated acute type B dissection. A systematic review and meta-analysis. *Ann Cardiothorac Surg* 2014; **3** (3): 234–46.

29. Rohlffs F, Tsilimparis N, Diener H, *et al.* Chronic type B aortic dissection: indications and strategies for treatment. *J Cardiovasc Surg* (Torino). 2015; **56** (2): 231–38.

30. Valentine RJ, Boll JM, Hocking KM, *et al.* Aortic arch involvement worsens the prognosis of type B aortic dissections. *J Vasc Surg* 2016; **64** (5): 1212–18.

31. Tsai TT, Isselbacher EM, Trimarchi S, *et al.* International Registry of Acute Aortic Dissection. Acute type B aortic dissection: does aortic arch involvement affect management and outcomes? Insights from the International Registry of Acute Aortic Dissection (IRAD). *Circulation* 2007; **116** (11 Suppl): I150–56.

32. Nauta FJ, Tolenaar JL, Patel HJ *et al.* Impact of retrograde arch extension in acute type B aortic dissection on management and outcomes. *Ann Thorac Surg* 2016; **102** (6): 2036–43.

33. Kuratani T. Best surgical option for arch extension of type B dissection: the endovascular approach. *Ann Cardiothorac Surg* 2014; **3** (3): 292–99.

34. Kim JB, Sundt TM 3rd. Best surgical option for arch extension of type B aortic dissection: the open approach. *Ann Cardiothorac Surg* 2014; **3** (4): 406–12.

# The natural history and predictors of type B aortic dissections

## D Böckler, MS Bischoff and M Ante

### Introduction

Knowledge of the natural history of vascular disease is crucial and particularly important when considering the treatment of asymptomatic patients. The spontaneous course and the incidence of disease associated complications or death needs to be understood so that the risk of these events can be balanced against the potential risks and benefits of treatment. Data from the International Registry of Acute Aortic Dissection (IRAD) registry, single-centre studies and the two randomised controlled trials INSTEAD (Investigation of stent grafts in aortic dissection)/INSTEAD XL (INSTEAD extended for late follow-up) and ADSORB (Acute dissection stent grafting or best medical treatment) have provided a better understanding of the natural history of acute type B aortic dissections.[1–5]

In the 2016 guidelines from the European Society for Vascular Surgery (ESVS),[6] best medical treatment remained the first-line treatment option for uncomplicated acute type B dissections. Intervention is accordingly reserved for patients who present with complications such as malperfusion or aortic rupture. From the IRAD-registry, Suzuki et al reported a 14-day mortality around 8% (Figure 1) for patients with uncomplicated dissections.[7] However, on the other hand, 20–50% of uncomplicated dissections will progress and chronically expand and, therefore, require intervention to prevent death due to rupture.[8] The estimated rupture rate increases to 30% once the aortic diameter reaches 6cm, and mortality is considered to be 20–40% at five years.[9–11]

Certain clinical factors—such as refractory pain and hypertension—are well known to be associated with increased in-hospital mortality.[12] Furthermore, identifying predictors of poor prognosis on imaging is potentially useful for selecting patients for whom a more aggressive management may be beneficial.[13]

The following chapter focuses on knowledge about the spontaneous course of type B aortic dissection and on predicting factors of progression, aneurysmal degeneration and late aortic events of type B dissections based on initial computed tomography (CT) scan imaging.

### Insights from the IRAD registry

The IRAD registry identified factors associated with increased in-hospital mortality that where taken were taken into consideration for risk stratification and

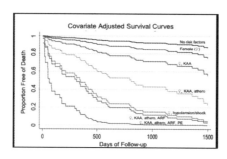

**Figure 1:** Influence of comorbidities on survival (ARF=atrial fibrillation; PE=pulmonary embolism).

decision-making. It also analysed patients with acute dissections, the majority of whom had hypertension and acute chest/back pain. In-hospital mortality was 13%, with most deaths occurring within the first week. Another publication, by Trimarchi *et al*, reported an in-hospital mortality of 6.1%.[14] Factors associated with increased in-hospital mortality on univariate analysis were hypotension/shock, widened mediastinum, periaortic haematoma, excessively dilated aorta (≥6cm), in-hospital complications of coma/altered consciousness, malperfusion, acute renal failure, and surgical management (all P<0.05). A risk prediction model with control for age and gender showed that hypotension/shock (odds ratio [OR] 23.8; P<0.0001), absence of chest/back pain on presentation (OR 3.5; P=0.01), and branch vessel involvement (OR 2.9, P=0.02)—referred to as "the deadly triad"—are independent predictors of in-hospital death.[9] Comorbidities have negative impact on survival (Figure 1).[15,16]

## Data from randomised controlled trials

The two prospective randomised trials on uncomplicated dissection—the ADSORB and the INSTEAD trials—give further information on its natural course. In ADSORB, 61 patients were randomised to undergo thoracic endovascular aortic repair (TEVAR) and best medical therapy (30) or to best medical therapy alone (31). Patients with malperfusion and rupture were excluded. During the first 30 days, no deaths occurred in either group but there were three crossovers from the best medical therapy to the best medical therapy and TEVAR group—all due to progression of disease within one week.

Incomplete false lumen thrombosis was found in 13 patients (43%) in the TEVAR plus best medical therapy group compared with 30 (97%) in the best medical therapy alone group (p<0.001). The false lumen reduced and true lumen increased in size in the best medical therapy plus TEVAR group (p<0.001). In conclusion, uncomplicated aortic dissection can be safely treated with a stent graft. Remodelling with thrombosis of the false lumen and reduction of its diameter is induced by the stent graft, but long-term results are needed.[5]

The INSTEAD trial, which enrolled 136 patients with chronic dissection, failed to show an improvement in two-year survival and adverse event rates with TEVAR. However, it did find that stent graft repair was associated with expansion of the true lumen compared with those treated medically. Furthermore, at five years, stent graft repair was associated with lower all-cause and aortic-related mortality than was medical treatment alone.[3]

INSTEAD-XL also showed improved aortic-related survival and delayed disease progression at five years. The risk of all-cause mortality (11.1% *vs.* 19.3%; p=0.13), aorta-specific mortality (6.9% *vs.* 19.3%; p=0.04) and progression (27% *vs.* 46.1%;

p=0.04) after five years was lower with TEVAR than with best medical treatment alone. Results showed a benefit of TEVAR regarding all-cause mortality (0% vs. 16.9%; p=0.0003), aorta-specific mortality (0% vs. 16.9%; P=0.0005) and progression (4.1% vs. 28.1%; P=0.004) between two and five years; in patients who received TEVAR, stent graft-induced false lumen thrombosis was observed in 90.6% of cases (p<0.0001). The conclusion of the trialists was that TEVAR is recommended for patients with stable type B dissection with suitable anatomy in addition to best medical treatment.[4]

## Perspective from a single-centre experience

A Swedish single-centre study prospectively analysed aneurysm formation, necessity of surgery, incidence of rupture and mortality in patients with conservatively treated acute aortic dissection.[2]

Follow-up included blood pressure control, clinic visits with physical examination, chest X-ray and spiral CT or magnetic resonance (MR) imaging at three and six months and annually thereafter. Sixty-six patients were followed for a mean of 79 months (range 22–179). The survival rate was 82% at five years and 69% at 10 years. Eighty-five percent of patients remained free from dissection-related death at five years and this figure was 82% at 10 years. Ten patients (15%) developed aneurysm (>6cm) of the dissected aorta. Three of these 10 patients died from aortic rupture and two underwent elective surgical repair. Of 56 patients without aneurysm, one died from rupture and one died suddenly of an unknown cause. One patient was treated with an endovascular stent graft. Five patients sustained a new type A aortic dissection, of which all but one were fatal. In 26 patients, the initial dissection was categorised as intramural haematoma. Twelve of these patients had, in addition to the haematoma, areas with localised dissection/ulcer-like projection. This was found to be a predictor of aortic events (dissection-related death, rupture, new type A aortic dissection, aneurysm formation) during follow-up, as was an initial diameter of >4cm at the first CT scan during the acute event. The authors concluded that patients with acute type B dissection treated conservatively had a low incidence of aneurysm formation and rupture during the chronic phase.

The same authors prospectively investigated quality of life in patients who received best medical therapy alone and compared them with the Swedish general population.[17] There were only minor differences in functioning and well-being between the patients and the general population—patients reported similar emotional well-being, cognitive functioning, quality of sleep, overall general health and quality of social relations as their normative counterparts. However, the patients' perception of their current health, prior health, perceived resistance to illness and health concern was worse than that of the normative population. Female patients also reported worse physical functioning and a lower satisfaction with their physical functioning than male patients or female counterparts in the normative population. In conclusion, patients with uncomplicated type B aortic dissection who are initially managed conservatively differ little from a normative Swedish population. This study supports conservative management of patients and challenges the indication of prophylactic stent graft in acute and subacute type B aortic dissection.

## Predictors for progression and aortic expansion in acute type B aortic dissection

Evangelista *et al* demonstrated that patients with a large entry tear located in the proximal part of the dissections are a high-risk subgroup. Optimal cut-off value of entry size for prediction of aortic complications was >10mm (hazard ratio [HR] 5.8; p>0.001).[18]

Loewe and Weiss identified a new predictor with primary entry tear at the concavity of the distal aortic arch. There was a significant difference with regard to complications (convexity 21% vs. concavity 61%; p=0.003) and time of appearance (convexity nine days vs. concavity zero days; p 0.02).[19,20]

Kato *et al* performed univariate and multivariate factor analyses to determine the predictors for chronic-phase enlargement (≥60mm).[21] The predictors for aortic enlargement were maximum aortic diameter of >40mm during the acute phase (p<0.001) and a patent primary entry site in the thoracic aorta (p=0.001). The rates of freedom from aortic enlargement for patients with large aortic diameter (≥40mm) during the acute phase and a patent primary entry site in the thorax at one, three, and five years were 70%, 29%, and 22%, respectively. No aortic enlargement was observed in the other patients throughout the entire follow-up period. These data suggest that patients with type B aortic dissection who have a large aortic diameter (≥40mm) and a patent primary entry site should be treated early during the acute phase. Same predictors were confirmed by other groups.[22–24]

Song *et al* wrote that a large false lumen diameter of >22mm at the upper descending thoracic aorta on the initial CT scan predicts late aneurysm dilatation and adverse outcomes (p<0.001). Aneurysmal dilatation occurred in 28%, with the highest growth rates in the upper descending aorta of 3.43+3.66mm/year. Additionally, Marfan syndrome and maximum diameter in the mid-descending thoracic aorta were independent predictors.[24]

The influence of the false lumen status, including partial false lumen thrombosis, was investigated by two groups. First, Tanaka *et al* demonstrated that the need for intervention was higher in patients with patent false lumen, but also showed that intervention did not alter long-term mortality. Furthermore, requirement of intervention was 0% in patients with complete thrombosis, 16% in partial thrombosis and 26% in patent false lumen.[25] Second, Tsai *et al* (in contrast to Tanaka *et al)* demonstrated that partial thrombosis of the false lumen, as compared with complete patency, is a significant independent predictor of post-discharge mortality (HR 2.69, 95% CI 1.45–4.98; p 0.002).[26]

Additionally, they found that the three-year mortality rate for patients with a patent false lumen was 13.7+7.1%, 31.6+12.4% for those with partial thrombosis, and 22.6+22.6% for those with complete thrombosis (median follow-up 2.8 years; p=0.003). These findings are explained by the creation of a blind sac due to obstructed re-entry tears and elevated mean and diastolic blood pressure levels.

Bernhard *et al* also showed that patency of descending aorta false lumen is responsible for progressive aortic dilation.[27]

Marui *et al* developed the "fusiform index" that expresses the degree of fusiform dilatation of the proximal descending aorta during the acute phase of aortic type B dissection to investigate whether late aortic events can be predicted with this index, and the authors then investigated whether late aortic events can be predicted with this index. The fusiform index is calculated by maximum diameter of the proximal descending aorta at the pulmonary level divided by diameter of the distal arch plus diameter of the descending aorta at the pulmonary level. A fusiform index value of >0.64 was considered to be the threshold for late aortic events.[28]

Lavingia *et al* concluded, in a five-year retrospective single centre study, that volumetric analysis of the initial index CT scan can predict growth. A true lumen volume/false lumen volume ratio <0.8 was highly predictive for requiring an intervention (sensitivity, 69%; specificity, 84%: positive predictive value, 71%; negative predictive value, 81%, odds ratio 12.2, 95% CI 5-26; P<0.001).[29]

Our own unpublished data of a retrospective two-centre study confirmed that significant aortic expansion is observed in every second uncomplicated type B aortic dissection under best medical therapy at one year. There is a correlation between the numbers of predictors and the annual growth rate. CT-based predictors may help to define type B aortic dissection-patients at risk for expansion and who may benefit from early endovascular repair. Further studies with larger cohorts and longer follow-up are warranted.

## Conclusion

According to growing evidence on natural history, endovascular therapy is increasingly considered to be an alternative to medical management in selected cases of acute uncomplicated type B dissection. Several groups identified predicting image-based factors and were able to define high-risk subgroups of patients who may benefit from earlier and more aggressive therapy. Further retrospective and prospective studies are needed in order to fully understand and confirm independent predictors of adverse outcome.

### Summary

- Type B aortic dissection is a heterogeneous disease that produces dissimilar clinical subsets, each of which can have specific natural course and outcomes.

- There are few long-term data for natural history of type B aortic dissection, with mid- and long-term survival under best medical therapy between 80% and 90% at five years.

- Aortic expansion >65mm is very rare, and fate of abdominal aortic segment still unknown.

- Overall survival in randomised controlled trials is better with TEVAR than with best medical therapy alone.

- Imaging-based predictors for acute and late adverse events have been reported in retrospective single-centre series.

- These predictors of progression are increasingly being implemented in clinical decision-making

- There is a trend towards early intervention in subgroups of patients at higher risk for aortic expansion.

# References

1. Hagan PG, Nienaber CA, Isselbacher EM, *et al.* The International Registry of Acute Aortic Dissection (IRAD): new insights into an old disease. *JAMA* 2000; **283** (7): 897–903.

2. Winnerkvist A, Lockowandt U, Rasmussen E, Rådegran K. A prospective study of medically treated acute type B aortic dissection. *Eur J Vasc Endovasc Surg* 2006; **32** (4): 349–55.

3. Nienaber CA, Rousseau H, Eggebrecht H, *et al.* Randomized comparison of strategies for type B aortic dissection: the INVestigation of STEnt Grafts in Aortic Dissection (INSTEAD) trial. *Circulation* 2009; **120** (25): 2519e28.

4. Nienaber CA, Kische S, Rousseau H, *et al.* Endovascular repair of type B aortic dissection: long-term results of the randomized investigation of stent grafts in aortic dissection trial. *Circ Cardiovasc Interv* 2013; **6**: 407–16.

5. Brunkwall J, Kasprzak P, Verhoeven E, *et al.* Endovascular repair of acute uncomplicated aortic type B dissection promotes aortic remodelling: 1 year results of the ADSORB trial. *Eur J Vasc Endovasc Surg* 2014; **48** (3): 285–91.

6. Riambau V, Böckler D, Brunkwall J, *et al.* Management of descending thoracic aorta diseases clinical practice guidelines of the European Society for Vascular Surgery (ESVS). *Eur J Vasc Endovasc Surg* 2017; **53**: 4e52.

7. Suzuki T, Mehta RH, Ince H, *et al.* International Registry of Aortic Dissection. Clinical profiles and outcomes of acute type B aortic dissection in the current era: lessons from the International Registry of Aortic Dissection (IRAD).Circulation 2003; **108 [Suppl II]:** II312–II 317.

8. Fattori R, Tsai TT, Myrmel T, *et al.* Complicated acute type B dissection: is surgery still the best option? A report from the International Registry of Acute Aortic Dissection. *JACC Cardiovasc Interv* 2008; **1**: 395–402.

9. Sueyoshi E, Sakamoto I, Uetani M. Growth rate of affected aorta in patients with type B partially closed aortic dissection. *Ann Thorac Surg* 2009; **88**: 1251–57.

10. Kato M, Bai H, Sato K, *et al.* Determining surgical indications for acute type B dissection based on enlargement of aortic diameter during the chronic phase. *Circulation* 1995; **92** (Suppl): II107–12.

11. Onitsuka S, Akashi H, Tayama K, *et al.* Long-term outcome and prognostic predictors of medically treated acute type B aortic dissections. *Ann Thorac Surg* 2004; **78:** 1268–73.

12. Estrera AL, Miller CC, Goodrick J, *et al.* Update on outcomes of acute type B aortic dissection. *Ann Thorac Surg* 2007; 83 **(2)**: S842–45.

13. Böckler D, Ante M, Bischoff MS. Predictors of chronic type B dissections,  in Charing Cross 2016 – Vascular and Endovascular Challenges Update – Book, Editor RM Greenhalgh, BIBA Publishing 2016.

14. Trimarchi S, Tolenaar JL, Tsai TT, *et al.* Influence of clinical presentation on the outcome of acute B aortic dissection: evidences from IRAD. *J Cardiovasc Surg* (Torino) 2012; **53** (2): 161–68.

15. Tolenaar JL, Froehlich W, Jonker FH, *et al.* Predicting in-hospital mortality in acute type B aortic dissection: evidence from International Registry of Acute Aortic Dissection. *Circulation* 2014; **130 (**11 Suppl 1): S45–50.

16. Winnerkvist A, Brorsson B, Rådegran K. Quality of life in patients with chronic type B aortic dissection. *Eur J Vasc Endovasc Surg* 2006; **32** (1): 34–37.

17. Evangelista A, Salas A, Ribera A, *et al.* Long-term outcome of aortic dissection with patent false lumen: predictive role of entry tear size and location. *Circulation* 2012; **125** (25): 3133–41.

18. Loewe C, Czerny M, Sodeck GH, *et al.* A new mechanism by which an acute type B aortic dissection is primarily complicated, becomes complicated, or remains uncomplicated. *Annals of Thoracic Surgery* 2012; **93** (4): 1215–22.

19. Weiss G, Wolner I, Folkmann S, *et al.* The location of the primary entry tear in acute type B aortic dissection affects early outcome. European Journal of Cardiothoracic Surgery 2012; **42(3):** 571–76.

20. Kato M, Bai H, Sato K, *et al.* Determining surgical indications for acute type B dissection based on enlargement of aortic diameter during the chronic phase. *Circulation* 1995; **92** (9)Supplement II: 107–12.

21. Onitsuka S, Akashi H, Tayama K, *et al.* Long-term outcome and prognostic predictors of medically treated acute type B aortic dissections. *Annals Thoracic Surgery* 2004; **78** (4): 1268–73.

22. Takahashi J, Wakamatsu Y, Okude J, *et al.* Maximum aortic diameter as a simple predictor of acute type B aortic dissection. Annals of Thoracic & Cardiovascular Surgery 2008; **14** (5): 303–10.

23. Kudo T, Mikamo A, Kurazumi H, *et al.* Predictors of late aortic events after Stanford type B acute aortic dissection. *J Thorac Cardiovasc Surg* 2014; **148**: 98–104.

24. Song JM, Kim SD, Kim JH, *et al.* Long-term predictors of descending aorta aneurysmal change in patients with aortic dissection. Journal of the American College of Cardiology 2007; **50** (8): 799–804.

25. Tanaka A, Sakakibara M, Ishii H, *et al.* Influence of the false lumen status on clinical outcomes in patients with acute type B aortic dissection. *Journal of Vascular Surgery* 2014; **59** (2): 321–26.

26. Tsai TT, Evangelista A, Nienaber CA, *et al.* International Registry of Acute Aortic Dissection. Partial thrombosis of the false lumen in patients with acute type B aortic dissection. *N Eng J Med* 2007; **357** (4): 349–59.
27. Bernard Y, Zimmermann H, Chocron S, *et al.* False lumen patency as a predictor of late outcome in aortic dissection. *Am J Cardiol* 2001; **87** (12): 1378–82.
28. Marui A, Mochizuki T, Koyama T, Mitsui N. Degree of fusiform dilatation of the proximal descending aorta in type B acute aortic dissection can predict late aortic events. *Journal of Thoracic & Cardiovascular Surgery* 2007; **134** (5): 1163–70.
29. Lavingia KS, Larion S, Ahanchi SS, *et al.* Volumetric analysis of the initial index computed tomography scan can predict the natural history of acute uncomplicated type B dissections. *J Vasc Surg* 2015; **62** (4): 893–99.

# Migration after thoracic endovascular aortic repair

P Geisbüsch, D Skrypnik, M Ante, M Trojan and
D Böckler

## Introduction

Thoracic endovascular aortic repair (TEVAR) is now accepted as a first-line treatment for most thoracic aortic pathologies.[1–4] The standardisation of the procedure, technical evolution in endograft design and imaging modalities—as well as a reduction in invasiveness—have led to an increasing amount of TEVAR procedures being performed worldwide.[5,6] However, the inherent complications of the procedure include early and late endoleaks, material fatigue (particularly with the early generation stent grafts), and stent graft migration.[7]

While late migration of thoracic aortic grafts (i.e. during follow-up) seems to be a relatively infrequent event, when it does occur, it can increase the risk of potentially life-threatening conditions such as late endoleak formation and the associated risk of aortic rupture and subsequent need for reintervention.[1,8–12] Therefore, identifying patients at risk of migration and monitoring them during follow-up before a potentially life-threating complication arises is important.

At present, data regarding the incidence and risk factors for late migration is sparse. Also, several definitions and approaches for reporting migration have been published—making comparisons of the reported results difficult.[1,13] The aim of this chapter is, therefore, to outline the current standards for reporting migration, the course of a centreline-based analysis, and to present the current evidence regarding late stent-graft migration. Additionally, we give an overview about the incidence and risk factors for migration during our experience with more than 500 TEVAR patients.

## Measuring and reporting migration

In 2002, Chaikof et al provided a strict definition of graft migration: a graft shift of more than 10mm relative to a primary anatomical landmark or any shift that leads to symptoms or that requires reintervention.[14] However, Fillinger et al published the current reporting standards for TEVAR in 2010 and these standards include graft migration screening parameters.[7] These parameters should be assessed on 3D-centerline reconstruction on spiral high-resolution computed tomography (CT) scans: the ostium of the left carotid artery and the coeliac trunk give anatomical landmarks from which the centreline measurement to the proximal and distal end of the endograft should be started (Figure 1). Proximal and distal distances help to differentiate between

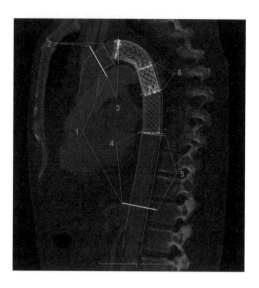

**Figure 1:** Assessment of graft position to identify migration according to the reporting standards: (1) Distance from left common carotid artery (LCCA) to coeliac trunc (CT) (2) LCCA to most proximal visualisation of the stent; (3) LCCA to most proximal point where the full circumference of the stent is first seen; (4) CT to most distal visualisation of the stent; (5) CT to most distal point where the full circumference of the stent is first seen; (6) Overlapping segments of multiple stent grafts.

graft migration (when both tip- and circumference-distance exceed 10mm) and graft angulation (when tip- or circumference-distance exceed 10mm but not both).

In case of an increase of distal or proximal distances (or both) for more than 10mm from the aortic arch branches, adjudicative analysis concerning nearest fixed landmarks (calcifications, bones, surgically clips or implanted prosthesis) is recommended. If a relevant shift is shown, migration should be considered as ascertained (Figure 2).

The distance between the left common carotid artery and coeliac trunk also provide an opportunity to review aortic elongation and to differentiate it from graft migration. To assess aortic configuration, Chen *et al* proposed the tortuosity index (Figure 3), which is determined by dividing the curved length along a centreline by the straight distance between proximal and distal landing zones.[15] A high tortuosity index has been shown to be associated with an increased risk for type III endoleaks.[16] Despite these definitions, there is a diversity of reporting and assessing algorithms for TEVAR, which make research results difficult to collect and analyse.[1,17]

## Incidence and risk factors for migration

Late migration of TEVAR is reported in 0.7–7.5% of cases.[2,4,9,18] The wide range of reported incidences is most likely attributable to the differences in patient cohorts and especially in the frequency of associated risk factor for migration.

### Risk factors

Altnji *et al* used a finite element method to investigate factors that might influence device (nitinol-stent) migration in a thoracic aortic aneurysm model.[19] Their analysis showed that a short length of the proximal landing zone (<18mm) is associated with an increased risk of migration, which is confirmed by clinical studies in the infrarenal segment.[20,21] Additionally, the simulation results showed that large oversizing (>25%) might increase the risk for late migration in the thoracic aorta, especially in patients with severely angulated necks.[19] This is in line with the clinical observation that large oversizing might lead to stent graft infolding, thereby stent graft collapse and potential migration. Endovascular aneurysm repair (EVAR) studies have shown that >30% oversizing is associated with a significant higher risk for device migration (14% vs.

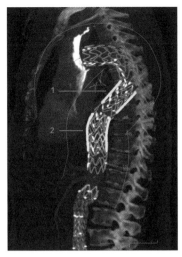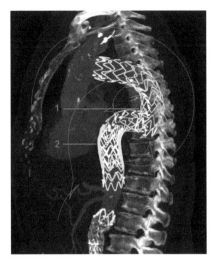

**Figure 2:** Late migration in the first overlapping zone after TEVAR for an asymptomatic thoracic aortic aneurysm with multiple stent graft, leading to complete device separation and reperfusion of the aneurysm (1 = first overlapping zone; 2= second overlapping zone). (A) Postoperative CT and (B) CT in 54 months after the implantation.

0.9%; p<0.002)[22] and the simulation also confirmed the influence of the quality of the proximal landing zone as a risk factor for device related complications.[23]

Aortic elongation seems another logical risk factor for device shift for several reasons. For example, multiple devices are typically required in elongated, diseased aortas, which increases the risk for migration in stent graft overlapping zones and causes device separation.[24]

In our experience, identifying migration between multiple endografts before complications (separation/endoleak) occur can be particularly difficult. Furthermore, aortic elongation of the non-stented aortic segment has been described in up to 31% of the patients.[25] As the stent graft usually adjusts on the outer curve of the aorta, this elongation can cause dislodgement from the primary landing zone with subsequent endoleak and device shift. Additionally, the first-generation endografts seem to be more prone to migration. Resch *et al* report, in their series of early TEVAR cases, that device shift occurred in 30% of the cases during follow-up.[26]

## Heidelberg experience

At our institution, patient data were prospectively gathered from a TEVAR database for analysis. Using the cumulated research, a retrospective evaluation for late migration was performed by three independent reader (in accordance with the aforementioned reporting standards).[7] Patients presenting with traumatic aortic rupture, penetrating atherosclerotic ulcer, intramural haematoma, aortic aneurysm and aortic dissection were included in the study. All hybrid and branched procedures were excluded. The resulting analysis was performed on 123 patients who underwent TEVAR between 2005 and 2015 and who had a follow-up CT angiography scan with minimum follow-up of six month. Migration was found in nine patients (7.3%), which is in line with the aforementioned series.

All device migrations occurred in patients with thoracic aortic aneurysm (6/37; 16.2%) and aortic dissections (3/39; 7.7%), but this pathology was not found to be an independent risk factor for migration. In our series, six patients (66%) with

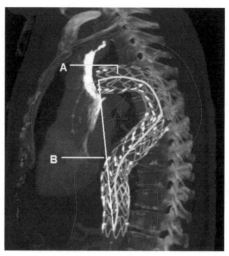

**Figure 3:** Assessment of tortuosity index to quantify global aortic elongation (Chen *et al* 2014). Tortuosity Index (TI) = A/B. (A) Centreline distance between landing zones; (B) Direct distance between landing zones in LAO-projection.

device migration had multiple endografts and aortic elongation was shown to be an independent risk factor for device migration (p=0.003). Also, the rate of tortuosity of patients with migrated device was not found to be significantly different from that of patients with non-migrated devices (p=0.17).

## Conclusion

Late migration after TEVAR is relative infrequent but it can predispose patients to potentially life-threatening conditions, such an endoleak and aortic rupture (and subsequent reintervention). It can be avoided through understanding graft migration and optimisation of the follow-up protocol. Patients with short, unhealthy proximal and distal landing zones, multiple stent grafts and global aortic elongation seem to be at a higher risk for late migration and should thus be carefully evaluated during follow-up.

## Summary

- The body of evidence regarding migration after TEVAR is low.

- Current reporting standards for migration after TEVAR exist and provide the opportunity to uniformly assess stent-graft position, report migration and differentiate it from graft angulation or aortic elongation, which might help to improve data in the future.

- Late migration after TEVAR is relatively infrequent (0.7–7.5%), but can be life-threating in case of development of endoleak with late consecutive aneurysm rupture.

- Reported predisposing factors for late endograft migration are: length (<18mm) and character of proximal landing zone, large (>30%) oversizing, aortic elongation and the use of multiple endografts.

# References

1. Canaud L, Marty-Ane C, Ziza V, *et al*. Minimum 10-year follow-up of endovascular repair for acute traumatic transection of the thoracic aorta. *J Thorac Cardiovasc Surg* 2015; **149** (3): 825–29.

2. Matsumura JS, Melissano G, Cambria RP, *et al*. Five-year results of thoracic endovascular aortic repair with the Zenith TX2. *J Vasc Surg* 2014; **60** (1): 1–10.

3. Abraha I, Romagnoli C, Montedori A, Cirocchi R. Thoracic stent graft *versus* surgery for thoracic aneurysm. *The Cochrane Database of Systematic Reviews* 2016(6): Cd006796.

4. Morales JP, Greenberg RK, Morales CA, *et al*. Thoracic aortic lesions treated with the Zenith TX1 and TX2 thoracic devices: intermediate- and long-term outcomes. *J Vasc Surg* 2008; **48** (1): 54–63.

5. Scali ST, Goodney PP, Walsh DB, *et al*. National trends and regional variation of open and endovascular repair of thoracic and thoracoabdominal aneurysms in contemporary practice. *J Vasc Surg* 2011; **53** (6): 1499–505.

6. Criado FJ. The TEVAR Landscape in 2012: A status report on thoracic endovascular aortic repair. *Endovascular Today* 2011; **11**: 34–47.

7. Fillinger MF, Greenberg RK, McKinsey JF, Chaikof EL. Reporting standards for thoracic endovascular aortic repair (TEVAR). *J Vasc Surg* 2010; **52** (4): 1022–33

8. O'Neill S, Greenberg RK, Resch T, *et al*. An evaluation of centerline of flow measurement techniques to assess migration after thoracic endovascular aneurysm repair. *J Vasc Surg* 2006; **43** (6): 1103-10.

9. Makaroun MS, Dillavou ED, Wheatley GH, Cambria RP. Five-year results of endovascular treatment with the Gore TAG device compared with open repair of thoracic aortic aneurysms. *J Vasc Surg* 2008; **47** (5): 912–18.

10. Ricotta JJ. Endoleak management and postoperative surveillance following endovascular repair of thoracic aortic aneurysms *J Vasc Surg* 2010; **52** (4 Suppl): 91–9s.

11. Rolph R, Duffy JM, Waltham M. Stent graft types for endovascular repair of thoracic aortic aneurysms. T*he Cochrane Database of Systematic Reviews* 2015; **9**: Cd008448.

12. Geisbusch P, Hoffmann S, Kotelis D, *et al*. Reinterventions during midterm follow-up after endovascular treatment of thoracic aortic disease. *J Vasc Surg* 2011; **53**(6): 1528–33.

13. Piffaretti G, Negri S, Ferraro S, *et al*. Delayed graft dislocation after thoracic aortic endovascular repair. *Kathmandu Univ Med J* 2014; **12** (46): 97–100.

14. Chaikof EL, Blankensteijn JD, Harris PL, al. Reporting standards for endovascular aortic aneurysm repair. *J Vasc Surg* 2002; **35** (5): 1048–60.

15. Chen CK, Liang IP, Chang HT, *et al*. Impact on outcomes by measuring tortuosity with reporting standards for thoracic endovascular aortic repair. *J Vasc Surg* 2014; **60** (4): 937–44.

16. Ueda T, Takaoka H, Raman B, *et al*. Impact of quantitatively determined native thoracic aortic tortuosity on endoleak development after thoracic endovascular aortic repair. A*m J Roentgenol* 2011; **197**(6): W1140–6.

17. Kasirajan K, Morasch MD, Makaroun MS. Sex-based outcomes after endovascular repair of thoracic aortic aneurysms. *J Vasc Surg* 2011; **54** (3): 669–75.

18. Hassoun HT, Mitchell RS, Makaroun MS, *et al*. Aortic neck morphology after endovascular repair of descending thoracic aortic aneurysms. *J Vasc Surg* 2006; **43**(1): 26–31.

19. Altnji HE, Bou-Said B, Walter-Le Berre H. Morphological and stent design risk factors to prevent migration phenomena for a thoracic aneurysm: a numerical analysis. *Med Eng Phys* 2015; **37**(1): 23–33.

20. Fulton JJ, Farber MA, Sanchez LA, *et al*. Effect of challenging neck anatomy on mid-term migration rates in AneuRx endografts. *J Vasc Surg* 2006; **44** (5): 932–37.

21. Zarins CK, Bloch DA, Crabtree T, *et al*. Stent graft migration after endovascular aneurysm repair: importance of proximal fixation. *J Vasc Surg* 2003; **38** (6): 1264–72.

22. Sternbergh WC, Money SR, Greenberg RK, Chuter TA. Influence of endograft oversizing on device migration, endoleak, aneurysm shrinkage, and aortic neck dilation: results from the Zenith Multicenter Trial. *J Vasc Surg* 2004; **39** (1): 20–26.

23. Wyss TR, Dick F, Brown LC, Greenhalgh RM. The influence of thrombus, calcification, angulation, and tortuosity of attachment sites on the time to the first graft-related complication after endovascular aneurysm repair. *J Vasc Surg* 2011; **54** (4): 965–71.

24. Hansen CJ, Bui H, Donayre CE, *et al*. Complications of endovascular repair of high-risk and emergent descending thoracic aortic aneurysms and dissections. *J Vasc Surg* 2004; **40** (2): 228–34.

25. Chaer RA, Makaroun MS. Late failure after endovascular repair of descending thoracic aneurysms. *Semin Vasc Surg* 2009; **22** (2): 81–86.

26. Resch T, Koul B, Dias NV, *et al*. Changes in aneurysm morphology and stent-graft configuration after endovascular repair of aneurysms of the descending thoracic aorta. *J Thorac Cardiovasc Surg* 2001; **122**(1): 47–52.

# Juxtarenal consensus update—Pathways of care

# Intervention methods & outcomes

# Rationale for infrarenal *versus* suprarenal choice

## C Brinster and R Milner

## Introduction

Endovascular aortic repair (EVAR) has revolutionised the treatment of abdominal aortic aneurysms. Although first-generation aortic stent grafts were, at times, challenging to use and limited by a variety of anatomical constraints, continuous technological innovation has led to increased anatomic applicability of currently available devices. These advances, in addition to a steadily increasing comfort level with performing EVAR among vascular specialists, have led to a continually increasing number of aortic stent grafts placed over the past 10 years.[1] Despite this rapid technological progress, prohibitive proximal neck anatomy continues as a common limitation to successful EVAR.

## Endograft fixation in the challenging aortic neck

The vast majority of patients with infrarenal abdominal aortic aneurysms have neck anatomy that is suitable for endovascular repair, and comprehensive series in recent years attest to the long-term performance of currently available devices when used within their respective individual instructions for use (IFU).[2,3] As devices have become more sophisticated and operator experience has grown over time, however, IFU boundaries have been pushed with increasing comfort and regularity. In fact, a review of the current literature demonstrates that 20–40% of EVARs are performed outside the respective device IFU.[2,4] Although aortic endograft use outside the delineated IFU is the subject of ongoing debate, several series have demonstrated that EVAR can be performed safely in these situations—especially if only one of the aforementioned anatomical constraints is present.[5-7] The long-term durability of endograft use outside the recommended IFU has not yet been firmly established, but given the continued increase in the number of EVAR procedures performed worldwide, more frequent endograft use outside the IFU can be anticipated.

Juxtarenal aortic aneurysms present a unique challenge to endovascular therapy, and optimal treatment strategies remain controversial. The very short or absent infrarenal neck found with juxtarenal aortic aneurysms often excludes standard EVAR from the treatment paradigm. The use of concomitant chimney grafts placed in parallel to the standard main body during EVAR to maintain perfusion to the renal or visceral branches has gained popularity as an alternative to open surgical aortic repair or fenestrated EVAR in the treatment of juxtarenal aortic aneurysms.

The increasing use of EVAR outside the IFU for infrarenal abdominal aortic aneurysms and the development of chimney EVAR for juxtarenal aortic aneurysms refocus attention on the long-standing question of proximal endograft fixation. This chapter will serve to review the relevant literature regarding the choice of infrarenal or suprarenal fixation for standard EVAR, especially in the setting of the short proximal neck, and for chimeny EVAR in the treatment of juxtarenal aortic aneurysms.

## Infrarenal fixation in the short neck during EVAR

Nearly all vascular specialists would agree that some form of active fixation with EVAR is mandatory to avoid stent graft migration over time, and several large series have demonstrated the hazards of EVAR in the short neck as compared to EVAR within device specific IFU.[5,8,9] The EUROSTAR (European collaborators on stent/graft technologies for aortic aneurysm repair) registry was established in 2006 and examined 3,499 patients to delineate outcome following EVAR based on infrarenal neck length. The study was divided into three groups according to infrarenal neck length: >15mm (group A); 11–15mm (group B); and ≤10mm (group C). Proximal type I endoleak within 30 days occurred in 10.9% of group C compared to only 2.6% of group A. After 48 months of follow-up, the incidence of proximal endoleaks was higher in groups B (9.6%) and C (11.3%) when compared to group A (3.4%).[8] AbuRahma and colleagues later demonstrated similar results in a series of 238 patients divided into three groups: those with proximal neck lengths ≥15mm, patients with necks 10–14mm, and those with neck lengths <10mm. They found that early type Ia endoleak occurred in 12%, 42%, and 53% of patients, respectively. The authors concluded that EVAR could be performed in patients with very short proximal necks, although the risk of type Ia endoleak and need for adjuvant proximal aortic extension cuffs were significantly higher in these patients when compared to those treated within the respective device IFU.[5]

There exists of paucity of data directly comparing outcomes with infrarenal *vs.* suprarenal fixation in the setting of the short infrarenal aortic neck. Hager and colleagues sought to clarify this issue in a study of 84 patients who underwent EVAR with short neck length defined as <15mm.[1] The Excluder device (Gore), which features active infrarenal fixation, was used to treat 60 of these patients, and the Zenith (Cook Medical), featuring suprarenal fixation, was used to treat the remaining 24 patients. They reported no statistically significant difference in endograft migration or in early or late type Ia endoleak among patient groups treated with infrarenal *vs.* suprarenal fixation. The authors concluded that, when other hostile neck parameters do not exist, EVAR with infrarenal fixation can be executed safely in patients with short, straight infrarenal aortic necks. Additionally, they observed no statistically significant difference in outcome when these patients were compared to those treated by EVAR with suprarenal fixation.

## Suprarenal fixation in the short aortic neck

Patients with short, angulated, or otherwise hostile infrarenal aortic necks are at increased risk for postoperative type Ia endoleak, stent graft migration, and for the need for reintervention following EVAR.[8] In order to prevent these complications and the need for secondary procedures, many have advocated for active fixation in the suprarenal aorta in patients with short or large diameter proximal aortic

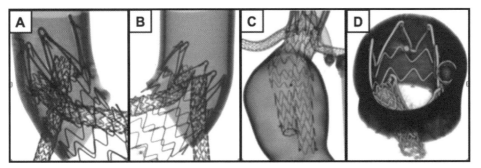

**Figures 1:** Medtronic Endurant II (A) 26mm and (B) 36mm main body with proximal extent of chimney stents above the sealing fabric but below the suprarenal fixation of the device. (C) Micro CT images with anteroposterior two-dimensional and (D) superior three-dimensional views demonstrating the bilateral chimney stents and main body endograft with suprarenal fixation.

necks.[6,10,11] Numerous recent studies have evaluated outcomes following EVAR with suprarenal fixation in these circumstances.

Lee and colleagues reported that EVAR with suprarenal fixation and aggressive use of supplemental proximal aortic cuffs as needed was preferential to the use of infrarenal fixation alone in a group of 75 patients with challenging infrarenal neck anatomy who were at prohibitive risk for open surgery.[10] After excluding patients with concomitant severe neck angulation from their cohort, Matsagakis *et al* examined a group of 19 patients with very short (<10mm) necks treated with the Endurant II endograft (Medtronic), which features suprarenal fixation.[7] This group was compared to 38 patients with aortic necks ≥10mm that were matched for age, sex, and maximal aneurysm diameter and also treated with the Endurant. Over a follow-up interval of 24 months, the investigators observed no difference between the two groups in technical success, postoperative morbidity, freedom from reintervention, or aneurysm related mortality. Although more patients in the very short neck group required intraoperative proximal aortic cuff placement (21% *vs.* 3%), no type I endoleak was observed in either group during the follow-up period. Finally, Gallitto and colleagues reported excellent results in a series of 60 patients undergoing EVAR with aneurysm necks <10mm in length.[6] All EVAR was performed with suprarenal fixation, with either the Endurant (n=28) or Zenith (n=32) device, after the patients were deemed too high risk for open surgical or fenestrated EVAR. Over a follow-up period of 51 months, the longest reported in the literature for EVAR in the treatment of very short neck aneurysms, five-year survival was 70% and freedom from reintervention was 90%. These results are commensurate with those widely reported in the literature for standard EVAR within device specific IFU.[6] These series suggest that EVAR with suprarenal fixation can be accomplished in short and very short aortic necks with high initial technical success and mid-term outcomes that compare favourably to those seen with EVAR performed within the IFU.

## Renal function following EVAR with suprarenal fixation

The presence of bare stent struts that cross the ostia of the renal arteries has led to concern regarding potential renal dysfunction after implantation of devices with suprarenal fixation. Several studies in recent years have sought to evaluate this phenomenon, with the majority concluding that there exists no real difference in renal function following EVAR with suprarenal fixation when compared to outcomes following EVAR with infrarenal fixation. Although individual reports have shown an increased rate of renal parenchymal infarction,[12] decreased creatinine clearance at one year,[13] or decreased estimated glomerular filtration rate at one year[14] with suprarenal fixation as compared to infrarenal fixation, none has demonstrated that these changes result in any tangible clinical change or lasting dysfunction among suprarenal fixation patients.

Three meta-analyses examining this phenomenon have been performed to include available published data through 2014.[15–17] A total of 53 studies and over 12,000 patients were evaluated in these three studies, which compared suprarenal and infrarenal fixation and their respective effects on postoperative renal function. No difference was found in any of the three meta-analyses regarding risk for renal dysfunction following EVAR with suprarenal *vs.* infrarenal fixation.

## Suprarenal *versus* infrarenal fixation for chEVAR

Optimal treatment of juxtarenal aortic aneurysms remains controversial. The short or absent neck of these aneurysms often precludes the use of standard EVAR devices. The broader use of fenestrated EVAR has allowed endovascular treatment of more complex juxtarenal aortic pathology, but fenestrated EVAR is technically complex, expensive, and not immediately available off-the-shelf, as custom grafts take four to six weeks to construct. Additionally, fenestrated EVAR is not anatomically feasible in every patient.

First reported in 2003, the chimney EVAR technique has gained increasing acceptance in of juxtarenal abdominal aortic aneurysms.[18] The goal of chimney EVAR is to increase the length of the proximal landing zone by stenting the necessary renal and visceral vessels in parallel to the main body endograft, thereby preserving antegrade perfusion to target organs while extending the proximal seal zone into the pararenal aorta. The chimney EVAR technique can also be used as a salvage manoeuvre when these aortic branches are inadvertently covered during routine EVAR.[19,20]

Several large studies have reported promising immediate and mid-term results following chimney EVAR for juxtarenal aneurysms. Most recently, the PROTAGORAS study reported 100% technical success with 187 chimney stents placed in 128 patients during chimney EVAR, with only two patients (1.6%) developing late type Ia endoleak and requiring reintervention.[21] Overall 30-day and mid-term mortality were low at 0.8% and 17.2%, respectively. During a mean follow-up of 25 months, chimney graft patency was 95.7% and freedom from reintervention was 93.1%. The authors sought to establish a standardised technique of chimney EVAR by using one main body endograft with suprarenal fixation. The Endurant stent graft, which features suprarenal fixation, was used in all 128 cases. The investigators concluded that standard use of the Endurant and suprarenal fixation for chimney EVAR is associated with high technical success, significant aneurysm sac regression, and low incidence of secondary procedures after two-year radiologic follow-up.

The PERICLES (Performance of the chimney technique for the treatment of complex aortic pathologies) registry evaluated 517 patients treated with 898 total stents during chimney EVAR.[22] The reported technical success was similar to that described in the PROTAGORAS study at 97.1%. Overall 30-day mortality was 4.9%, and mortality at three years was 25.1%. Patency of the chimney grafts was 94.1%. A total of 119 patients in US centres and 398 in European centres were treated during the study period. US centres preferentially used the Zenith (54%) and European centres the Endurant (62%) as the main body endograft component. Notably, these results were achieved using main body endografts with suprarenal fixation in over 70% of patients. When summarising the study data, the authors recognised the preferential selection of endografts with suprarenal fixation, citing a collective desire to use a device that would both secure the chimney grafts in place in the pararenal aorta and actively fix the main body in the challenging proximal aortic neck. In a review of the registry, a lead investigator reported that univariate analysis of type Ia endoleak demonstrated that grafts with suprarenal fixation outperformed those with infrarenal fixation, but that this discrepancy was not apparent with multivariate analysis.[22]

## Our approach to chimney EVAR: Suprarenal fixation

The advantage of main body suprarenal fixation during chimney EVAR is the inherent separation of the fixation component from the sealing component found in this type of endograft. By using a main body with suprarenal fixation, chimney stents can be landed above the fabric of the main body device but below the points of active fixation. Each chimney graft is deployed with a target 15–20mm overlap with the aortic endograft. Ideally, chimney grafts extend 10–15mm cephalad to the proximal extent of the main body endograft fabric. An effort is made to land the proximal chimney graft below the barbed suprarenal component of the device to avoid potential compromise of active fixation with subsequent endoleak and stent graft migration. This configuration maintains overall device fixation, even in the setting of potential gutter endoleaks along the proximal aspect of the main body seal zone (Figures 1A and 1B). By contrast, because main body endografts that rely on infrarenal fixation both fix and seal at the same anatomic level, there exists a greater potential for concomitant type Ia endoleak and device migration with the development of gutter endoleaks. Micro- and standard computed tomography (CT) imaging have demonstrated the successful interaction between chimney stents and endografts with suprarenal fixation (Figures 1C and 1D). The reported data from large, carefully examined registries and the radiographic findings on both micro and standard CT scan imaging confirm the efficacy of chimney EVAR with suprarenal fixation in carefully selected patients with juxtarenal aortic aneurysms. Further long-term studies are needed for widespread standardisation, and certainly before this technique is widely used as an elective treatment for juxtarenal abdominal aortic aneurysms.

## Conclusion

As technology evolves and operator experience increases, more patients will undergo EVAR and chimney EVAR in the treatment of abdominal aortic aneurysms with complex neck anatomy. Devices that feature suprarenal fixation have demonstrated favourable results in the short and mid-term when used to treat selective patients with short or absent infrarenal aortic necks. Meticulous attention to detail in patient selection, preoperative planning, and intraoperative technique are required. Long-term studies are needed to fully evaluate the durability of these techniques before widespread clinical acceptance and use are realised.

## Summary

- Infrarenal and suprarenal fixation perform well in the long term when EVAR is performed within device-specific IFU.

- EVAR with suprarenal fixation can be performed safely in select patients with very short (<10mm) proximal aortic necks in the absence of other hostile neck characteristics.

- Based on all currently available evidence, renal function does not differ significantly following EVAR with suprarenal versus infrarenal fixation.

- Endografts that feature suprarenal fixation are uniquely suited to perform well with chimney EVAR.

- Further large-scale studies are needed to fully evaluate the durability of these techniques before broad clinical applicability is achieved.

## References

1. Hager ES, Cho JS, Makaroun MS, *et al.* Endografts with suprarenal fixation do not perform better than those with infrarenal fixation in the treatment of patients with short straight proximal aortic necks. *J Vasc Surg* 2012; **55** (5): 1242–46.
2. Schanzer A, Greenberg RK, Hevelone N, *et al.* Predictors of abdominal aortic aneurysm sac enlargement after endovascular repair. *Circulation* 2011; **123** (24): 2848–55.
3. Cambria RP. Endovascular repair of abdominal aortic aneurysm: no cause for alarm. *Circulation* 2011; **123** (24): 2782–83.
4. Katsargyris A, Verhoeven EL. Endovascular strategies for infrarenal aneurysms with short necks. *J Cardiovasc Surg* (Torino) 2013; **54** (1 Suppl 1): 21–26.
5. AbuRahma AF, Campbell J, Stone PA, *et al.* The correlation of aortic neck length to early and late outcomes in endovascular aneurysm repair patients. *J Vasc Surg* 2009; **50** (4): 738–48.
6. Gallitto E, Gargiulo M, Freyrie A, *et al.* Results of standard suprarenal fixation endografts for abdominal aortic aneurysms with neck length. *J Cardiovasc Surg* (Torino) 2015. Epub.
7. Matsagkas M, Kouvelos G, Peroulis M, *et al.* Standard endovascular treatment of abdominal aortic aneurysms in patients with very short proximal necks using the Endurant stent graft. *J Vasc Surg* 2015; **61** (1): 9–15.
8. Leurs LJ, Kievit J, Dagnelie PC, *et al.* Influence of infrarenal neck length on outcome of endovascular abdominal aortic aneurysm repair. *J Endovasc Ther* 2006; **13** (5): 640–48.
9. Abbruzzese TA, Kwolek CJ, Brewster DC, *et al.* Outcomes following endovascular abdominal aortic aneurysm repair (EVAR): an anatomic and device-specific analysis. *J Vasc Surg* 2008; **48**(1): 19–28.
10. Lee JT, Ullery BW, Zarins CK, *et al.* EVAR deployment in anatomically challenging necks outside the IFU. *Eur J Vasc Endovasc Surg* 2013; **46**(1): 65–73.
11. Thomas B, Sanchez L. Proximal migration and endoleak: impact of endograft design and deployment techniques. *Semin Vasc Surg* 2009; **22** (3): 201–06.
12. Bockler D, Krauss M, Mansmann U, *et al.* Incidence of renal infarctions after endovascular AAA repair: relationship to infrarenal *versus* suprarenal fixation. *J Endovasc Ther* 2003; **10** (6): 1054–60.
13. Kouvelos GN, Boletis I, Papa N. Analysis of effects of fixation type on renal function after endovascular aneurysm repair. *J Endovasc Ther* 2013; **20** (3): 334–44.
14. Saratzis A, Sarafidis P, Melas N, *et al.* Suprarenal graft fixation in endovascular abdominal aortic aneurysm repair is associated with a decrease in renal function. *J Vasc Surg* 2012; **56**(3): 594–600.
15. Sun Z, Stevenson G. Transrenal fixation of aortic stent-grafts: short- to midterm effects on renal function—a systematic review. *Radiology* 2006; **240**(1): 65–72.

16. Walsh SR, Boyle JR, Lynch AG, *et al.* Suprarenal endograft fixation and medium-term renal function: systematic review and meta-analysis. *J Vasc Surg* 2008; **47** (6): 1364–70.
17. Miller LE, Razavi MK, Lal BK. Suprarenal *versus* infrarenal stent graft fixation on renal complications after endovascular aneurysm repair. *J Vasc Surg* 2015; **61** (5): 1340–9.e1.
18. Greenberg RK, Clair D, Srivastava S, *et al.* Should patients with challenging anatomy be offered endovascular aneurysm repair? *J Vasc Surg* 2003; **38**(5): 990–96.
19. Criado FJ. Chimney grafts and bare stents: aortic branch preservation revisited. *J Endovasc Ther 2007*; **14** (6): 823–24.
20. Lee JT, Greenberg JI, Dalman RL. Early experience with the snorkel technique for juxtarenal aneurysms. *J Vasc Surg* 2012; **55** (4): 935–46; discussion 945–6.
21. Donas KP, Torsello GB, Piccoli G, *et al.* The PROTAGORAS study to evaluate the performance of the Endurant stent graft for patients with pararenal pathologic processes treated by the chimney/snorkel endovascular technique. *J Vasc Surg* 2016; **63** (1): 1–7.
22. Donas KP, Lee JT, Lachat M, *et al.* Collected world experience about the performance of the snorkel/chimney endovascular technique in the treatment of complex aortic pathologies: the PERICLES registry. *Ann Surg* 2015; **262** (3): 546–53.

# Thoracoabdominal and pararenal four-vessel fenestrated-branched reconstruction with low mortality

GS Oderich, G Sandri, M Ribeiro, A Direrrich, J Wigham, J Hofer and TA Macedo

## Introduction

Fenestrated and branched endovascular aortic repair continues to evolve since the first case performed by John Anderson in 1998.[1] Contemporary reports from large aortic centres worldwide have shown high technical success (>95%), with mortality in the range of 1–5% for pararenal and 5–10% for thoracoabdominal aortic aneurysms.[2–9] Improvements in preoperative planning, patient selection, implantation techniques and perioperative care have lowered mortality and paraplegia.

Device design has changed substantially in the last decade. Early experiences used one or two renal fenestrations and a scallop for the superior mesenteric artery in patients with juxtarenal aortic aneurysms.[7,10] With time, the indications of fenestrated and branched endovascular aortic repair were broadened to include more complex aneurysms involving the mesenteric arteries, which required placement of sealing stents in the distal thoracic aorta. Because of the risk of disease progression, which can compromise the repair and its targets, several centres including ours have adopted a policy of using more stable segments for sealing zones above the superior mesenteric artery and coeliac axis.[7,11]

## Device design

Aneurysm morphology is determined by high resolution computed tomography (CT) angiography datasets. A minimum proximal sealing zone of at least 25mm was selected in normal supra-coeliac aortic segments, defined by parallel aortic wall with no evidence of thrombus, calcium or diameter enlargement >10%. Options for vessel incorporation are doublewide coeliac axis scallops (20x20mm), large (8x8mm) or small (6x6mm) fenestrations and directional branches (8mm or 6mm). Specific device design varies depending on aneurysm extent, vessel angulation and

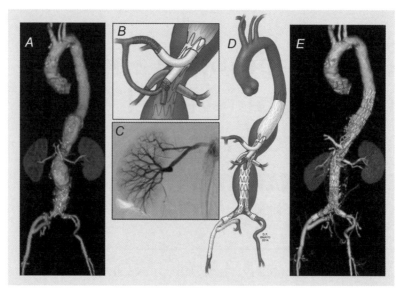

**Figure 1:** (A) Preoperative CT angiography of a patient with type III thoracoabdominal aortic aneurysm. (B) The patient was treated by a patient-specific stent graft with two directional branches for the coeliac artery and superior mesenteric artery, and two renal fenestrations. Selective angiography of the (C) right renal fenestrated branch (D) Illustration and (E) postoperative CT angiography demonstrate complete repair with no endoleak.

inner aortic diameter, and it includes either patient-specific devices with up to five fenestrations or branches, or off-the-shelf T-branch multibranch stent grafts (Figure 1). Selection of design is tailored depending on aneurysm extent and diameter of the aortic lumen. For renal targets, fenestrations are preferred whenever possible, except when aortic inner diameter is large. In these cases, directional renal branches are used if the aortic lumen is >40mm and vessel orientation is down-going without excessive tortuosity. The most common design for pararenal aneurysms is four fenestrations or three fenestrations with a doublewide coeliac scallop. For thoracoabdominal aortic aneurysms, the most common designs are four fenestrations for extent IV, and a combination of directional branches and fenestrations for extent I–III aneurysms.[12–13]

## Target vessel stenting

Alignment stents are standardised for fenestrations and branches, with no alignment stent for doublewide scallops. All fenestrations are aligned using balloon-expandable iCAST covered stents (Atrium; Maquet). Directional branches are stented using either a Viabahn (Gore) or Fluency (Bard) stent graft, which will be reinforced distally by a bare metal self-expandable stent.

## Prevention of spinal cord injury

A standardised protocol is used to prevent spinal cord injury and has been reported elsewhere (Figure 2).[14] The protocol includes permissive hypertension, routine cerebrospinal fluid drainage for all patients with >2 sealing stents above the coeliac axis, staging of extensive thoracoabdominal aortic aneurysms with prior thoracic

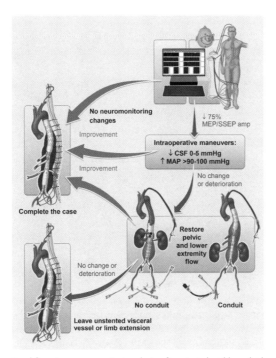

**Figure 2:** Standardised protocol for using neuromonitoring during fenestrated and branched endovascular aortic repair.

endovascular aortic repair (TEVAR), intraoperative neuromonitoring with motor evoked and somatosensory evoked potential monitoring, and early limb reperfusion.

## Technique

Fenestrated and branched endovascular aortic repair is performed by a dedicated aortic team (led by the senior author of this chapter) in a hybrid endovascular room using the GE Discovery IGS 740 unit. Most patients are operated on under general endotracheal anaesthesia using a total percutaneous femoral approach and left brachial approach. Fusion imaging and cone-beam CT is routinely used to locate the target vessels and for final assessment. Once the target vessels are located using fusion, the aortic device is oriented extra-corporeally, introduced via the femoral approach and deployed with perfect apposition between the fenestrations and the target renal arteries.

Most devices are designed with pre-loaded catheters for the coeliac axis and superior mesenteric artery. The catheters allow guidewires to be advanced and snared via the brachial approach. The aortic stent graft is deployed to the level of the renal arteries, and access is sequentially established into the coeliac axis and superior mesenteric artery using brachial access and the preloaded wires (Figure 3). Stiff guidewires are positioned into these vessels and a sheath is advanced into the superior mesenteric artery. The remainder of the aortic device is deployed below the renal arteries and both renal artery fenestrations are sequentially catheterised via the femoral approach. The diameter-reducing ties are removed, the aortic device is completely deployed, and the delivery system removed. Renal artery stenting is done using balloon-expandable covered stents, which are flared to 10mm. At this

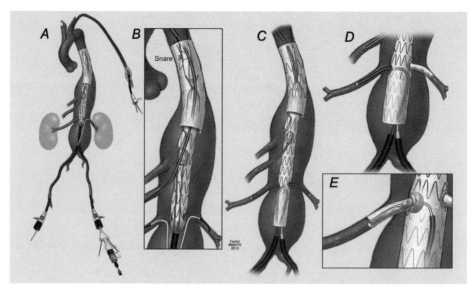

**Figure 3:** (A) A two branch-two fenestration stent graft design has been used to treat complex thoracoabdominal aortic aneurysms. The procedure is performed usually using bilateral femoral and left brachial approach. A proximal thoracic component is deployed first if needed. Pre-catheterisation of at least one of the renal arteries is used to locate the target vessels using on-lay CT. The branched component is deployed up to the level of the renal fenestrations . (B) Using pre-loaded catheters, guidewires are snared from the brachial approach, and the coeliac axis and superior mesenteric artery are catheterised from above. (C) A sheath is typically placed into the superior mesenteric artery (C). The device is unsheathed completely and the renal fenestrations and renal arteries are catheterised via the femoral approach. Hydrophilic sheaths are advanced into both renal arteries over 0.035-inch Rosen guide-wires. (D) Sequential renal artery stenting is performed using balloon-expandable covered stents, (E) which are flared using a 10mm angioplasty balloon.

point the author's preference is to place the distal bifurcated device and iliac limbs, restoring flow into both lower extremities (Figure 4). The procedure is completed by placement of the superior mesenteric artery and coeliac stents, followed by completion angiography and cone-beam CT.

## The Mayo Clinic experience

Patients treated by fenestrated and branched endografts at the Mayo Clinic were enrolled in a prospective, single-centre, non-randomised trial registered at the ClinicalTrials.Gov (NCT 1937949 and NCT2089607).[15] Participation required informed consent approved by the Institutional Review Board and compliance with the study protocol. Follow-up consists of clinical examination, laboratory studies, and imaging before discharge and at one, six, and 12 months and annually thereafter for the first five years. Imaging was independently evaluated by a dedicated group of vascular radiologists. Clinical data entry and case report forms were independently monitored for compliance with regulatory guidelines. Adverse events and causes of death were independently reviewed and adjudicated by a clinical event committee and data safety monitoring board.

# Results

## Clinical characteristics

There were 127 patients enrolled in the study, including 91 male (72%) and 36 female (28%), with mean age of 75±10 years. Aneurysm classification was pararenal in 47 (37%), type IV thoracoabdominal aortic aneurysms in 42 (33%) and type I– III thoracoabdominal aortic aneurysms in 38 patients (30%), including five type I, 18 type II and 15 type III. The maximum aneurysm diameter averaged 59±17mm. Patients in the three groups had similar demographics, cardiovascular risk factors, American Society of Anesthesiologists, and total Society for Vascular Surgery scores. History of prior aortic repair was more frequent in patients with type I– III thoracoabdominal aortic aneurysms (55%, P<0.001). The most prevalent risk factors were cigarette smoking in 88%, hypertension in 87%, hypercholesterolaemia in 87%, ischaemic cardiomyopathy in 53%, chronic obstructive pulmonary disease in 37% and Stage III–V chronic kidney disease in 17%.

## Stent graft design

A total of 496 renal mesenteric arteries (123 coronary arteries, 126 superior mesenteric arteries, 120 right renal, 120 left renal arteries, seven other) were incorporated by 352 fenestrations, 125 directional branches and 19 doublewide scallops with a mean of 3.9 vessels per patient. Among patients treated for pararenal aneurysms, 181 target vessels were incorporated using 160 fenestrations, 19 doublewide scallops and two directional branches. For type IV thoracoabdominal aortic aneurysms, there were 165 vessels incorporated by 143 fenestrations (87%) and 22 directional branches (13%), whereas for type I–III thoracoabdominal aortic aneurysms there were 150 vessels incorporated by 49 fenestrations (33%) and 101 directional branches (67%). Three patients (2%) had four internal iliac artery branch devices.

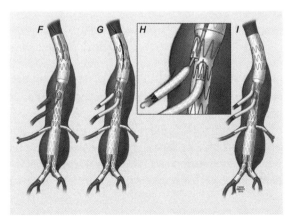

**Figure 4:** (F) The bifurcated component and iliac limbs are deployed after placement of the renal stents. Flow is restored into both lower limbs. (G) The procedure is completed by placement of the superior mesenteric artery and coeliac self-expandable stents. (H) Note that each stent is extended distally with a bare metal self-expandable stent. (I) Final illustration depicts complete repair.

## Procedure details

All procedures were performed in a hybrid endovascular room with a fixed imaging unit using general endotracheal anaesthesia. Cerebrospinal fluid drainage was used in 69%, neuromonitoring in 71%. Technical success was achieved in 99.6% of targeted renal mesenteric vessels (494 of 496). There were no fenestrations left without a stent. Two patients (1.6%) required occlusion of renal artery targets by coil embolisation due to inadvertent disruptions caused by small vessel diameter and excessive tortuosity. Estimated blood loss was 477–517ml, and was significantly higher for type I–III thoracoabdominal aortic aneurysms (P=0.03).

## Early outcomes

There were no 30-day, in-hospital or aneurysm-related deaths. Twenty-seven patients (21%) had major adverse events, with identical rates in the three groups. The most common major adverse events were decline in estimated glomerular filtration rate (eGFR) 50% in 9%, 1L blood loss in 8%, myocardial infarction in 7%, respiratory failure requiring reintubation in 3%, stroke in 3%, ischaemic colitis in 2% and paraplegia in 1.5%. There were two patients with paraplegia, with one having complete recovering and the other having permanent disability (0.8%). One patient (0.8%) required temporary, new-onset dialysis.

## Late outcomes

Mean follow-up was 9.2±7 months (range 1–26). A total of 403 follow-up CT angiography studies were analysed with a mean of 3.2 studies per patient. There were 11 late deaths, all due to non-aortic related causes, including cardiac events in five patients, respiratory failure in three and malignancy, subdural haematoma after a fall, or indeterminate cause in one patient each. Patient survival at one year was 96±2% for the entire cohort with no difference between patients with pararenal (89±5%) or thoracoabdominal aortic aneurysms (100%). There were no ruptures or conversions to open conventional repair.

## Reinterventions

Reinterventions were needed in 23 patients (18%), including 15 patients (12%) who had aortic-related and eight (6%) who had non aortic-related procedures. Indications for aortic reintervention were treatment of endoleaks in eight patients (two type I, two type II and III and four type III), target vessel stenosis or kinks in four, iliac stenosis or occlusion in two, and severe aortic stent infolding in one. All aortic reinterventions were performed using a percutaneous approach and were technically successful. Non-aortic reinterventions included treatment of access site complications or laparotomy for bowel resection in four patients each. Freedom from aortic-related reintervention was 86±4% at one year, with no difference (P=0.438) for pararenal (90±5%), Extent IV (93±5%) and Extent I-III thoracic aneurysms (71±11%).

## Endoleaks, sac changes, migration and integrity issues

Fifty-nine patients (46%) had endoleaks identified by follow up CT angiography, including type I endoleak in three patients (2%), type II endoleak in 43 (34%), type III endoleaks in 10 (8%) and type IV endoleak in one patient. Two patients had type Ic endoleaks due to insufficient distal branch sealing zones. One patient was treated for chronic dissection and had a known type Ia endoleak in the proximal thoracic stent that had been placed at an outside institution, which was revised by proximal arch extension after fenestrated and branched endovascular aortic repair. All type I endoleaks resolved with reintervention. Type III endoleaks occurred in 10 patients (8%) due to insufficient seal at reinforced fenestrations in eight (6%) or inadequate overlap of aortic component in two (2%). Type II endoleaks were observed in all patients except for two, one of whom had successful coil embolisation.

## Target vessel stenosis, kinks and occlusion

Ten patients (8%) had seven stenoses and four occlusions of target vessels, including one patient with bilateral renal in-stent stenosis. Occlusions were attributed to an unrecognised kink in one patient, heparin-induced thrombocytopaenia in one, and no identifiable cause in two patients. All occlusions occurred in renal artery stents, with a rate of 3% for fenestrations and 5% for directional branches. Primary target vessel patency was 94±1% and secondary target vessel patency was 97±2% at one year, with no difference in primary patency (96±1% *vs.* 94±3%; p=0.841) or secondary patency (98±1% *vs.* 97±2%; p=0.493) for fenestrations *vs.* branches, respectively. For renal targets, primary patency was 94±1% for fenestrations and 82±9% for directional branches (p=0.188). Secondary patency was 97±1% and 89±6%, respectively (p=0.137).

## Branch instability

Freedom from branch instability was 93±2% at one year for all targeted vessels, and was lower for renal targets (89±3%) compared to coronary artery or superior mesenteric targets (93±2%; p=0.024). There was no difference in freedom from branch instability for fenestrations (93±3%) compared to directional branches (92±2%) for all targets at one year (p=0.509).

## Renal function deterioration

Freedom from renal function deterioration was 89±4% at one year, with no significant difference (p>0.05) for patients with pararenal (97±3%), type IV (87±7%) and type I–III thoracoabdominal aortic aneurysms (80±8%). There were no patients on permanent dialysis. Chronic kidney disease staging remained stable in most patients.

## Discussion

This study represents the interim results of a prospective, non-randomised analysis of endovascular repair of pararenal or thoracoabdominal aortic aneurysms using fenestrated and branched stent grafts. A wide range of designs was used to adapt to the patient anatomy, reflecting real-world use of branch technology with broader indications including failed aortic repairs, chronic dissections and variations of four-vessel anatomy. The observations of high technical success (99.6%), no mortality and low rate of major adverse events (21%), type Ia endoleak, permanent paraplegia or temporary dialysis, support the safety and effectiveness of fenestrated and branched stent grafts to treat complex aortic aneurysms, beyond what has already been demonstrated in the US Zenith fenestrated study for juxtarenal aneurysms.[9]

The strategy of using supra-coeliac sealing zones was based on evidence of late neck enlargement and type I endoleaks with fenestrated and branched endovascular aortic repair performed with less extensive coverage.[7,16] Although there is a valid concern that more fenestrations may increase the risk of complication, recent studies including ours indicate that these repairs are safe.[4,7,10–11] Paraplegia is still the most feared complication of thoracoabdominal aortic aneurysm repair. Some reports have shown remarkably high rates of spinal cord injury in up to 50% of patients.[5] Using our specific protocol that included selective staged procedures, routine cerebrospinal fluid drainage, neuromonitoring and early limb reperfusion; 4% of our patients developed any spinal cord injury and 1.5% had paraplegia, which was permanent in only one patient (0.8%).[15] Other recent series have also shown marked improvement in paraplegia rates in the range of 0%–2.5%.[2,4–9] A common factor in these reports is that operators have overcome their steep learning curve and adopted routine adjuncts to optimise collateral spinal network perfusion, based on experimental evidence of spinal cord collateral adaptation after staged arterial coverage.

Branch instability, particularly in the renal arteries, continues to be a focus of research. For fenestrated branches, freedom from branch instability was 88% at one year and 70% at five years, which compares favourably to our rate of 93% at one year.[3] Several experts propose using fenestrations for all renal arteries because of their low occlusion rates (<2%) compared to directional branches (5–10%).[1–14] However, several of the prior reports used rigid bridging stent grafts for branches. We have standardised renal branch constructions by using Viabahn stent grafts and found no difference in the rate of occlusion for fenestrations (2%) or branches (5%). One problem of using renal fenestrations is the higher risk of type III endoleaks, which reaches up to 15%.

## Summary

- Fenestrated and branched endovascular aortic repair of complex aortic aneurysms continues to evolve with improvements in device design, implantation techniques and adjunctive manoeuvres to decrease mortality and paraplegia.

- Supra-coeliac sealing zones may prevent future complications associated with progression of aortic disease.

- Our results shows high technical success, low rate of major adverse events and no aneurysm rupture, conversion or mortality, supporting the safety and efficacy of fenestrated and branched endografts using supra-coeliac sealing zones.

## References

1. Anderson JL, Berce M, Hartley DE. Endoluminal aortic grafting with renal and superior mesenteric artery incorporation by graft fenestration. *J Endovasc Ther* 2001; **8**: 35.

2. Kasprzak PM, Gallis K, Cucuruz B, *et al*. Editor's choice--Temporary aneurysm sac perfusion as an adjunct for prevention of spinal cord ischaemia after branched endovascular repair of thoracoabdominal aneurysms. *Eur J Vasc Endovasc Surg* 2014; **48:** 258–65.

3. Mastracci TM, Greenberg RK, Eagleton MJ and Hernandez AV. Durability of branches in branched and fenestrated endografts. *J Vasc Surg* 2013; **57:** 926–33.

4. Maurel B, Delclaux N, Sobocinski J, *et al*. The impact of early pelvic and lower limb reperfusion and attentive peri-operative management on the incidence of spinal cord ischemia during thoracoabdominal aortic aneurysm endovascular repair. *Eur J Vasc Endovasc Surg* 2015; **49** (3): 248–54.

5. Dias NV, Sonesson B, Kristmundsson T, *et al*. Short-term outcome of spinal cord ischemia after endovascular repair of thoracoabdominal aortic aneurysms. *Eur J Vasc Endovasc Surg* 2015; **49**: 403–09

6. Eagleton MJ, Follansbee M, Wolski K, *et al*. Fenestrated and branched endovascular aneurysm repair outcomes for type II and III thoracoabdominal aortic aneurysms. *J Vasc Surg* 2016; **63** (4): 930–42.

7. Verhoeven E, Katsargyris A. SS17. Comparison of standard double fenestrated EVAR vs triple or quadruple fenestrated EVAR in the treatment of complex aortic aneurysms. VAM 2016 Abstracts. *J Vasc Surg* 2016; **63**(6S): 136S.

8. Banga P, Oderich GS, Reis de Souza L, *et al*. Neuromonitoring, Cerebrospinal Fluid Drainage, and Selective Use of Iliofemoral Conduits to Minimize Risk of Spinal Cord Injury During Complex Endovascular Aortic Repair. *J Endovasc Ther* 2016; **23**: 139–49.

9. Oderich GS, Greenberg RK, Farber M, *et al*. Zenith Fenestrated Study Investigators. Results of the United States multicenter prospective study evaluating the Zenith fenestrated endovascular graft for treatment of juxtarenal abdominal aortic aneurysms. *J Vasc Surg* 2014; **60** (6):1420–28.

10. O'Callaghan A, Greenberg RK, Eagleton MJ, *et al*. Type Ia endoleaks after fenestrated and branched endografts may lead to component instability and increased aortic mortality. *J Vasc Surg*. 2015; **61** (4): 908–14.

11. O'Callaghan A, Mastracci, TM, Eagleton MJ. Staged endovascular repair of thoracoabdominal aortic aneurysms limits incidence and severity of spinal cord ischemia. *J Vasc Surg* **61:** 347–54.

12. Martin-Gonzalez T, Mastracci T, Carrell T, *et al*. Mid-term outcomes of renal branches *versus* renal fenestrations for thoraco-abdominal aneurysm repair. *Eur J Vasc Endovasc Surg* 2016.

13. Mastracci TM, Carrell T, Constantinou J, *et al*. Effect of branch stent choice on branch-related outcomes in complex aortic repair. *Eur J Vasc Endovasc Surg* 2016; **51**(4): 36–42.

14. Panuccio G, Bisdas T, Berekoven B, *et al*. Performance of Bridging Stent Grafts in Fenestrated and Branched Aortic Endografting. *Eur J Vasc Endovasc Surg* 2015; **50** (1): 60–70.

15. Oderich GS, Ribeiro M, Hofer J, *et al*. Prospective, nonrandomized study to evaluate endovascular repair of pararenal and thoracoabdominal aortic aneurysms using fenestrated-branched endografts based on supraceliac sealing zones. *J Vasc Surg* 2016. Epub.

# Custom EVAR–a step between EVAR and fenestrated EVAR

F Fanelli, A Cannavale, M Gazzetti and M Santoni

## Introduction

Endovascular aneurysm repair (EVAR) has replaced traditional open surgery in a large number of centres to treat infrarenal abdominal aortic aneurysms because this minimally invasive technique offers a procedure with little risk of morbidity and mortality.[1–3]

However, approximately 50% of patients are found to be not suitable for EVAR due to their aortic anatomical configuration—some of them with a very short (<1cm) or very tortuous proximal neck, which is not usable as landing zone for the aortic stent graft. Thus, proximal neck adequacy and endograft seal zone have been identified as key predictors of long-term outcomes and success after EVAR.[3]

Mid-term outcome of infrarenal EVAR in complex anatomy has meanwhile become a matter of great concern in recent studies.

Aneurysms with short infrarenal necks or those extending to the level of the renal arteries represent a challenging cohort for standard EVAR devices. Also a distal landing zone, at the level of the iliac arteries, is not suitable for standard EVAR because of a very large diameter or due to aneurysm extension down towards the iliac bifurcation.

When treating patients with inadequate proximal and distal necks, it is necessary to improve the sealing zone of the stent graft and move it to a healthier portion of the aorta or of the iliac vessels.

Additionally, EVAR cannot be performed when an accessory inferior renal artery is present because, as reported in previous studies, embolisation of this branch is required to avoid a type II endoleak during the follow-up.

A high risk of renal failure has to be considered because accessory renal arteries are frequently responsible for <35% of renal parenchyma vascularisation.[4] As a consequence, renal activity may be compromised after EVAR procedure especially in elderly patients.[5]

Strict inclusion criteria have characterised EVAR from the very beginning of its introduction, but nowadays the number of patients who are candidates for this endovascular treatment is steadily increasing. At present, infrarenal EVAR is even offered to patients who do not completely fulfil the anatomic requirements because this procedure is justly perceived as being minimally traumatic.

To safely extend the use of this minimally invasive treatment to challenging cases, several options have been proposed and recently actively introduced. The first attempt has been based on the use of the so-called "chimney technique", especially in cases of short proximal necks. With this technique, a supra-renal fixation—in

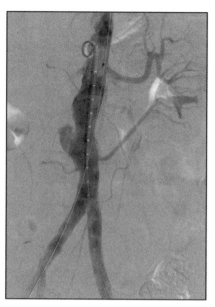

**Figure 1:** Digital subtraction angiography showed the presence of a dissected aneurysm of the abdominal aorta. An accessory inferior right renal artery is clearly visible.

a healthy portion of the aorta—can be achieved by placing two stent grafts into the renal arteries and landing into the aortic lumen in parallel with the aortic main body. This technique is still open to several discussions regarding long-term durability and the increased risk of type I endoleak.

Lee *et al*[6] have reported their experience using the "snorkel technique" for juxtarenal aneurysms in 56 patients. Technical success of snorkel placements was 98.2%. Thirty-day mortality was 7.1%. Postoperative imaging revealed one renal snorkel graft occlusion at three months (98.2% overall primary patency). Seven (25%) early endoleaks were noted on the first follow-up computed tomography (CT). The secondary intervention rate was 3.6%.

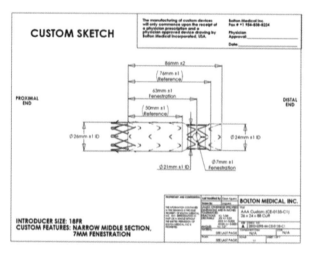

**Figure 2:** For this reason, a custom-made aortic stent graft (Bolton Medical) was planned.

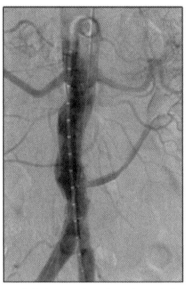

**Figure 3:** Final angiogram after stent graft deployment showed complete exclusion of the aortic disease. Moreover, the accessory renal artery and both main renal arteries look patent with a good flow.

The use of EVAR in more complex aneurysm anatomy has become really widespread over the past decade with the introduction of fenestrated EVAR or branched EVAR devices.[7-11] They enable operators to exclude the aneurysmatic sack keeping patent all the abdominal branches such as the superior mesenteric artery, the renal arteries and the accessory renal arteries (Figures 1–3). By using such devices, a better sealing is achieved because the landing zone is secured in a straight and healthy portion of the aorta.

Shahverdyan *et al*[12] have reported their experience in 48 fenestrated EVAR procedures using the Anaconda custom-made device (Vascutek). The primary technical success rate was 94% with three unsuccessful cannulations of the renovisceral arteries. The 30-day mortality was 4%. Two occlusions of the right renal stent/artery were detected.

Fenestrated EVAR and branched EVAR can also allow the treatment of thoracoabdominal aneurysms ensuring a less invasive treatment even in the presence of this complex pathology.

Gallito *et al*[13] reported their experience in 30 patients affected by thoracoabdominal aneurysms treated with custom-made (73%) and off-the-shelf (23%) endografts. Postoperative cardiac and pulmonary complications occurred in two cases each. Renal function worsening (≥30% of the baseline level) was observed in four cases (13%). The 30-day mortality was 6.6%, with a survival rate of 85% at 12 months and of 68% at 24 months.

Even though these grafts are customised to suit patients individually, planning and manufacturing have led to significant treatment delays—subjecting patients to the risk of rupture during the waiting period. This is one of the reasons why this new technology is not available in acute settings.

The manufacturing process of a customised graft is time- and labour-consuming. The delivery time takes from six to eight weeks depending on the device complexity.

## Conclusion

Fenestrated EVAR is now an established alternative to hybrid and chimney techniques. However, specific criteria and prerequisites are mandatory for the use and improvement of this procedure. Precise deployment of the fenestrated stent graft is essential for a successful visceral vessel revascularisation. Accurate sizes of stent grafts and customisation, a high level of technical skill and facilities with modern imaging techniques—including 3D road mapping and dedicated hybrid rooms—are equally required.

It is a general hope that in the near future, customisation time can be reduced to offer a better service, even to patients at high risk of rupture.

## Summary

- When treating patients with inadequate proximal and distal necks, it is necessary to improve the sealing zone of the stent graft and move it to a healthier portion of the aorta or of the iliac vessels.

- The use of EVAR in more complex aneurysm anatomy has become really widespread over the past decade with the introduction of fenestrated or branched devices.

- Fenestrated EVAR and branched EVAR can allow a pretty safe treatment of thoracoabdominal aneurysms.

## References

1. ReschTA, Dias NV, SobocinskiJ, et al. Development of off-the-shelf stent grafts for juxtarenal abdominal aortic aneurysms. *European Journal of Vascular and Endovascular Surgery* 2012; **43**: 655e–60.
2. Haulon S, Amiot S, Magnan PE, et al. An analysis of the French multicentre experience of fenestrated aortic endografts: Medium-term outcomes. *Ann Surg* 2010; **251** (2): 357e–62.
3. Resch T. Pararenal aneurysms: currently available fenestrated endografts. *J Cardiovasc Surg* 2013; **54** (1 Suppl 1): 27–33.
4. Manning BJ, Agu O, Richards T, et al. Early outcome following endovascular repair of pararenal aortic aneurysms: triple- *versus* double- or single-fenestrated stent grafts. *J Endovasc Ther* 2011; **18** (1): 98e–105.
5. Azzaoui R, Sobocinski J, Maurel B, et al. Anatomic study of juxtarenal aneurysms: impact on fenestrated stent grafts. *Ann Vasc Surg* 2011; **25** (3): 315e–21.
6. Lee JT, Greenberg JI, Dalman RT. Early experience with the snorkel technique for juxtarenal aneurysms. *J Vasc Surg* 2012; **55** (4): 935–46.
7. Lee JT, Lee GK, Chandra V, et al. Comparison of fenestrated endografts and the snorkel/chimney technique. *J Vasc Surg* 2014; **60**: 849–57.
8. Lachat M, Veith FJ, Pfammatter T, et al. Chimney and periscope grafts observed over 2 years after their use to revascularise 169 renovisceral branches in 77 patients with complex aortic aneurysms. *J Endovasc Ther* 2013; **20**: 597–605.
9. Wilson A, Zhou S, Bachoo P, et al. Systematic review of chimney and periscope grafts for endovascular aneurysm repair. *Br J Surg* 2013; **100**: 1557–64.
10. Katsargyris A, Oikonomou K, Klonaris C, et al. Comparison of outcomes with open, fenestrated, and chimney graft repair of juxtarenal aneurysms: Are we ready for a paradigm shift? *J Endovasc Ther* 2013; **20**: 159–69.
11. Georgiadis GS, Van Herwaarden JA, Antoniou GA, et al. Fenestrated stent grafts for the treatment of complex aortic aneurysm disease: A mature treatment paradigm. *Vasc Med* 2016; **21** (3): 223–38.
12. Shahverdyan R, Gray D, Gawenda M, et al. Single centre results of total endovascular repair of complex aortic aneurysms with custom-made Anaconda fenestrated stent grafts. *Eur J Vasc Endovasc Surg* 2016; **52** (4): 500–508.
13. Gallitto E, Gargiulo M, Freyrie A, et al. Endovascular repair of thoraco-abdominal aortic aneurysm in high-surgical risk patients: Fenestrated and branched endografts. *Ann Vasc Surg* 2016. Epub.

# Radiation dose awareness in aortic interventions

# Radiation protection in the endosuite and the importance of correct use of shields

S Bruce, K Mani, A Wanhainen and L Jangland

## Introduction

Today's complex endovascular procedures, with long fluoroscopy time and multiple X-ray images, may result in high radiation doses to the patient and to healthcare personnel; in fact, vascular surgeons and interventional radiologists receive the highest individual doses in healthcare.[1–3] This review will focus on radiation safety to personnel working with endovascular procedures, measures to control the dose, and different types of radiation shields.

## Basic concepts, quantities and units

The objective of the following description is to help the reader to get a practical, rather than a theoretically stringent, understanding of the quantities and concepts used in this field.

### Cancer and genetic effects

Cancer and genetic effects (stochastic effects, late effects) increase linearly with dose. According to the International Commission on Radiological Protection (ICRP), there is no magnitude of dose that is known to be completely safe. This is why all medical use of X-rays need to be justified and the dose need be as low as reasonably achievable (the ALARA principle). Younger persons, especially children, are more radiosensitive than older people. Tissues with a fast cell division (bone marrow, colon, lung, stomach, breast and gonads) are more radiosensitive than tissues with slow cell division.[4]

### Tissue reactions

Tissue reactions (deterministic effects, early effects), i.e. harmful reactions, occur for high doses above specific threshold levels. The higher the dose, the more severe reaction is. Examples of tissue reactions relevant in endovascular procedures are skin reaction on patients, for example hair loss and skin erythema, and cataract for personnel.[4]

### Absorbed dose

Absorbed dose is the amount of energy that is deposited by ionising radiation in a mass of some material, with the unit Joule/kg (=Gray). The SI unit is Gray (Gy).[4]

### Equivalent dose

Equivalent dose is used to express the biological effect in a specific organ or tissue taken into account that the effect varies dependent on the type of radiation used, i.e. alpha-particles are 20 times more harmful than X-rays. Equivalent dose cannot be measured directly but are most often estimated from direct measurements with personal dosimeters. The SI unit is Sievert (Sv).[4]

### Effective dose

Effective dose is used to estimate the risk of cancer and genetic effects. Effective dose is the sum of the equivalent doses to each organ multiplied by their specific weighing factor, to account for the radiosensitivity of each organ. Effective dose may reasonably be applied to medical exposures remembering that effective dose is based on population-average kinetic models and reference individuals (e.g. a 70kg adult). It cannot be used for risk estimates for individual patients since patient-specific parameters (weight, age, sex, individual radiosensitivity, etc.) are not included in the model. The SI unit is Sv.[4]

### Radiation dose at IRP

Radiation dose at the interventional reference point (IRP) is the cumulative radiation dose (sum of the dose in all projections) at a position 15cm from the isocenter towards the X-ray tube. The quantity is commonly given by the system as "skin dose" and is used to estimate the peak skin dose related to possible skin injury. Appropriate estimation of peak skin dose includes taking into account the different positions of the C-arm relative to the patient during the procedure. The SI unit is Gy.[5]

### Dose area product

Dose area product (DAP) is the product of the area of the irradiated surface and the radiation dose within this area.[6] Knowledge of the DAP and projection of the X-ray beam can be used to estimate the effective dose by using tabulated conversions factors (in mSv per Gy/m²).[7] Dose area product is usually measured with an ion-chamber integrated in the housing of the X-ray tube. The SI unit is $Gy*m^2$.

## Justification, optimisation and dose limits (based on the ALARA principle)

Justification: all medical exposures shall be justified. This means that every exposure should be expected to do more good than harm to the patient (expected positive medical outcome of the procedure *vs.* radiation risk for the patient). Responsibility for the justification decision of a particular procedure falls on the relevant medical practitioner.[4]

Optimisation: radiation dose to the patient should always be kept to a minimum without jeopardising the medical outcome of the procedure. Optimisation includes the settings of the radiological equipment as well as the practical performance of the procedure.[4]

Dose limits (legal limits): These are only used for personnel and not applied to patients. The limit for effective dose is set to ensure that no individual will be exposed to an unacceptable radiation risk in his/her employment. There are limits for specific tissues, skin, lens of the eye and extremities since these tissues will

## Occupational radiation safety in vascular surgery

| Radiation shield | Scope of protection | Whom | Pro and cons, comments | |
|---|---|---|---|---|
| (A) Ceiling-suspended shields | Upper body & eyes | Table side personnel* | + High degree of protection, varies with projection (50-90%)<br><br>- May be difficult to position, interfere with some procedures | |
| (B/C) Table mounted shields | Lower body | Table side personnel* | + High degree of protection (~60 %)<br><br>- Possible interference with sterile draping | |
| (D) Shielding placed on the patient | Upper body & eyes | Table side personnel* | + Intermediate degree of protection (~50%)<br><br>- If positioned in the primary field interference with automatic exposure control (dose rise)<br>- Minor increase of patient dose | |
| Ceiling suspended/ Floor standing personal garments | Central body | Operator | + High degree of protection (~95%)<br><br>- Possible conflict with other ceiling suspended/floor mounted equipment<br>- May affect sterility and interfere the surgeons mobility | |
| Lead aprons and thyroid shields | Central body and thyroid | All personnel | + High degree of protection (~95%)<br>+ Always works when used<br>Should be individually tailored to maximize comfort | |
| Eye shields, glasses or visors | Eye lens | Table side personnel* | + Eye lens must have protection<br><br>- Highly variable degree of protection (~ 10-50 %)<br>- May be uncomfortable<br>Must be used routinely in combination with ceiling mounted shield | |

## Occupational radiation safety in vascular surgery

| Radiation shield | Scope of protection | Whom | Pro and cons, comments | |
|---|---|---|---|---|
| Head shields | Brain | Table side personnel* | - Lack of consensus of necessity | |
| Hand shields, gloves | Fingers | Operator | - Low degree of protection, ~25% in the primary field<br>- Might give false sense of security<br>- Will interfere with automatic exposure control | |
| Floor standing mobile shields | Whole body | Anesthesia staff and other stationary personnel | + Very high degree of protection (~ 98%)<br>- Must be adequately positioned | |

*ie operator and operator assistant personnel*

not necessarily be protected against radiation induced tissue reactions by the limit of effective dose. The recommended annual dose limits are; effective dose 20mSv, equivalent dose to the eye 20mSv (In 2011 ICRP changed their recommendation on the threshold dose for cataract from 3Gy to 0.5Gy and the annual limit for personnel from 150mSv to 20mSv based on recent research of personnel exposed to lower dose levels) and to the skin and extremities 500mSv.[4]

Dose constraints are set locally and depend on the circumstances of the exposure. If a constraint is exceeded some planned actions will take place. As an example of a dose constraint can be set as a monthly effective dose for personnel working in the endosuite representing the highest expected dose. Exceeding the dose constraint will lead to an investigation of the working situation. For patients, dose constraints on skin dose should be set and if exceeded follow-up of possible radiation induced skin reactions will be initiated.[4]

# Image formation and scattered radiation

The X-ray beam from the tube (the primary beam) penetrates the patient with the following outcome:

1. Part of the radiation will be absorbed in the patient, as a rule of thumb, about two thirds
2. Part of the radiation will be scattered (change direction). This is also referred to as secondary radiation, approximately one third of the radiation
3. Part of the radiation will pass straight through the patient without any interaction, will reach the detector and form the image. This is approximately a single per cent or less.

Dense structures, like bone, will absorb a larger fraction of the radiation compared to soft tissue. This "absorption difference" between structures is measured at the detector and is the fundamental basis for the X-ray image. With thicker material, a larger amount of radiation will be absorbed. The automatic exposure control (AEC; also called automatic brightness control—ABC) will automatically keep the dose to the detector constant by adjusting the tube output (e.g. kV, mA, S and filtration). AEC will thereby compensate for patients of different sizes that require different amount of radiation (to achieve similar image quality). As a rule of thumb, a 3–5cm thicker patient will double the beam intensity and the patient dose. Oblique projections, especially steep projections, therefore result in much higher radiation doses compared to an anteroposterior projection.

The amount of scattered radiation will increase with higher radiation intensity and larger irradiated volumes. Scattered radiation from the patient is the principal source of exposure to the personnel. Consequently, measures that reduces patient dose will reduce the dose to the personnel as well. Scattered radiation will to some extent reach the detector and increase the noise in the image and thereby degrade the low contrast.

# Measures to control personnel radiation doses

Reducing the dose to the patient decreases scattered radiation and is, therefore, the basis in radiation safety for the personnel. A prerequisite is the operator's knowledge and practical experience of the X-ray system, what features are available and when to use them. In the X-ray system there are protocols for different organs and procedures that may vary in radiation dose settings as well as image processing. Within each protocol, it is often possible to adjust some of the parameters and change the dose settings and the image quality. During an endovascular procedure the need for good image quality varies. For most of the procedure, a low-dose setting with reduced image quality is adequate. It is, therefore, essential that the default setting starts at low pulse frequency and low dose level and that better image quality features are selected when required.

## Positions in the room

The scattered radiation diverges from its source (the irradiated part of the patient) and the dose decreases rapidly with the squared distance (the inverse squared law). If you double the distance from the patient, the dose will decrease to a quarter (25%); if you triple the distance, the dose will decrease to a ninth (11%). An efficient and easy measure to decrease personnel doses is to minimise the number of persons close to the patient, minimise the time being close to the patient and to take a step back when possible, for example during radiation-intense acquisition.

There will be much more scattered radiation on the tube side of the patient than on the detector side due to the higher intensity of the primary beam on the tube side. If possible personnel should be positioned at the detector side when lateral projection is used.

### Acquisition images

Fluoroscopy is normally used to see moving objects, i.e. to navigate and position guidewires, catheters and stents. Acquisition is used to record sequences of high quality diagnostic images, i.e. images for archiving and digital subtraction angiography (DSA). As a rule of thumb, the dose per image (per pulse) is in magnitude of 10 times higher for acquisition than fluoroscopy. Decreasing the number of acquisition images is certainly very dose efficient. This can be achieved by shorter sequences, reduced image frequency or by archiving a high-dose level fluoroscopy sequence instead of an acquisition sequence.

### Fluoroscopy pulse frequency

The pulse frequency determines the rate of new images shown at the screen. With lower pulse rate the video will appear draggier. For most of the procedure, the pulse rate can be relatively low without interfering with the quality of the procedure (at our institution 4p/s is used). The X-ray system usually displays total fluoroscopy time, regardless of the pulse frequency. A 50% shorter fluoroscopic time—with the same pulse frequency—will decrease the dose by 50%. A 50% lower pulse frequency—for the same fluoroscopic time—will decrease the dose by 50%.

### Dose level

There are usually different dose levels that can be chosen (typically low, normal and high). Higher dose levels results in less noisy images but increase radiation. For thicker patients higher dose levels might be needed to get adequate images. For some X-ray systems, a change in "dose level" can in fact be a change in pulse rate and/or other dose features instead of just the dose per pulse.

### Beam collimation

By collimating the field size, the irradiated patient volume decreases. The dose to the personnel decreases and the image improves with less scattered radiation to the detector. To work with a small field size and see less anatomy is often a matter of habit. Beam collimation is an easy and effective measure in saving both patient and personnel doses. A 50% smaller area decreases the doses by 50%.

### Field of view

A smaller field of view will result in a magnified and more detailed image and an increase of the dose in the field. Decreasing the field of view should not be equated with the use of collimation; the field area is decreased in both cases, but the dose rate in the field will remain the same when collimation is used while it will increases with magnification. In a hybrid room, a large image screen should be used so that magnification is not needed due to too small images. Some X-ray systems provide digital zoom where the image will be enlarged at the screen while the dose settings will remain the same.

## Passive radiation shields

Passive shields can be divided in shields positioned between the personnel and the patient (source of scatter) and personal protective devices. It is essential that the design of the endosuite includes thorough selection of type of shields and planning of their position to minimise interference. Personal protective devices should be individually selected to achieve maximum protection and comfort.

It is important to realise that the passive shields are complementary to each other and to other measures in reducing radiation. The protection with different eyewear varies depending not only on the eyewear and its fitting to the face but also with the variation of radiation geometry depending on the imaging projections used. To achieve an adequate protection of the eyes use of the ceiling mounted shield is vital and personal protective eyewear should only be seen as complementary to that.[8–10] The floor standing shield is a complement to personal protective garments.

In the figure, a number of passive shields with some essential characteristics are summarised.[8–15]

## Management

The radiation safety programme includes obvious parts such as design of the facility, choice of the radiological equipment, quality assurance, radiation dose monitoring and protective devices. The medical physicist involved in the programme must be familiar with the clinical aspects of the procedures performed at the facility.[3] Their involvement should include quality insurance of equipment, dose monitoring, optimisation of procedures and education, both lectures and practical training. In the optimisation process of the equipment, it is of great importance to include the manufacturer since adjustments of the X-ray system and image processing parameters interact with each other in a complex manner. The vascular surgeon, as responsible for all aspects of patient safety in the endosuite, must be actively involved in managing radiation dose to maximise safety for the patient and all personnel. Successful management of radiation safety programme in interventional radiology is, therefore, a collaborative effort including vascular surgeons, medical physicists, radiologists, nurses, X-ray technicians and manufacturers.

Radiation safety training programmes should be mandatory for all personnel working in the endosuite and included as an important part in the formal training of vascular surgery residents.[2,16]

### Summary

- Endovascular surgery is a radiation-intense occupation.
- Education in radiation safety is imperative.
- Measures to decrease patient dose will decrease the dose to personnel.
- Use available protective shielding whenever possible.
- Radiation safety is multidisciplinary.

# References

1. Bartal G, Vano E, Paulo G, Miller DL. Management of Patient and Staff Radiation Dose in Interventional Radiology: Current Concepts. *Cardiovasc Intervent Radiol* 2014; **37**: 289–98.
2. ICRP. Radiological Protection in Fluoroscopically Guided Procedures outside the Imaging Department; 2010.
3. Sailer AM, Schurink GWH, Bol ME, *et al.* Occupational Radiation during endovascular Aortic repair. *CardioVascular and Interventional Radiology* 2015; **38**: 827–32.
4. ICRP. The 2007 Recommendations of the International Commission on Radiological Protection; 2007.
5. Commission IE. Medical electrical equipment - Part 2-43:particular requirements for the safety of x-ray equipment for interventional procedures. IEC report 60601. 2000.
6. Huda W. Kerma-area product in diagnostic radiology. *American Journal of Roentgenology* 2014; **203** (6): 565–69.
7. Compagnone G, Giampalma E, Domenichelli S, et al. Calculation of conversion factors for effective dose for various interventional radiology procedures. *Medical Physics* 2012; **39** (5): 2491–98.
8. Cousin A, Lawdahl R, Chakraborty D, Koehler R. The case for radioprotective eyewear/facewear. Practical implications and suggestions. *Investigative Radiology* 1987; **22**: 688–92.
9. Maeder M, Brunner-La Rocca H, Wolber T, *et al.* Impact of a lead glass screen on scatter radiation to eyes and hands in interventional cardiologists. *Catheter Cardiovascular Intervention* 2006; 67: 18–23.
10. Thornton R, Dauer L, Altamirano J, *et al.* Comparing strageties for operator eye protection in the interventional radiology suite. *Journal of Vascular Interventional Radiology* 2010; **21**: 1703–07.
11. ouguin A, Goldstein J, Bar O, Goldstein J. Brain and neck tumors among physicians performing interventional procedures. *American Journal of Cardiology* 2013; **111**: 1368–72.
12. Murphy J, Darragh K, Walsh S, Hanratty C. Efficiancy of the RADPAD protective drape during real world complex percutaneous coronary intervention procedures. *American Journal of Cardiology* 2011; **108**: 1408–10.
13. Marichal D, Anwar T, Kirsch D, *et al.* Comparision of a suspended radiation protection system *versus* standard lead apron for radiation exposure of a simulated interventionalist. *Journal of Vascular Inteventional Radiology* 2011; **22**: 437–42.
14. Wagner L, Mulhern O. Radiation-attenuating surgical gloves: effects on scatter and secondary electron production. *Radiology* 1996; **22**: 45–48.
15. Balter S. Promoting fluroscopic personal radiation protection equipment: unfamilarity, facts and fears. Radiation Protection Dosimetry.
16. Bardolini S, Carsten C, Cull D, *et al.* Radiation safety education in vascular surgery training. *Journal of Vascular Surgery* 2014; **59**: 860–64.

# Measurement of radiation exposure to operators

MM Li and CV Riga

## Introduction

There has been a paradigm shift in recent years towards the endovascular approach in the management of arterial disease. However, a negative by-product of fluoroscopically-guided procedures is the exposure to ionising radiation. With the increasing complexity and regularity of endovascular workload, current vascular interventionalists may expect to have a much higher lifetime radiation exposure than their predecessors.

In 2007, the International Commission on Radiological Protection (ICRP) defined the safe dose limit for occupational exposure as 20mSv per year for the body and 150mSv per year for the eye lens.[1] However, the yearly eye lens dose limit was subsequently reduced to 20mSv in 2011.[2] This recent revision of the guidelines highlights the importance and urgent need for improved radiation awareness.

## Adverse effects of radiation

The adverse effects of ionising radiation can be classified into deterministic (cataracts, skin damage) and stochastic (cancer, teratogenicity) effects. Deterministic effects are those that are dose dependent and usually have a threshold above which they occur. Stochastic effects increase in likelihood with increased exposure, although the severity is independent of dose.[3]

The adverse effects of high-level radiation exposure are well-documented through population studies from those affected by the Chernobyl nuclear power plant disaster and from atomic bomb survivors.[4] However, the long-term effects of low-level radiation exposure experienced by vascular interventionalists are not fully understood, and the safety thresholds are unclear. Nuclear industry workers are similarly continually exposed to low levels of radiation; a large cohort study in this population found an association between lifetime exposure and solid cancer mortality.[5] Amongst endovascular interventionalists, high-profile cases and worrying reports of left-sided brain and neck tumours have emerged; probably the direct results of long-term radiation exposure, since the left side of the head is known to be more exposed and is not routinely shielded by protective equipment.[6,7]

Cataracts are also another significant consequence to consider. The tissue of the eye lens is highly radiosensitive, with lens opacification and subsequent cataract formation occurring with cumulative radiation exposure. Radiation exposure to the eye lens in endovascular surgery is not insignificant,[8] and studies of interventional cardiology personnel have found them to be at increased risk of radiation-induced cataract formation.[9,10] The thyroid gland is also radiosensitive, and exposure to radiation at a younger age appears to increase the risk of later developing thyroid cancer.[11]

## Measuring radiation exposure

Previous studies of healthcare-related radiation have primarily focused on patient, rather than occupational, radiation exposure. The current literature reports varying doses for the principal operator undertaking common endovascular procedures. For endovascular aneurysm repair (EVAR), the average operator dose per case has been reported at 0.05mSv,[12,13] but also as high as 0.11mSv.[14] A much lower dose of 0.006mSv has also been reported with the use of a mobile C-arm rather than a fixed fluoroscopy unit.[13] Reported exposure for thoracic endovascular aortic repair (TEVAR) and fenestrated EVAR have been similarly varied: 0.06–0.42mSv for TEVAR[12,14,15] and 0.13—0.36 for fenestrated EVAR,[14,16–18] which perhaps reflects the heterogeneity of cases in more complex endovascular work. Nonetheless, radiation exposure for fenestrated EVAR and TEVAR both appear to be higher than for conventional EVAR.[12,14] Reported radiation doses appear higher with increasing publication date, reflecting perhaps the increasing levels of radiation operators are exposed to as they take on a more complex endovascular work and higher caseloads.

It is not only the principal operator who receives a high dose of radiation, however. The assistant and anaesthetist are exposed to lower, though still substantial, levels of radiation.[12] One study on fenestrated EVAR found the anaesthetist's dose to be more than double that of the principal operator.[17]

Acute C-arm angulation has been identified as a significant factor affecting radiation exposure. In a study on fenestrated EVAR and branched EVAR, the degree of left anterior oblique angulation and digital subtraction angiography (DSA) acquisition time in this position were strong predictors of head radiation exposure.[16] Positioning in the operating theatre has also been identified as a significant factor affecting the level of radiation exposure. A study on fenestrated EVAR observed the highest doses for those standing at the head end of the table. Visceral vessel (superior mesenteric artery, coeliac artery) cannulation was identified as a procedural stage with high radiation exposure (0.08mSv), which was also significantly higher than for renal artery cannulation (0.03mSv). The axillary/brachial approach often used in visceral vessel cannulation involves standing at the head of the table, which, in addition to use of oblique C-arm angulation, may explain the high level of radiation exposure in this step.[18]

## Reducing radiation exposure

The ALARA—as low as reasonably achievable—principle aims to optimise radiation protection by keeping the likelihood of exposure, number of people exposed, and magnitude of doses as low as possible.[1] Effective methods for dose reduction include: use of pulsed rather than continuous fluoroscopy, a low dose setting, minimising DSA acquisitions, collimation, magnification, and table height adjustment.[19,20] The importance of simple shielding using lead gowns, thyroid shields and protective eyewear should also not be underestimated: 0.5mm lead garments will attenuate the absorbed dose by 90%, and thyroid shields are important in preventing radiation-induced thyroid cancer.[19] Use of leaded safety glasses will also significantly reduce the dose to the eye lens.[21]

Radiation awareness is also a key factor in reducing exposure. Staff education on good operating practice for dose reduction was found to be an effective measure in reducing radiation exposure, with subsequent improvement in table height elevation. Appropriate table height reduces the distance from the patient to the image detector, thus reducing scatter radiation.[22] Use of ceiling-mounted shields is also effective, particularly during DSA acquisitions, which produce higher radiation doses than fluoroscopy. A study using a phantom model found that ceiling-mounted shields were able to protect from 80% of scatter radiation in interventional cardiology procedures.[23] Scatter radiation decreases as distance from the source increases, so stepping away from the table during DSA acquisitions is also effective in reducing radiation exposure.[16]

Radiation-absorbing surgical drapes have also been proposed as a way to reduce scatter radiation, reducing the dose to the principal operator by 55%.[24] Another, more extreme, option is the ZeroGravity suit—a suspended lead apron and face shield that offers full body radiation protection and also eliminates the orthopaedic stress of regular lead garments.[25]

The use of novel technology may represent the way forward in terms of achieving significant and sustained radiation reduction. Image fusion uses computed tomography (CT) and live fluoroscopy to provide a three-dimensional roadmap to facilitate endovascular navigation. Using image fusion, much lower figures for operator exposure have been reported compared to conventional techniques: 0.004mSv for EVAR, 0.002mSv for TEVAR, 0.009mSv for fenestrated EVAR.[19] The ideal situation would be for no exposure at all, however. Endovascular robotic systems may be the answer. Remote navigation systems enable the operator to perform procedures seated completely away from the source of radiation, and has shown promise in current early clinical experience. There is potential for use in procedural stages known to be at risk of high radiation levels, such as visceral vessel cannulation.[26]

# Conclusion

Radiation exposure for endovascular procedures is significant. The cumulative effects of long-term exposure, despite being within recommended safety limits, remain a tangible hazard for endovascular workers. Staff education regarding radiation protection and awareness is essential. Novel technologies such as image fusion and endovascular robotics may represent the future in terms of radiation reduction.

## Summary

- The effects of ionising radiation can be deterministic (dose-dependent, e.g. cataracts) or stochastic (no threshold for occurrence, eg. cancer).

- Radiation exposure for complex endovascular procedures, such as TEVAR and fenestrated EVAR is significant.

- Oblique C-arm angulation, operator positioning, and procedural stage are factors affecting the occupational radiation exposure.

- Use of the ALARA principle, effective shielding, and staff education are important methods for radiation reduction.

- Novel technologies such as image fusion and remote robotic navigation may represent the way forward.

# References

1. ICRP. The 2007 Recommendations of the International Commission on Radiological Protection. Ann ICRP 2007; **37:** 2–4.
2. ICRP. Statement on tissue reaction. shttp://www.icrp.org/docs/ICRP Statement on Tissue Reactions.pdf (accessed 29 December 2016).
3. Stecker MS, Balter S, Towbin RB, *et al.* Guidelines for patient radiation dose management. *J Vasc Interv Radiol* 2009; **20:** S263–73.
4. Sholl LM, Barletta JA, Hornick JL. Radiation-associated neoplasia: clinical, pathological and genomic correlates. Histopathology 2017; **70:** 70–80.
5. Richardson DB, Cardis E, Daniels RD, *et al.* Risk of cancer from occupational exposure to ionising radiation: retrospective cohort study of workers in France, the United Kingdom, and the United States (INWORKS). *BMJ* 2015; **351:** h5359
6. BIBA Medical. Working with radiation is like keeping a pet tiger in your living room. Vascular News 2015; **67:** 1–2
7. Roguin A, Goldstein J, Bar O, *et al.* Brain and neck tumors among physicians performing interventional procedures. *Am J Cardiol* 2013; **111:** 1368–72.
8. Attigah N, Oikonomou K, Hinz U, *et al.* Radiation exposure to eye lens and operator hands during endovascular procedures in hybrid operating rooms. *J Vasc Surg* 2016; **63:** 198–203.
9. Jacob S, Boveda S, Bar O, *et al.* Interventional cardiologists and risk of radiation-induced cataract: Results of a French multicenter observational study. Int J Cardiol 2013; **167:** 1843–47.
10. Vano E, Kleiman NJ, Duran A, *et al.* Radiation cataract risk in interventional cardiology personnel. *Radiat Res* 2010; **174:** 490–95.
11. Ron E, Lubin JH, Shore RE, *et al.* Thyroid cancer after exposure to external radiation: A pooled analysis of seven studies. *Radiat Res* 1995; **141:** 259.
12. Patel AP, Gallacher D, Dourado R, *et al.* Occupational radiation exposure during endovascular aortic procedures. *Eur J Vasc Endovasc Surg* 2013; **46:** 424–30.
13. Kalef-Ezra JA, Karavasilis S, Kouvelos G, *et al.* Endovascular abdominal aortic aneurysm repair: methods of radiological risk reduction. *J Cardiovasc Surg* (Torino) 2011; **52:** 769–78.
14. Sailer AM, Schurink GWH, Bol ME, *et al.* Occupational Radiation Exposure During Endovascular Aortic Repair. *Cardiovasc Intervent Radiol* 2015; **38:** 827–32.
15. Panuccio G, Greenberg RK, Wunderle K, *et al.* Comparison of indirect radiation dose estimates with directly measured radiation dose for patients and operators during complex endovascular procedures. *J Vasc Surg* 2011; **53:** 885–894.e1; discussion 894.
16. Albayati MA, Kelly S, Gallagher D, *et al.* Editor's choice--Angulation of the C-arm during complex endovascular aortic procedures increases radiation exposure to the head. *Eur J Vasc Endovasc Surg* 2015; **49:** 396–402.
17. Mohapatra A, Greenberg RK, Mastracci TM, *et al.* Radiation exposure to operating room personnel and patients during endovascular procedures. *J Vasc Surg* 2013; **58:** 702–09.

18. Li M, Bicknell C, Cheung S, *et al.* Occupational radiation exposure during FEVAR: A stage-by-stage analysis. Presented at the Charing Cross Symposium 2016.
19. Hertault A, Maurel B, Midulla M, *et al.* Editor's choice – minimizing radiation exposure during endovascular procedures: basic knowledge, literature review, and reporting standards. *Eur J Vasc Endovasc Surg* 2015; **50:** 21–36.
20. Haqqani OP, Agarwal PK, Halin NM, *et al.* Minimizing radiation exposure to the vascular surgeon. *J Vasc Surg* 2012; **55:** 799–805.
21. Thornton RH, Dauer LT, Altamirano JP, *et al.* Comparing strategies for operator eye protection in the interventional radiology suite. *J Vasc Interv Radiol* 2010; **21:** 1703–07.
22. Kirkwood ML, Arbique GM, Guild JB, *et al. Surgeon* education decreases radiation dose in complex endovascular procedures and improves patient safety. *J Vasc Surg* 2013; **58:** 715–21.
23. Fetterly KA, Magnuson DJ, Tannahill GM, *et al.* Effective use of radiation shields to minimize operator dose during invasive cardiology procedures. *JACC Cardiovasc Interv* 2011; **4:** 1133–39.
24. Kloeze C, Klompenhouwer EG, Brands PJM, *et al.* Editor's choice--Use of disposable radiation-absorbing surgical drapes results in significant dose reduction during EVAR procedures. *Eur J Vasc Endovasc Surg* 2014; **47:** 268–72.
25. Marichal DA, Anwar T, Kirsch D, *et al.* Comparison of a suspended radiation protection system *versus* standard lead apron for radiation exposure of a simulated interventionalist. *J Vasc Interv Radiol* 2011; **22:** 437–42.
26. Bonatti J, Vetrovec G, Riga C, *et al.* Robotic technology in cardiovascular medicine. *Nat Rev Cardiol* 2014; **11:** 266–75.

# Cellular markers of radiation damage during EVAR

## AS Patel, T El-Sayed, A Smith and B Modarai

## Introduction

The health risks associated with medical radiation exposure have become a focus of discussion, with the risk of contracting cancer a particular concern. Endovascular aneurysm repair (EVAR) carries a significant burden of radiation exposure for both the operator and the patient.[1–3] The follow up study of the EVAR 1 trial recently reported an increased incidence of cancer in the cohort of patients treated by EVAR compared with those treated by open repair, possibly a consequence of radiation exposure during endovascular interventions and the diagnostic/surveillance imaging required.[4] The patient is exposed to a higher dose than the operator for a single intervention, but the latter sustains frequent, low-dose exposures over a career that often spans many years. Emerging evidence points to a higher incidence of malignancy, including brain and breast cancer, in interventionists performing fluoroscopically-guided procedures[5–7] but robust epidemiological data that would allow one to draw definitive conclusions are lacking. Anecdotal evidence does, however, suggest an alarming trend of atypical cancers developing at an earlier age in high volume complex EVAR operators than in the general population.

It would be prudent to assume that there is a linear, no-threshold relationship between exposure and risk of malignant transformation, meaning that there is no amount of radiation exposure that is considered risk free and that the greater the exposure, the greater the increase in risk. Standard physical radiation dosimeters currently used by operators crudely record cumulative exposure in an isolated body area, and the "safe" exposure limits defined using these tools may not apply universally as they do not take into account individual susceptibility to DNA damage. A better understanding of the hazards of occupational radiation exposure may be gained by using sensitive tools that measure the biological consequences of low dose radiation exposure at a cellular level for each individual exposed.

## Cytogenetic markers of radiation damage

Ionising radiation energises nucleic acids in the cell and generates reactive oxygen/nitrogen species, damaging the cellular DNA structure by causing base pair alterations, nucleotide modifications and single/double strand DNA breaks.[8] The immediate response to DNA damage is activation of a cell cycle checkpoint response that initiates specific signalling and repair mechanisms, but "misrepair" can still occur despite this protective trigger and lead to characteristic chromosomal aberrations such as micronuclei and dicentric chromosomes.[9]

Micronuclei are chromosomal fragments lost from the cell nucleus during mitosis that can be found in the cytoplasm; the frequency of micronuclei in cells can be determined using the cytokinesis block micronucleus assays or flourescence *in situ* hybridisation (FISH).[10] They are more frequently detected in lymphocytes isolated from hospital workers chronically exposed to low-dose occupational radiation.[11] Peripheral blood lymphocytes are commonly used for cytogenetic analysis of the effects of radiation exposure as they are particularly radiosensitve and are relatively easy to sample and process.[12]

Dicentric chromosomes, possessing two centromeres that are formed through the abnormal fusion of separate chromosome fragments, are more specifically associated with radiation exposure than micronuclei. Background levels of the latter are influenced by diet, exposure to environmental mutagens, age and gender.[13] Dicentric chromosomes can be detected on cells during metaphase. Although the dicentric assay requires cells to be cultured for 48 hours under mitosis inhibiting conditions (as well as an individual dose-response calibration), the technique provides an accurate estimation of radiation exposure.[10] Higher frequencies of dicentrics have been detected in interventional cardiologists and radiologists compared with control populations not involved in fluoroscopically guided intenventions.[14]

Techniques such as FISH can be used to detect chromosomal translocations in lymphocytes.[15] Translocations can be present years after occupational radiation exposure and can be passed on from irradiated stem cells to descendent lymphocytes.[16] Recently, a biodosimetric technique has been developed that combines FISH with micronuclei assays, resulting in a semi-automated, high throughput and sensitive method for biological assessment of the effects of radiation exposure.[17] This technique has shown that despite recording low physical radiation doses based on

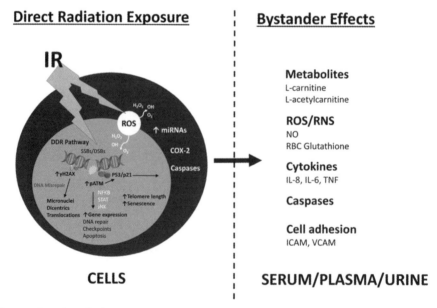

**Figure 1:** Biomarkers of radiation-induced DNA damage. Exposure to ionising radiation can cause DNA damage in cells via direct energy transfer and production of reactive oxygen species. This activates the DNA damage response pathway and upregulates a range of genomic and proteomic markers that can be detected within cells, including γ-H2AX and pATM. Misrepair of damaged DNA can produce chromosomal aberrations such as micronuclei, dicentrics and translocations. Radiation-exposed cells generate a range of metabolites, reactive oxygen/nitrogen species, cytokines, apoptotic enzymes and cell adhesion markers that can be detected in the serum, plasma and/or urine.

their standard dosimeters readings, interventional radiologists and cardiologists demonstrate relatively high levels of chromosomal damage, further outlining the limitations of physical dosimetry when compared with biodosimetry.[17]

## Genetic biomarkers of radiation exposure

*In vitro* gene expression studies on irradiated cells have identified biomarkers of exposure that include genes with a role in DNA repair (DDB2, XRCC4), cell cycle checkpoints (CDKN1A, CCNB1, GADD45A) and apoptosis (BAX, PUMA).[18] Several of these genes have been found to be differentially expressed in lymphocytes of patients after computed tomography (CT) angiography.[19] These data have implications for patients who undergo complex endovascular aortic repair and subsequently require regular CT surveillance. It is important to note that genomic biomarkers can be affected by age, gender and smoking. There is also increasing interest in the use of microRNAs (miRNAs), noncoding RNAs that post-transcriptionally regulate gene expression, for detecting the effects of radiation exposure.[20] These biomarkers are stable, have low inter-individual variability and can be measured in samples of serum and plasma. Work in rodent models has shown that specific miRNA signatures reflect exposure to radiation,[20, 21] including miR-34-a-5p and miR-182-5p that are also upregulated in human lymphocytes following exposure to ionising radiation[18] and may be promising novel biomarkers.

## Protein biomarkers of radiation exposure

An alternative to the genetic approaches described above is to analyse changes in protein expression in cells that are exposed to radiation. The formation of double strand DNA breaks triggers the phosphorylation of the histone protein H2AX to form γ-H2AX; these foci can be measured using flow cytometry or immunofluorescence microscopy, allowing detection of radiation-induced DNA damage at levels lower than 1mGy.[22] Subsequent to this phosphorylation event, several other proteins are phosphorylated, including protein 53 (p53) and ataxia-telangiectasia mutated (ATM). Although phosphorylation of H2AX does not exclusively reflect double strand DNA breaks, it is a very useful marker as it is independent of cell-cycle, strongly correlated with repair kinetics and independent from the repair pathway. These proteins are, however, only useful for measuring the acute, transient response to radiation induced DNA damage with peak phosphorylation occurring 0.5 to two hours after exposure. As a result, they are especially useful when samples are collected at multiple time points within appropriate time windows and may be particularly useful for demonstrating individual sensitivity against low-dose radiation. Raised expression of γ-H2AX, p53 and pATM has been detected in patients after cross-sectional imaging and fluoroscopically-guided cardiovascular procedures.[12] Our group recently found increased levels of γ-H2AX and pATM in circulating lymphocytes of interventionists who carry out complex endovascular procedures (unpublished data). The levels of both markers vary between individuals exposed to similar radiation doses, a phenomenon that may reflect individual variation in sensitivity to radiation induced DNA damage. This may mean that radiation exposure doses that are considered safe vary between individuals.

Nuclear magnetic resonance (MR) and mass spectrometry-based metabolomics have emerged as a powerful approach for identifying biomarkers of radiation exposure in pre-clinical *in vitro* and *in vivo* studies sampling urine, saliva, and serum. Preclinical studies have found that changes in metabolites—such as as L-carnitine and L-acetylcarnitine in urine[23] and products of nicotinate and nicotinamide metabolism in saliva[24]—can be detected after exposure to radiation. The sheer complexity of both the metabolome and proteome make studies aiming to identify sensitive and specific biomarkers following exposure to radiation highly challenging. Nevertheless, use of high-throughput technologies and advanced multilevel computational methods is likely to help identify a distinct metabolomic signature that quantifies the biological effect of radiation exposure in samples of bodily fluid from patients and operators.[25]

## Systemic biochemical markers of radiation exposure

There is now increasing recognition of the so called radiation-induced bystander effect—the induction of biological effects in neighbouring cells which have not been directly exposed to radiation, but receive signals from nearby cells that have had a radiation hit.[26] The bystander effect is mediated by reactive oxygen species[8] that are transmitted from radiation damaged cells to radiation naïve cells via cell-cell contact (usually via gap junctions) or released into the extracellular space. Additionally, inflammatory cytokines released by exposed cells can bind to nearby cells and activate downstream pathways (JAK-STAT, NFkB and MAPK), resulting in production of COX-2 and nitric oxide.[26] In cardiologists, chronic low-dose exposure to radiation results in a significant increase in serum reactive oxygen species levels and caspase-3 levels (a marker of cellular apoptosis) in lymphocytes, sensitising these cells to radiation-induced apoptosis. This response is associated with an increase in the levels of the scavenging antioxidant, glutathione, in circulating red cells in an attempt to minimise the damage incurred by higher levels of reactive oxygen species. The bystander effect also involves activation of gene products that modulate the immune system, including cell adhesion molecules (ICAM1, VCAM1), cytokines/chemokines (CCL5, interleukin-1A, B and 6, TNF), cell receptors (CD14, CD40 and ILR2) and transcription factors (NFKB and STAT3).[27]

Several studies have reported that the bystander effect increases the risk of cardiovascular disease in patients treated with radiotherapy, including those irradiated for Hodgkin's lymphoma and breast cancer.[28–31] Although the mechanism of radiation-induced cardiovascular disease is not yet fully known, it is currently believed that acceleration of atherosclerosis is the primary mechanism. In ApoE-/- mice, genetically predisposed to atherosclerosis when fed a high-fat diet, low-dose radiation promotes atherosclerosis, particularly after repeated exposure.[32] It may be possible to further elucidate the mechanism responsible for this phenomenon by analysing the function of cells, including leucocytes and endothelial cells, that are important in the development of atherosclerotic disease. For example, *in vitro* studies have shown that chronic radiation exposure results in activation of the p53/p21 pathway in endothelial cells causing premature senescence.[33] Low-dose irradiation also induces detrimental effects in the pathways that control oxidative stress, fatty acid metabolism and cholesterol synthesis in human endothelial cells.[34] It is believed that oxidative stress induced DNA damage results in cell senescence and a shortening of telomere length, both of which are associated with increased risk of cardiovascular disease.[35] A recent analysis carried out on clinical staff working in interventional cardiac catheterisation laboratories suggested that age and radiation exposure are independent determinants of reduced telemore length in their leucocytes.[36]

# Conclusion

Conventional dosimetry fails to account for the biological consequences of radiation exposure and any inter-individual differences in susceptibility to deleterious effects. A number of genetic and protein based cellular markers, some of which readily lend themselves to high throughput sampling, have been associated with radiation induced damage. These markers merit further investigation in both patients and operators after EVAR to refine our understanding of the health risks associated with low dose radiation exposure and develop strategies for mitigating against this risk.

## Summary

- Current methods for recording radiation exposure to patients and operators during EVAR do not reflect individual susceptibility to this exposure and its biological consequences.

- Circulating lymphocytes are radiosensitive cells that readily express cellular markers associated with radiation exposure.

- Measuring cellular chromosomal aberrations, DNA repair proteins such as γ-H2AX, circulating microRNAs, caspases and telomere length may allow a biodosimetric assessment of the effects of radiation exposure.

# References

1. Howells P, Eaton R, Patel AS, *et al*. Risk of radiation exposure during endovascular aortic repair. *Eur J Vasc Endovasc Surg* 2012; **43**: 393–97.
2. Patel AP, Gallacher D, Dourado R, *et al*. Occupational radiation exposure during endovascular aortic procedures. *Eur J Vasc Endovasc Surg* 2013; **46**: 424–30.
3. Albayati MA, Kelly S, Gallagher D, *et al*. Angulation of the C-arm during complex endovascular aortic procedures increases radiation exposure to the head. *Eur J Vasc Endovasc Surg* 2015; **49**: 396–402.
4. Patel R, Sweeting MJ, Powell JT, Greenhalgh RM, *et al*. Endovascular *versus* open repair of abdominal aortic aneurysm in 15-years' follow-up of the UK endovascular aneurysm repair trial 1 (EVAR trial 1): a randomised controlled trial. *Lancet* 2016; **388**: 2366–74.
5. Roguin A, Goldstein J, Bar O, Goldstein JA. Brain and neck tumors among physicians performing interventional procedures. *Am J Cardiol* 2013; **111**: 1368–72.
6. Yoshinaga S, Hauptmann M, Sigurdson AJ, *et al*. Nonmelanoma skin cancer in relation to ionizing radiation exposure among U.S. radiologic technologists. *Int J Cancer* 2005; **115**: 828–34.
7. Rajaraman P, Doody MM, Yu CL, *et al*. Cancer Risks in U.S. Radiologic Technologists Working With Fluoroscopically Guided Interventional Procedures, 1994-2008. *Am J Roentgenol* 2016; **206**: 1101–08.
8. Reisz JA, Bansal N, Qian J, *et al*. Effects of ionizing radiation on biological molecules--mechanisms of damage and emerging methods of detection. *Antioxid Redox Signal* 2014; **21**: 260–92.
9. Sancar A, Lindsey-Boltz LA, Unsal-Kaçmaz K, Linn S. Molecular mechanisms of mammalian DNA repair and the DNA damage checkpoints. *Annu Rev Biochem* 2004; **73**: 39–85.
10. Manning G, Rothkamm K. Deoxyribonucleic acid damage-associated biomarkers of ionising radiation: current status and future relevance for radiology and radiotherapy. *Br J Radiol* 2013; **86**: 20130173.
11. Sari-Minodier I, Orsière T, Auquier P, *et al*. Cytogenetic monitoring by use of the micronucleus assay among hospital workers exposed to low doses of ionizing radiation. *Mutat Res* 2007; **629**: 111–21.
12. Lee WH, Nguyen PK, Fleischmann D, Wu JC. DNA damage-associated biomarkers in studying individual sensitivity to low-dose radiation from cardiovascular imaging. *Eur Heart J* 2016; **37**: 3075–80.

13. Willems P, August L, Slabbert J, *et al.* Automated micronucleus (MN) scoring for population triage in case of large scale radiation events. Int J Radiat Biol 2010; **86:** 2–11.

14. Zakeri F, Hirobe T. A cytogenetic approach to the effects of low levels of ionizing radiations on occupationally exposed individuals. *Eur J Radiol* 2010; **73:** 191–95.

15. Tucker JD. Low-dose ionizing radiation and chromosome translocations: a review of the major considerations for human biological dosimetry. Mutat Res 2008; **659:** 211–20.

16. Little MP, Kwon D, Doi K, *et al.* Association of chromosome translocation rate with low dose occupational radiation exposures in U.S. radiologic technologists. Radiat Res 2014; **182:** 1–17.

17. Vral A, Decorte V, Depuydt J, *et al.* A semi-automated FISH-based micronucleus-centromere assay for biomonitoring of hospital workers exposed to low doses of ionizing radiation. Mol Med Rep 2016; **14:** 103–10.

18. Kabacik S, Manning G, Raffy C, *et al.* Time, dose and ataxia telangiectasia mutated (ATM) status dependency of coding and noncoding RNA expression after ionizing radiation exposure. Radiat Res 2015; **183:** 325–37.

19. Nguyen PK, Lee WH, Li YF, *et al.* Assessment of the Radiation Effects of Cardiac CT Angiography Using Protein and Genetic Biomarkers. JACC Cardiovasc Imaging 2015; **8:** 873–84.

20. Cui W, Ma J, Wang Y, Biswal S. Plasma miRNA as biomarkers for assessment of total-body radiation exposure dosimetry. PLoS One 2011; **6:**e22988.

21. Acharya SS, Fendler W, Watson J, *et al.* Serum microRNAs are early indicators of survival after radiation-induced hematopoietic injury. Sci Transl Med 2015; **7:** 287ra69.

22. Rothkamm K, Löbrich M. Evidence for a lack of DNA double-strand break repair in human cells exposed to very low x-ray doses. Proc Natl Acad Sci U S A. 2003; **100:** 5057–62.

23. Pannkuk EL, Laiakis EC, Authier S, *et al.* Global Metabolomic identification of long-term dose-dependent urinary biomarkers in nonhuman primates exposed to ionizing radiation. Radiat Res 2015; **184:** 12133.

24. Laiakis EC, Strawn SJ, Brenner DJ, Fornace AJ. Assessment of Saliva as a Potential Biofluid for Biodosimetry: A Pilot Metabolomics Study in Mice. Radiat Res 2016; **186:** 92–97.

25. Laiakis EC, Mak TD, Anizan S, *et al.* Development of a metabolomic radiation signature in urine from patients undergoing total body irradiation. Radiat Res 2014; **181:** 350–61.

26. Nikitaki Z, Mavragani IV, Laskaratou DA, *et al.* Systemic mechanisms and effects of ionizing radiation: A new 'old' paradigm of how the bystanders and distant can become the players. Semin Cancer Biol 2016; **37–38:**77–95.

27. Georgakilas AG, Pavlopoulou A, Louka M, *et al.* Emerging molecular networks common in ionizing radiation, immune and inflammatory responses by employing bioinformatics approaches. Cancer Lett 2015; **368:** 164–72.

28. Bhatti P, Sigurdson AJ, Mabuchi K. Can low-dose radiation increase risk of cardiovascular disease? *Lancet* 2008; **372:** 697–99.

29. Little MP, Tawn EJ, Tzoulaki I, *et al.* A systematic review of epidemiological associations between low and moderate doses of ionizing radiation and late cardiovascular effects, and their possible mechanisms. Radiat Res 2008; **169:** 99–109.

30. Galper SL, Yu JB, Mauch PM, *et al.* Clinically significant cardiac disease in patients with Hodgkin lymphoma treated with mediastinal irradiation. Blood 2011; **117:** 412-18.

31. Taylor CW, McGale P, Darby SC. Cardiac risks of breast-cancer radiotherapy: a contemporary view. Clin Oncol (R Coll Radiol). 2006; **18:** 236-46.

32. Mitchel RE, Hasu M, Bugden M, *et al.* Low-dose radiation exposure and protection against atherosclerosis in ApoE(-/-) mice: the influence of P53 heterozygosity. Radiat Res 2013; **179:** 190–99.

33. Yentrapalli R, Azimzadeh O, Barjaktarovic Z, *et al.* Quantitative proteomic analysis reveals induction of premature senescence in human umbilical vein endothelial cells exposed to chronic low-dose rate gamma radiation. Proteomics 2013; **13:** 1096–107.

34. Pluder F, Barjaktarovic Z, Azimzadeh O, *et al.* Low-dose irradiation causes rapid alterations to the proteome of the human endothelial cell line EA.hy926. Radiat Environ Biophys 2011; **50:** 155–66.

35. Fyhrquist F, Saijonmaa O, Strandberg T. The roles of senescence and telomere shortening in cardiovascular disease. Nat Rev Cardiol 2013; **10:** 274–83.

36. Andreassi MG, Piccaluga E, Gargani L, *et al.* Subclinical carotid atherosclerosis and early vascular aging from long-term low-dose ionizing radiation exposure: a genetic, telomere, and vascular ultrasound study in cardiac catheterization laboratory staff. JACC Cardiovasc Interv 2015; **8:** 616–27.

# Recent use of reduced contrast with CT scans for patients with aneurysm and renal insufficiency

GF Torsello, C Bremer and GB Torsello

## Introduction

Endovascular aneurysm repair (EVAR) and thoracic endovascular aortic repair (TEVAR) require high-resolution computed tomography (CT) angiography for adequate preoperative planning. CT angiography is also the standard imaging method to identify issues of the major vessels and in endoleak detection.[1] In order to reliably detect these, large amounts of contrast media are needed, which in turn can induce deterioration of renal function in patients after EVAR.[2] The administration of iodinated contrast medium is known to cause contrast-induced nephropathy, especially in patients with pre-existing chronic kidney disease,[3] which has in turn similar risk factors as aortic aneurysmal disease.

For patients with chronic or acute renal disease (glomerular filtration rate[GFR]<60ml/min/1.73m2) contrast-enhanced duplex ultrasound, native CT or magnetic resonance (MR) angiography have been proposed as possible diagnostic alternatives.[4] However, in the case of aneurysm-related symptoms or high suspicion of endoleaks, detection of the underlying lesion and planning of the next therapeutic step can be demanding. This is particularly difficult in patients after use of stainless steel devices.

## Imaging protocol for EVAR patients with renal insufficiency

Our protocol for patients with renal disease consists of (A) hydration with N-acetyl-cysteine prior to- and after the investigation, (B) consulting of the institution's nephrologist and (C) CT angiography with intra-arterially injected contrast medium.

### Intra-arterial CT angiography technique

Before the CT angiography, the left brachial artery is punctured and a 4Fr sheath is placed. After the administration of 5,000 units of heparin, a standard wire (Terumo) is used to place a 4Fr straight angiographic catheter (Radiofocus, Terumo) at the level of the proximal descending aorta. The catheter is fixated to the skin and a sterile drape is wrapped around the angio catheter and the 4Fr sheath.

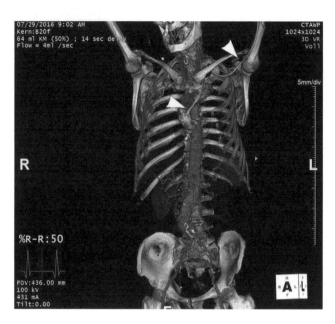

**Figure 1:** 3D reconstruction of a transarterial CT angiography. Note the transbranchically advanced angiography highlighted by the arrows.

A low dose heparin infusion is connected to both sheath and the angio catheter to avoid clotting on the way to the tomography. Depending on patient's body weight, 20–40ml of contrast agent is used. We have developed a protocol to allow optimal bolus timing so that an arterial or venous contrast phase may be achieved (Figure 1).

After the CT angiography, the patient returns to the ward and both sheath and angio catheter are removed and a circular compression bandage is used to close the puncture site.

## Experience with the transarterial CT angiography

To our knowledge, there is no literature available on this technique. We are currently reviewing our experience with transarterial CT angiography. Since January 2011, we performed 79 transarterial CT angiographies in patients with abdominal aortic aneurysms. Except for eight cases, all patients were female and the mean age was 74.9 years. In 45 cases, the CT angiography was performed preoperatively and postoperatively in others.

In order to assess the incidence of contrast-induced nephropathy, we retrospectively analysed pre-examination serum creatinine levels and GFR and compared these to the respective values routinely measured 24 hours after the examination.

To understand the diagnostic value of these examinations, we firstly assessed subjective image quality, rated independently by two experienced vascular surgeons and secondly measured attenuation values at the level of the superior mesenteric artery.

Access vessel complications such as thrombosis, haematoma, false aneurysm, dissection and peripheral nerve injury were recorded. Furthermore, we assessed the incidence of transient and permanent neurological disorders, interventions secondary to the examination as well as death resulting from the examination.

The incidence of contrast-induced nephropathy, defined as an increase of ≥0.5mg/dl serum creatinine or a decrease of ≥25% in GFR after contrast medium administration, in the examined patient population was 2.5% (2/79). The mean serum creatinine increase was 0.1±0.2mg/dl, the mean GFR decrease was 1.5±6.5%.

Subjective imaging quality was sufficient in 96.2% (76/79) of cases. In three cases, a sufficient contrast between the arterial vasculature and the surrounding tissue could not be achieved, either because the bolus timing or the amount of contrast was not sufficient.

The mean attenuation value of the aorta at the level of the superior mesenteric artery was 257±138 Hounsfield units. Arteries are considered to be adequately attenuated in case of 250 or more Hounsfield units.

There were three access vessel complications (3.8%), two puncture site haematomas which needed no further intervention and a false aneurysm of a left brachial artery which necessitated treatment.

We recorded no transient or permanent neurologic deficits, none of the patients died because of the examination.

## Conclusion

Transarterial CT angiography is a possible diagnostic tool in the evaluation of patients with aortic aneurysms with a low incidence of complications and satisfactory diagnostic quality.

## Summary

- Chronic kidney disease poses a challenge in the diagnosis and follow-up of aortic aneurysms.

- Alternatives to CT angiography as the diagnostic gold standard for EVAR planning and endoleak detection are in some cases not satisfactory.

- Transarterial CT angiography is an invasive, yet safe means of creating high-quality imaging in cases of complex aneurysmal disease.

## References

1. Moll FL, Powell JT, Fraedrich G, et al. Management of abdominal aortic aneurysms clinical practice guidelines of the European society for vascular surgery. Eur J Vasc Endovasc Surg 2011; 41 (Suppl 1): S1–S58. Epub 2011/01/11.
2. Gray D, Eisenack M, Gawenda M, et al. Repeated contrast medium application after EVAR and not the type of endograft fixation seems to have .deleterious effect on the renal function. J Vasc Surg 2017; 65 (1): 46–51.
3. Aubry P, Brillet G, Catella L, et al. Outcomes, risk factors and health burden of contrast-induced acute kidney injury: an observational study of one million hospitalizations with image-guided cardiovascular procedures. BMC Nephrol 2016; 17 (1): 167.
4. Cantisani V, Ricci P, Grazhdani H, Net al. Prospective comparative analysis of colour-Doppler ultrasound, contrast-enhanced ultrasound, computed tomography and magnetic resonance in detecting endoleak after endovascular abdominal aortic aneurysm repair. Eur J Vasc Endovasc Surg 2011; 41 (2): 186–92.

# Fusion imaging using a mobile C-arm to reduce radiation exposure. An alternative to fixed systems "for the people"

T Martin-Gonzalez, B Maurel and TM Mastracci

## Introduction

Endovascular aneurysm repair (EVAR) has evolved since it was first performed in 1991,[1] and today treatment for even complex aneurysm pathology can be performed using complex devices, such as fenestrated EVAR and branched EVAR devices.[2,3] This type of treatment is becoming increasingly common, associated with a low morbidity rate and good medium-term outcomes;[4,5,6] however, it also requires increased radiation and nephrotoxic contrast administration.[7,8]

Advanced imaging techniques, such as 3D fusion, significantly reduce radiation exposure and contrast use in EVAR as well as in complex endovascular procedures,[9] but until now have been limited to fixed imaging and hybrid rooms.

## Benefits of fusion imaging

The replacement of mobile C-arms for fixed imaging systems has been associated with a higher image quality, nevertheless, it comes with higher radiation.[10] Fixed imaging systems have larger detectors correlated to larger irradiated fields and higher capabilities and at the end, higher dose area products. On the other hand, flat panel fixed systems, compared with mobile imaging units, can generate more energy and improve heat dispersion, leading to a higher quality image with more contrast and less noise. Additionally, there is more focus on technical innovations, as fusion image guidance, allowing improvement in radiation dose and contrast amount, especially in the case of complex repairs.

In most proprietary systems, image fusion guidance is performed from acquisition of an unenhanced intraoperative cone-beam computed tomography (CT) study or from a preoperative contrast enhanced CT scan. In all the cases, those images are sent to a workstation where the 3D aortic volume is constructed and the overlap is performed using boney landmarks. This volume is synchronised to the table and gantry position and helps guide standard and complex EVAR.

There has been much interest in the recent published literature in the use of fusion imaging in hybrid operating theatres. Studies have demonstrated a significant reduction of injected contrast without a reduction in radiation

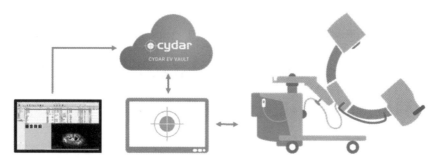

**Figure 1:** Workflow of the ROAM technique.

dose[11,12] using fusion, due to the increased dose from the preoperative cone-beam CT. In contrast, using a similar fusion technique, McNally *et al*[13] reported a significant reduction in radiation exposure, contrast use and overall procedure time. The Lille group,[14] performing fusion from orthogonal fluoroscopic views and a preoperative contrast enhanced CT scan, showed a reduction in dose area product as well as contrast dose, avoiding added radiation from a perioperative cone-beam CT.

In all the cases, close adherence to the "ALARA" (As low as reasonably achievable) principle is mandatory to reduce the X-ray radiation, including minimising fluoroscopy time, maximising collimation, use of protection barriers and optimising angulations.[15,16]

## Fusion in C-arms; the ROAM technique

The compelling disadvantage of current fusion techniques is that this application is available only in expensive and modern hybrid operating rooms, which are only accessible in selected centres. If the benefit of fusion imaging is truly going to have impact in the field of vascular surgery, it will need to be accessible in all imaging suites. We have been working with new digital, flat panel mobile C-arms to test the use of fusion imaging in lower cost imaging scenarios. We call this technique "ROAM"—real-time overlay for aneurysm repair on a mobile unit. The Cydar software is a new technology that provides image guidance by overlaying preoperative 3D vessel anatomy from the preoperative CT scans onto live fluoroscopic images. This software differs in that it is based in the cloud, and employs image matching techniques to continuously update the registration, and it works through a standard computer with its own monitor. This computer connects the video output of the live X-ray set to the cloud through the hospital network and functions with fixed fluoroscopic equipment as well as mobile C-arms.

The workflow is the same for fixed imaging units and mobile C-arms. First, a suitable CT scan is uploaded in advance of the procedure. The aortic volume is segmented and prepared to highlight target anatomic landmarks. Once the volume is ready, it can be selected to be used in the procedure and when the X-ray images appear, the 3D overlay starts automatically (Figure 1). The system deduces the patient position by automatically comparing vertebrae visible on X-ray to that on the preoperative CT scan. In order for the fusion to show up, at least two vertebrae must be visible on the screen. This system provides an accessory

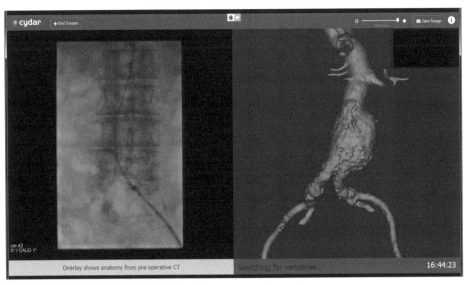

**Figure 2A:** Right mask turning to grey after a movement has been detected.

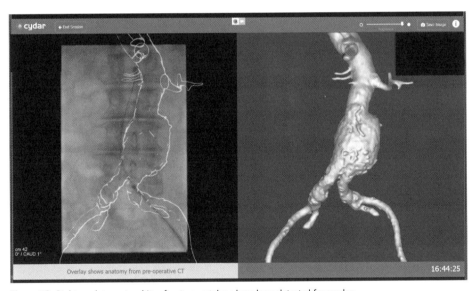

**Figure 2B:** Right mask turns to white after two vertebrae have been detected for overlay.

screen, which is split in two. On the right-hand side the volume appears in grey. In three to eight seconds of calculation, an updated overlay is projected on the left hand side of the Cydar screen, as a green outline superimposed onto the live X-ray fluoroscopy images, and the mask on the right hand side turns to green (white on Figure 2B). When a movement is detected from the table or the C-arm, the overlay automatically disappears and a new overlay updated with patient position is generated in about five seconds. During the calculation, the right mask turns to grey (Figures 2A and 2B).

In order to assess the accuracy of the mask, an angiography at the level of the renal arteries and/or a pre-catheterisation of the lowest renal artery is mandatory if

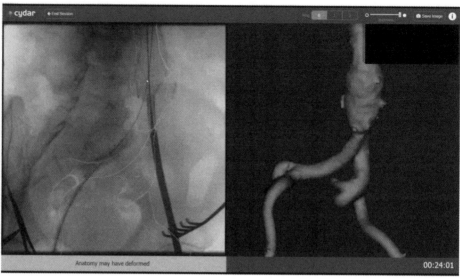

**Figure 3:** Iliac arteries position checked with a fluoro loop.

a standard EVAR is performed. In a case of a complex aortic endovascular repair, the pre-catheterisation of two or more target vessels can be performed to check the accuracy of the mask. At the level of the iliac arteries, the position will be checked with a fluoro loop (Figure 3).

However, this technique has some limitations. First, this is a body region covering eight vertebrae from T10 to L5, and remains uncertain in its ability to assist treatment of descending thoracic aortic aneurysms. Second, in the current iteration of the technology, the 3D overlays will only appear in a range of angles from 40 degrees left oblique to 40 degrees right oblique and 30 degrees cranial to 30 degrees caudal. Finally, as with most current fusion systems, even if the 3D overlays accurately represent preoperative anatomy, the mask is static, cannot be corrected in case of inaccuracy and does not show cardiac or respiratory movement. In addition, stiff wires and sheaths often straighten blood vessels, changing their shape and leading to significant deformation of native anatomy, not reflected in the overlay.

## Exploring the deformation in the literature

The compelling limitation of any fusion technique is the potential overlay inaccuracy due to deformation of the aorta after instrumentation. Sailer et al[17] identified three main reasons: the differences between the preoperative CT angiography and the cone-beam CT, the rigid coregistration especially at the level of the tortuous iliac arteries and in the distal elongated descending thoracic aorta, and the patient movement. Carrell et al[18] detected the maximum errors in the more angulated aortas after device insertion when they analysed the feasibility of an automated 2D–3D image registration system. Fukuda et al[19] showed overall positive results in terms of accuracy when the registration is done with boney structures as the landmark, being of 80% at the level of the lowest renal artery (less than 3mm) and 85% at the level of the iliac bifurcation. On the other hand, Maurel et al[20] found that the insertion of rigid material leads to significant displacement of the aorta and of the origin of the main aortic branches always needed an adjustment. This group promoted a correction tool based on digital subtraction angiography acquisition, as also described in Kauffman *et al.*[21]

## The gentrification of fusion imaging

The emphasis on new technologies, such as fusion guidance, developing to reduce the radiation and contrast doses,[13,14] are only available in high-cost operating theatres which are not affordable for a large proportion of the hospitals globally. As the technology develops for these hybrid suites, new iterative versions of both hardware and software are required to manifest its use in clinical care. This means that even modern imaging suites reach obsolescence for new technology much faster than in previous generations. By contrast, in the vast majority of cases, a mobile C-arm is the eligible X-ray system. In these systems, a higher radiation dose is mandatory to obtain the required appropriate image quality for complex procedures or challenging standard ones.

The new availability of the ROAM technique will allow a reduction in the radiation and contrast doses regardless of the X-ray system. This technology makes relevant the use of fusion image guidance, being available for all the hospital centres. Additionally, the advances in technology should be deployable with software upgrades, meaning that more costly hardware acquisitions will not be necessary to continue to offer patients the latest iteration of the technology.

A trial is running at the moment to demonstrate the reduction in radiation dose and contrast with this fusion and the results will be available soon.

## Conclusion

The new image technology allows a reduction radiation dose during endovascular procedure. At the beginning, fusion guidance image was only available for the expensive hybrid operating rooms; however, the new ROAM technique implements this technique in mobile C-arms, making useful fusion for everyone.

## Summary

- 3D fusion significantly reduces radiation exposure and contrast during endovascular procedures; however, it seems limited to the expensive hybrid rooms.

- A new software based in the cloud provides image guidance in mobile C-arms, the ROAM technique .

- The inaccuracy of the overlay due to deformation of the aorta remains the compelling limitation of the fusion techniques.

- The ROAM technique will allow a reduction in the radiation and contrast doses regardless the X-ray system.

# References

1. Parodi JC, Palmaz JC, Barone HD. Transfemoral intraluminal graft implantation for abdominal aortic aneurysms. *Ann Vasc Surg* 1991; **5** (6): 491–99.
2. Faruqi RM, Chuter TA, Reilly LM, *et al.* Endovascular repair of abdominal aortic aneurysm using a pararenal fenestrated stent-graft. J Endovasc Surg Off J Int Soc Endovasc Surg 1999; **6** (4): 354–58.
3. Chuter TA, Gordon RL, Reilly LM, *et al.* An endovascular system for thoracoabdominal aortic aneurysm repair. *J Endovasc Ther Off J Int Soc Endovasc Spec* 2001; **8** (1): 25–33.
4. Verhoeven ELG, Katsargyris A, Bekkema F, *et al.* Editor's Choice: Ten-year Experience with Endovascular Repair of Thoracoabdominal Aortic Aneurysms: Results from 166 Consecutive Patients. *Eur J Vasc Endovasc Surg Off J Eur Soc Vasc Surg* 2015; **49** (5): 524–31.
5. Martin-Gonzalez T, Pinçon C, Maurel B, *et al.* Renal Outcomes Following Fenestrated and Branched Endografting. *Eur J Vasc Endovasc Surg Off J Eur Soc Vasc Surg* 2015; **50**(4): 420–30.
6. Kristmundsson T, Sonesson B, Dias N, *et al.* Outcomes of fenestrated endovascular repair of juxtarenal aortic aneurysm. *J Vasc Surg* 2014; **59** (1): 115–20.
7. Solomon R, Dumouchel W. Contrast media and nephropathy: findings from systematic analysis and Food and Drug Administration reports of adverse effects. Invest Radiol 2006; **41** (8): 651–60.
8. Kirkwood ML, Arbique GM, Guild JB, *et al. Surgeon* education decreases radiation dose in complex endovascular procedures and improves patient safety. *J Vasc Surg* 2013; **58(3):** 715–21.
9. Hertault A, Maurel B, Pontana F, *et al.* Benefits of Completion 3D Angiography Associated with Contrast Enhanced Ultrasound to Assess Technical Success after EVAR. *Eur J Vasc Endovasc Surg Off J Eur Soc Vasc Surg* 2015; **49** (5): 541–48.
10. de Ruiter QMB, Reitsma JB, Moll FL, van Herwaarden JA. Meta-analysis of Cumulative Radiation Duration and Dose During EVAR Using Mobile, Fixed, or Fixed/3D Fusion C-Arms. *J Endovasc Ther Off J Int Soc Endovasc Spec* 2016; **23** (6): 944–56.
11. Bruschi A, Michelagnoli S, Chisci E, *et al.* A comparison study of radiation exposure to patients during EVAR and Dyna CT in an angiosuite vs. an operating theatre. *Radiat Prot Dosimetry* 2015; **163** (4): 491–98.
12. Tacher V, Lin M, Desgranges P, *et al.* Image guidance for endovascular repair of complex aortic aneurysms: comparison of two-dimensional and three-dimensional angiography and image fusion. *J Vasc Interv Radiol JVIR* 2013; **24(11):** 1698–706.
13. McNally MM, Scali ST, Feezor RJ, *et al.* Three-dimensional fusion computed tomography decreases radiation exposure, procedure time, and contrast use during fenestrated endovascular aortic repair. *J Vasc Surg* 2015; **61**(2): 309–16.
14. Hertault A, Maurel B, Sobocinski J, *et al.* Impact of hybrid rooms with image fusion on radiation exposure during endovascular aortic repair. *Eur J Vasc Endovasc Surg Off J Eur Soc Vasc Surg* 2014; **48**(4): 382–90.
15. Stecker MS, Balter S, Towbin RB, *et al.* Guidelines for patient radiation dose management. *J Vasc Interv Radiol* 2009; **20** (7 Suppl): S263–73.
16. Hertault A, Maurel B, Midulla M, *et al.* Editor's Choice - Minimizing Radiation Exposure During Endovascular Procedures: Basic Knowledge, Literature Review, and Reporting Standards. *Eur J Vasc Endovasc Surg Off J Eur Soc Vasc Surg* 2015; **50**(1): 21–36.
17. Sailer AM, de Haan MW, Peppelenbosch AG, *et al.* CTA with fluoroscopy image fusion guidance in endovascular complex aortic aneurysm repair. *Eur J Vasc Endovasc Surg Off J Eur Soc Vasc Surg* 2014; **47** (4): 349–56.
18. Carrell TWG, Modarai B, Brown JRI, Penney GP. Feasibility and limitations of an automated 2D-3D rigid image registration system for complex endovascular aortic procedures. *J Endovasc Ther Off J Int Soc Endovasc Spec* 2010; **17** (4): 527–33.
19. Fukuda T, Matsuda H, Doi S, *et al.* Evaluation of automated 2D-3D image overlay system utilizing subtraction of bone marrow image for EVAR: feasibility study. *Eur J Vasc Endovasc Surg Off J Eur Soc Vasc Surg* 2013; **46**(1): 75–81.
20. Maurel B, Hertault A, Gonzalez TM, *et al.* Evaluation of visceral artery displacement by endograft delivery system insertion. *J Endovasc Ther Off J Int Soc Endovasc Spec* 2014; **21** (2): 339–47.
21. Kauffmann C, Douane F, Therasse E, *et al.* Source of errors and accuracy of a two-dimensional/three-dimensional fusion road map for endovascular aneurysm repair of abdominal aortic aneurysm. *J Vasc Interv Radiol* 2015; **26** (4): 544–51.

# Abdominal aortic aneurysm consensus update— Pathways of care

# Screening, indications and imaging

# Cardiopulmonary exercise testing predicts perioperative mortality and long-term survival in abdominal aortic aneurysm patients

SW Grant, NA Wisely and CN McCollum

## Introduction

An accurate assessment of a patient's perioperative mortality risk and anticipated long-term survival is vital in elective abdominal aortic aneurysm repair as most patients are asymptomatic and only benefit from repair if it prevents premature death due to aneurysm rupture. Several methods of estimating both the short- and long-term risks for patients undergoing elective abdominal aortic aneurysm repair have been proposed, including risk prediction models, biomarkers, genetic testing and assessment of functional capacity.

While risk prediction models based on clinical registry data are probably the most widely studied and used method for estimating operative risk, assessment of functional capacity using cardiopulmonary exercise testing has increasingly been adopted over recent years. It was estimated in 2013, that more than 15,000 cardiopulmonary exercise tests were performed as part of preoperative assessment in England alone with upwards of a third of anaesthetic departments having a cardiopulmonary exercise testing service or in the process of establishing one.[1]

Cardiopulmonary exercise testing provides a gold standard objective assessment of a patient's functional capacity and several studies have demonstrated an association between measurements from cardiopulmonary exercise tests and outcomes after non-cardiac surgery.[2–4] While there are no data from randomised controlled studies, there are data from several observational studies that suggest cardiopulmonary exercise testing measures are associated with both short- and long-term outcomes after elective abdominal aortic aneurysm surgery.

## Cardiopulmonary exercise testing

Cardiopulmonary exercise testing involves the breath-by-breath measurement of respiratory oxygen uptake ($VO_2$), carbon dioxide production ($VCO_2$), and ventilation (VE) during exercise and recovery and allows an assessment of the integrative exercise responses of multiple organ systems. Exercise is usually performed using a treadmill or a cycle ergometer (Figure 1). Walking or running on a treadmill uses a larger muscle mass than a cycle ergometer meaning the maximum $VO_2$ achieved is on average higher. Patients' exercise ability on a cycle may also be reduced by musculoskeletal impairments such as joint replacements or poor quadriceps power and this may reduce their peak $VO_2$. However, the cycle ergometer is lower impact than the treadmill and hence generally better tolerated by older patients with arthritis or balance issues. The cycle ergometer is also less prone to noise artefacts and usually cheaper. An arm ergometer can also potentially be used in patients with lower limb disabilities although there is limited experience with this in the context of preoperative assessment.

While exercising, fast-responding oxygen and carbon dioxide sensors acquire respiratory data on a breath-by-breath basis and ventilatory flow is measured with a pneumotachograph. The patient may also undergo blood pressure measurements and continuous ECG monitoring can also be used to identify inducible cardiac ischaemia when ≥1 mm of ST-segment depression in two or more adjacent ECG leads is recorded.

After collecting resting data, a symptom-limited exercise test is performed by increasing the workload according to a defined protocol until the patient develops symptoms or is unable to continue. A number of specific protocols for increasing workload are available but the chosen protocol should ideally be tailored to the individual to achieve exercise duration of between eight and 12 minutes. A number of measures can be used to assess whether a maximal effort test has been performed including achieving 85% of the age predicted maximal heart rate or a respiratory exchange ratio (ratio of $VCO_2$ and $VO_2$) of ≥1.10.[5]

Many different variables can be derived from cardiopulmonary exercise testing with the most commonly used including, peak $VO_2$, $VO_2$ at anaerobic threshold, and the relationship between minute ventilation (VE) and $VCO_2$. Maximum $VO_2$ represents the limit of the cardiopulmonary system and is defined by the Fick equation as the product of cardiac output and arterial-venous oxygen difference at peak exercise. It is measured in litres of oxygen per minute adjusted for body weight. Peak $VO_2$ represents the highest $VO_2$ achieved during a test but this may not necessarily represent the limit of the cardiopulmonary system for that patient as the test may have been stopped early due to symptoms or muscle fatigue. True maximum $VO_2$ is defined by a sustained plateau in $VO_2$ that occurs during maximum effort. True $VO_2$ max is rarely achieved in patients who undergo cardiopulmonary exercise testing prior to major surgery and as a result, peak $VO_2$ is more commonly used.

Anaerobic threshold is the value of $VO_2$ at the point when oxygen demand exceeds oxygen supply to the tissues during incremental exercise. At this point, anaerobic glycolysis occurs and an increase in ventilation is required to eliminate the excess carbon dioxide produced during the buffering of lactic acid. Anaerobic threshold generally occurs at approximately 40–50% of peak VO2 in untrained individuals, but may not be observed in patients who are unable to complete a maximum effort test. Anaerobic threshold is generally reported in absolute terms but it can also be reported as a percentage of peak $VO_2$.

The relationship between minute ventilation and $VCO_2$ provides a measure of ventilatory efficiency and physiological lung dead space. $VE/VCO_2$ is generally measured at anaerobic threshold. Lower values of $VE/VCO_2$ suggest good ventilatory efficiency and low physiological lung dead space whereas high values of VE/VCO2

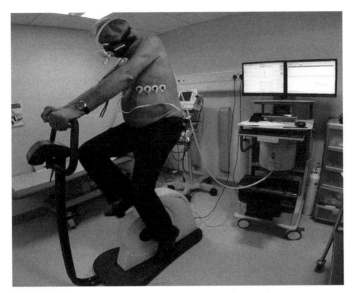

**Figure 1:** A patient performing a cardiopulmonary exercise testing test using a cycle ergometer.

suggest poor ventilatory efficiency and higher physiological lung dead space. Although numerous other variables can also be derived from cardiopulmonary exercise testing, the aforementioned three variables detailed are the most commonly analysed variables in preoperative assessment.

## Cardiopulmonary exercise testing and outcomes after abdominal aortic aneurysm repair

Risk prediction models are the most widely studied method of estimating risk in patients undergoing elective abdominal aortic aneurysm repair. Several risk prediction models were developed specifically for this purpose and have demonstrated good statistical performance on external validation.[6] These models tended to be developed using routinely collected data such as age, gender, comorbidities and routine preoperative laboratory investigations from large clinical registries. Cardiopulmonary exercise testing has not been routinely undertaken in most centres performing elective abdominal aortic aneurysm repair to date meaning that measures derived from these tests have not been included in the registries used to develop these models. However, several studies at centres that perform cardiopulmonary exercise testing prior to elective abdominal aortic aneurysm repair have demonstrated an association between the variables derived from cardiopulmonary exercise testing and either perioperative mortality or survival after elective abdominal aortic aneurysm repair.[7–10]

The earliest study on the association between cardiopulmonary exercise testing derived variables and outcomes specifically in elective abdominal aortic aneurysm repair was published in 1998 and analysed data from 30 patients who underwent cardiopulmonary exercise testing prior to elective abdominal aortic aneurysm repair.[7] The authors demonstrated that 70% of patients who developed perioperative

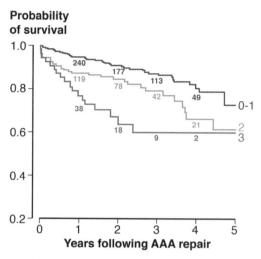

**Figure 2:** Survival after elective abdominal aortic aneurysm repair stratified by the number of subthreshold preoperative cardiopulmonary exercise testing measurements taken from Grant *et al*.[11] Initial numbers in each group were 293, 159 and 54 for patients with 0 or 1, 2 and 3 subthreshold cardiopulmonary exercise testing measurements respectively.

complications or died within a year of surgery had a peak $VO_2$ of <20 ml.kg-1. min.-1, compared with only 50% of patients who did not develop complications.[7]

Carlisle *et al* were the first to demonstrate an independent association between cardiopulmonary exercise testing derived variables and outcomes in elective abdominal aortic aneurysm repair. They analysed data from 130 patients who underwent cardiopulmonary exercise testing prior to elective abdominal aortic aneurysm repair with a 30-day mortality rate of 10.8%. On multivariable analysis, higher values of $VE/VCO_2$ and lower values of anaerobic threshold were found to be statistically associated with worse mid-term survival.[8] An association between anaerobic threshold and mid-term mortality was separately demonstrated in a study of 102 patients but it included both operated and non-operated patients.[9]

We were the first to report the independent association between cardiopulmonary exercise testing derived variables and perioperative mortality after elective abdominal aortic aneurysm repair in 2012.[10] Unlike all previous studies, our analysis included both open and endovascular aneurysm repair (EVAR) procedures. A total of 415 patients underwent cardiopulmonary exercise testing prior to elective abdominal aortic aneurysm repair in two vascular centres. EVAR was performed in 269 patients (64·8%) and open repair in 146 (35·2%).[10] The 30-day mortality rate for the cohort was 3.4%, with six deaths following EVAR and eight following open repair. The 90-day mortality rate was 4.6% due to five deaths between 30 and 90 days post EVAR. An anaerobic threshold below 10·2 ml.kg-1. min.-1, peak $VO_2$ less than 15ml/kg-1/min/-1, a $VE/VCO_2$ slope above 42 and inducible cardiac ischaemia were associated with both 30- and 90-day mortality on univariable analysis.[9] Preoperative anaemia and juxta/suprarenal abdominal aortic aneurysm were also associated with 90-day mortality. Multivariable logistic regression analysis demonstrated that an anaerobic threshold below 10.2ml/kg-1/min-1, open abdominal aortic aneurysm repair, inducible cardiac ischaemia and preoperative anaemia were independently associated with 30-day mortality. Peak

VO2 less than 15 ml/kg-1/min/-1, inducible cardiac ischaemia and preoperative anaemia were independently associated with 90-day mortality. Patients with at least two cardiopulmonary exercise testing-derived values below the defined abnormal thresholds had a significantly increased risk of both 30- and 90-day mortality.[10]

An updated analysis of this patient group in 2015 was the largest study to date on the relationship between cardiopulmonary exercise testing derived variables and survival after elective abdominal aortic aneurysm repair.[11] This analysis included data from an additional 91 patients with a median follow-up of 26 months and maximum follow-up of 67 months. There were a total of 90 deaths overall. The survival model was stratified on operation type with anaerobic threshold below 10.2ml/kg-1/min-1, peak $VO_2$ less than 15ml/kg-1/min/-1, a $VE/VCO_2$ slope above 42 all significantly associated with reduced mid-term survival on univariabe analysis. In addition to the cardiopulmonary exercise testing derived variables, age, diabetes, preoperative statin therapy, serum creatinine level, elevated serum urea, and haemoglobin level were all found to be associated with mid-term survival. The total number of cardiopulmonary exercise testing variables below the abnormal thresholds for each individual patient was also an important risk factor for reduced survival: patients with zero or one subthreshold cardiopulmonary exercise testing variables achieved a three-year survival of 86.4% compared with 59.9% in patients with three subthreshold cardiopulmonary exercise testing variables (Figure 2). On multivariable analysis, peak $VO_2$ less than 15ml/kg-1/min-1, $VE/VCO_2$ slope above 42, male gender, diabetes, not taking preoperative statins and low haemoglobin were independently associated with reduced mid-term survival. Due to a strong correlation between anaerobic threshold and peak $VO_2$, and because peak $VO_2$ is more likely to be achieved than anaerobic threshold, peak $VO_2$ rather than anaerobic threshold was included in the multivariable analysis.

In 2013, Goodyear et al assessed the impact of introducing a cardiopulmonary exercise testing programme on outcomes after elective abdominal aortic aneurysm repair. They analysed 128 patients over five years prior to the introduction of cardiopulmonary exercise testing and 230 patients over four years following the introduction of the test. Patients were deemed to have passed the test if they achieved an anaerobic threshold of more than 11 ml/kg-1/min/-1. This information was used in clinical decision making and the authors demonstrated that following the introduction of cardiopulmonary exercise testing to assist clinical decision making, the perioperative mortality for patients undergoing open abdominal aortic aneurysm repair was significantly lower (12.6% vs. 4%) and mid-term survival was improved.[12]

## Conclusion

There is consistent evidence that cardiopulmonary exercise testing derived variables are associated with outcomes after elective abdominal aortic aneurysm repair. The 2014 American College of Cardiology/American Heart Association guidelines on perioperative cardiovascular evaluation and management of patients undergoing non-cardiac surgery give cardiopulmonary exercise testing a class IIb (level of evidence B) and recommend that it is considered for patients undergoing high-risk procedures.[13] There are currently no incremental performance studies to determine whether cardiopulmonary exercise testing enhances the value of established risk prediction tools. There is some evidence to suggest that introducing a cardiopulmonary exercise testing programme can have a positive impact on outcomes after elective abdominal aortic aneurysm repair. The increased scrutiny on outcomes after elective abdominal aortic aneurysm repair and introduction of abdominal aortic aneurysm screening programmes focus attention on the role of cardiopulmonary exercise testing and risk-prediction models in the preoperative assessment of patients undergoing elective abdominal aortic aneurysm surgery.

## Summary

- Cardiopulmonary exercise testing is increasingly being used in the preoperative assessment of patients who are being considered for abdominal aortic aneurysm repair.

- Cardiopulmonary exercise testing involves the breath by breath measurement of respiratory oxygen uptake ($VO_2$), carbon dioxide production ($VCO_2$), and ventilation (VE) during exercise and provides a gold standard objective assessment of a patient's functional capacity.

- Peak $VO_2$, $VO_2$ at anaerobic threshold and the relationship between minute ventilation (VE) and $VCO_2$ are the most commonly studied cardiopulmonary exercise testing measures in patients with abdominal aortic aneurysm. Inducible cardiac ischaemia can also be assessed.

- There is consistent evidence that cardiopulmonary exercise testing derived variables are associated with outcomes after elective abdominal aortic aneurysm repair and there is some evidence to suggest that introducing a cardiopulmonary exercise testing programme can have a positive impact on outcomes after elective abdominal aortic aneurysm repair.

## References

1. Huddart S, Young EL, Smith R-L, *et al.* Preoperative cardiopulmonary exercise testing in England – a national survey. *Perioperative Medicine* 2013; **2**: 4.
2. Hennis PJ, Meale PM, Grocott MPW. Cardiopulmonary exercise testing for the evaluation of perioperative risk in non-cardiopulmonary surgery. *Postgraduate Medical Journal* 2011; **87** (1030): 550–57.
3. Moran J, Wilson F, Guinan E, *et al.* Role of cardiopulmonary exercise testing as a risk-assessment method in patients undergoing intra-abdominal surgery: a systematic review. *British Journal of Anaesthesia* 2016; **116** (2): 177–91.
4. Colson M, Baglin J, Bolsin S, Grocott MPW. Cardiopulmonary exercise testing predicts five-year survival after major surgery. *British Journal of Anaesthesia* 2012; **109** (5): 735–41.
5. Balady GJ, Arena R, Sietsema K, *et al.* Clinician's guide to cardiopulmonary exercise testing in adults. A scientific statement from the American Heart Association 2010; **122** (2): 191–225.
6. Grant SW, Hickey GL, Carlson ED, McCollum CN. Comparison of three contemporary risk scores for mortality following elective abdominal aortic aneurysm repair. *European Journal of Vascular and Endovascular Surgery* 2014; **48** (1): 38–44.
7. Nugent AM, Riley M, Megarry J, *et al.* Cardiopulmonary exercise testing in the pre-operative assessment. *Irish Journal of Medical Science* 1998; **167** (4): 238–41.
8. Carlisle J, Swart M. Mid-term survival after abdominal aortic aneurysm surgery predicted by cardiopulmonary exercise testing. *British Journal of Surgery* 2007; **94** (8): 966–69.
9. Thompson A, Peters N, Lovegrove R, *et al.* Cardiopulmonary exercise testing provides a predictive tool for early and late outcomes in abdominal aortic aneurysm patients. *Annals of The Royal College of Surgeons* of England 2011; **93** (6): 474–81.

10. Hartley RA, Pichel AC, Grant SW, *et al.* Preoperative cardiopulmonary exercise testing and risk of early mortality following abdominal aortic aneurysm repair. *British Journal of Surgery* 2012; **99** (11): 1539–46.

11. Grant SW, Hickey GL, Wisely NA, *et al.* Cardiopulmonary exercise testing and survival after elective abdominal aortic aneurysm repair. *British Journal of Anaesthesia* 2015; **114** (3): 430–36.

12. Goodyear SJ, Yow H, Saedon M, *et al.* Risk stratification by pre-operative cardiopulmonary exercise testing improves outcomes following elective abdominal aortic aneurysm surgery: a cohort study. *Perioperative Medicine* 2013; **2**: 10.

13. Fleisher LA, Fleischmann KE, Auerbach AD, *et al.* 2014 ACC/AHA guideline on perioperative cardiovascular evaluation and management of patients undergoing noncardiac surgery. A report of the American College of Cardiology/American Heart Association Task Force on Practice Guidelines *Circulation* 2014; **130** (24): e278–e333.

# The indications for the treatment of iliac aneurysms

## MT Laine, M Venermo and K Mani

## Introduction

Although there is occasional debate about the proper treatment threshold for abdominal aortic aneurysms, the evidence base, although old, supporting current guidelines is robust. However, the evidence base for the treatment threshold of other rarer—but not uncommonly encountered in clinical practice—types of aneurysms is less robust. This chapter aims to look at the evidence for the treatment of aneurysms of the iliac arteries. These aneurysms are the most common type of intra-abdominal aneurysms after abdominal aortic aneurysms, but still they only constitute a minority of intra-abdominal aneurysms.

In 1817, Sir Astley Cooper performed the first (reported) operation for an iliac artery aneurysm. He ligated the aorta of a man with a traumatic aneurysm of the external iliac artery.[1] The patient died 40 hours later—as was usually the case after ligating the aorta. Cooper said later, in his lectures, that he knew for "his own part" he would not hesitate to have his own aorta ligated "if it would save my life for only forty hours".[2] The first report of a common iliac artery aneurysm was by Valentine Mott, who described a successful ligation of the common iliac artery in 1827.[3] Since then, only sporadic reports of individual cases or small patient series have been reported.

## Definition

The Ad Hoc Committee on Reporting Standards of the Society for Vascular Surgery defined aneurysm as a focal dilatation of over 50% in diameter compared with the normal diameter of the corresponding artery based on measurements on healthy individuals.[4] Based on these data, the intervention thresholds for aneurysms in the common iliac artery are 1.8cm for men and 1.5cm for women, and are 0.8cm for internal iliac aneurysms in both sexes. The definitions used in the literature are varied and range from 1.5 to 2.5cm but do not usually differ between iliac vessels.

## Natural history

Richardson and Greenfield reported in 1988 that 3% of all atherosclerotic, non-cranial aneurysms were iliac artery aneurysms and 2.2% of all intra-abdominal were this type of aneurysm.[5] These numbers were derived from clinical practice before there was widespread use of imaging studies. In an autopsy study of 26,251 patients, 0.03% were found to have an isolated iliac artery aneurysm (seven in total, five common, one external and one internal) and 0.6% had an aortoiliac aneurysm compared with 3.2% who had an abdominal aortic aneurysm.[6] Overall, in this study, iliac aneurysms constituted almost 20% of all intra-abdominal aneurysms. The common iliac artery is the most frequent location of an iliac aneurysm and aortic aneurysm also often involve this vessel. The internal iliac artery, which is also known as the hypogastric artery, is the second most common location; isolated aneurysms, however, are most commonly found in this artery. Aneurysms rarely occur in the external iliac artery, which is likely due to embryological reasons because this artery develops from a different cell population than the common and internal iliac arteries. In a report from the Mayo Clinic, 86% of 438 patients with an aneurysm in the common iliac artery had a concomitant abdominal aortic aneurysm, 65% also had a contralateral common iliac artery aneurysm, 29% had an aneurysm of the internal iliac artery as well and only 3% had an aneurysm of the external iliac artery.[7] In a multicentre study of ruptured internal iliac aneurysms, 43% had a bilateral internal iliac aneurysm, 65% had a concurrent common iliac artery aneurysm, and 42% had a concurrent abdominal aortic aneurysm. Also, 37% had both common iliac and abdominal aortic aneurysms in addition to the ruptured internal iliac aneurysm.[8]

Reports on expansion rates of iliac aneurysm are varying. Santilli *et al* reported an expansion rate of 0.05—0.15cm/year for aneurysms <3cm and 0.25–0.28cm/year for those >3cm. Although 37.5% of aneurysms did not show any growth during follow-up (mean 31.4 months), all aneurysms between 4cm and 4.9cm did expand. Those that were over 5cm were urgently repaired.[9] Huang *et al* reported median expansion rate of 0.29cm/year with higher rates in patients with hypertension.[7]

The reported average diameter of ruptured iliac aneurysms is relatively large: mean diameter of 7.8cm reported by McCready and 7.5cm by Lowry and Kraft; Richardson and Greenfield described diameters ranging from 3.5cm to 18cm.[5,10,11] Aneurysms included in these studies were mostly common iliac artery aneurysms. Huang reported that the median diameter of ruptured common iliac aneurysm as 6cm (Figure 1); Laine *et al* reported mean diameter of ruptured internal iliac artery aneurysm as 6.8cm (Figure 2).[7, 8] In a review by Wilhelm *et al* of isolated internal iliac artery aneurysms, the mean diameter of ruptured aneurysm was 8.3cm and 7.6 for symptomatic aneurysms.[12]

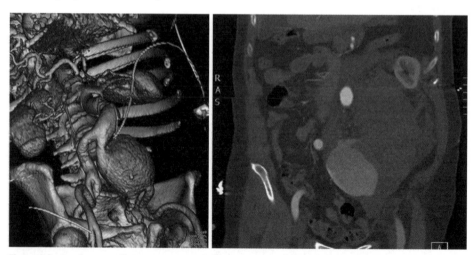

**Figure 1:** Ruptured common iliac artery aneurysm in 3D reconstruction (left) and 2D CT-image (right).

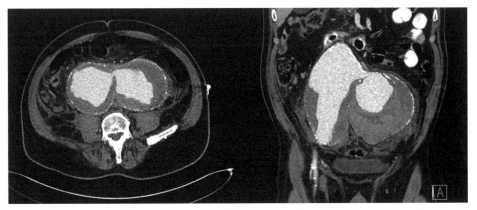

**Figure 2:** Bilateral aneurysms of common iliac artery, which was treated with open surgery due to rupture in the left common iliac artery; 12cm in maximum diameter.

## Indications for repair

The most commonly referenced indication for repair is a diameter of >3cm, which was first proposed by McCready *et al* in 1983.[10] Santilli *et al* proposed in 2000 that common iliac artery aneurysms larger than 3.5–4cm should be repaired.[9] Furthermore, Laine *et al* suggested that follow-up, without intervention, should be used for internal iliac artery aneurysms until they had a diameter of 4cm.[8] With symptomatic aneurysms, repair should be performed at a smaller diameter.

Iliac aneurysms can be symptomatic and in addition to pain, may cause symptoms due to compression of pelvic organs. Krupski *et al* reported 21 patients with symptoms in 57%, most commonly abdominal pain but also neurological symptoms, claudication and urinary symptoms.[13] Huang *et al* reported 29% of patients being symptomatic, most commonly abdominal pain. They also reported two patients with acute deep vein thrombosis and three arteriovenous fistulas out of the total 438 patients.[7] Santilli *et al* reported symptoms only in aneurysms >4cm in diameter.[9] Out of 55 patients, in a study by Richardson and Greenfield, 45% were asymptomatic—33% with acute pain reflecting rupture or expansion and 9% with chronic pain attributed to compression of nerve roots or abdominal viscera. Richard *et al* also reported that two patients with arteriovenous fistulas and these patients had dyspnoea and fatigue. Urological symptoms such as flank pain, urgency or frequency was reported in 7%.[5]

## Choice of repair

The historical choice for treating iliac artery aneurysms was ligation, but since development of vascular prosthesis, endoaneurysmorrhaphy and reconstruction have become first-line options. In the case of internal iliac artery, ligation is often still the only option. Just as EVAR has become the primary treatment method for abdominal aortic aneurysms, it has become the first-line option for iliac aneurysms. There are particular challenges to treating iliac artery aneurysms and aortoiliac aneurysms. Occluding the internal iliac artery is often done when there is an aneurysmatic common iliac artery to get a good landing zone in the external iliac artery (Figure 3). When there is a slightly aneurysmatic common iliac artery and a concomitant abdominal aortic aneurysm, a large diameter limb can be used to

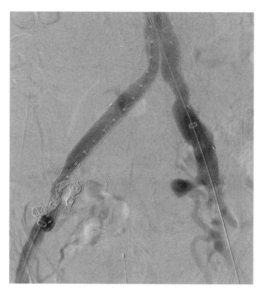

**Figure 3:** Aneurysm of the right common iliac artery has been treated with coil embolisation of the internal iliac artery and extending the stent graft down to external iliac artery. In the left side ectatic common iliac artery aneurysm has been treated with "bell-bottom" technique.

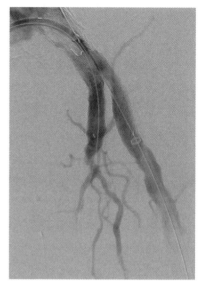

**Figure 4:** Use of Iliac branched stent graft preserves the internal iliac artery and thus the possible complications related to this are avoided.

achieve adequate sealing zone (Figure 3). This "bell-bottom" technique, however, has the downside of leaving the iliac aneurysm untreated, leading to continuing dilatation of the common iliac and a high risk for development of distal type I endoleak as well as rupture of the iliac aneurysm. Currently there are dedicated stent grafts for the treatment of common iliac aneurysm without compromising the internal iliac artery flow (Figure 4). These iliac branched stent grafts are available from three manufacturers: Zenith (Cook), Excluder (Gore) and E-iliac (Jotec).[14–16] Techniques using parallel grafts, chimneys and snorkels have also been described to achieve preservation of internal iliac flow.[17] EndoVascular Aneurysm Sealing (EVAS) with the Nellix (Endologix) device has also been used in treating iliac aneurysms.[18]

## Complications

Preservation of at least one internal iliac artery is preferable as its occlusion can lead to complications ranging from buttock claudication to ischaemia of the bowel or the spinal cord. Although extremely rare, there may be also fatal complications after occlusion of internal ilica artery, as reported by Jean-Baptiste *et al.* Buttock claudication was seen in 25.3% of patients 30 days after discharge. Those patients that had distal internal iliac artery occluded as well, due to an aneurysm, had a higher incidence of buttock claudication (43%). Claudication persisted at 18 months in 85%.[19] Chitragari *et al* reported buttock claudication in 21.2%, buttock necrosis in 5%, erectile dysfunction in 2.7%, colonic ischaemia in 7% and spinal cord ischaemia in 9% of vascular surgery patients with ligation or embolisation of internal iliac artery. Embolisation, especially distal embolisation, of the internal iliac artery was associated with more complications than proximal ligation.[20]

## Results of repair

Wilhelm *et al* reported in their largely historic review that the mortality after repair of ruptured internal iliac artery was 52.9%, after repair of symptomatic aneurysm 10.3% and 0% after asymptomatic repair.[12] Laine *et al* reported 30-day mortality of 12.7% after repair of ruptured internal iliac artery aneurysm, including both open (73%) and endovascular repair (27%). The five-year survival, however, was only 50.6%, the causes of death mainly being unrelated to the aneurysm.[8] Richardson and Greenfield reported operative mortality of 30%.[5] Huang *et al* reported 30-day mortality of 3%, 1% after elective repair and 27% after emergency repair; 10% were treated with EVAR. Clinically significant ischaemic colitis was seen in four patients and spinal cord ischaemia in two patients out of all 438 patients. Primary and secondary patency were 99.4% and 100%, respectively, without difference between open and endovascular repair. Hospital length of stay was significantly shorter in EVAR patients. Endoleak was seen in 31% of stent graft patients at discharge and in 20% at the last available imaging study (median follow-up 1.6 years). Incidence of buttock claudication was 5% after open repair and 34% after EVAR; although in open cases where internal iliac artery was ligated, incidence was 27%. Most patients reported improvement of symptoms during follow-up.[7]

Jongsma *et al* reported a 9.3% occlusion rate for the internal iliac branch during follow-up (mean using the Zenith Iliac branched stent graft device). Six of these 13 patients developed buttock claudication and 12.1% of patients required secondary interventions. Mortality was 1.4% and major complications were seen in 4.3%.[14] van Sterkenburg *et al* reported results for the Gore Excluder device. Their six-month primary patency of the internal iliac component as 94%. Reinterventions were required in 7.1% of patients.[17] The E-iliac device results were reported by Mylonas *et al.* At one year, survival was 98.5% with all internal iliac limbs open, although two common iliac and one external iliac occlusions occurred.[16] Krievins reported results for the Nellix system in treating common iliac artery aneurysms. The proposed advantage of the system is that it does not need a heathy landing zone in the common iliac artery. The internal iliac artery remained patent in 98% during the five-year follow up. It had to be occluded in three patients to extend the sealing zone into the external iliac artery. In cases in which the common iliac artery could only partially be excluded, they found that the annual growth rate of the aneurysm was actually higher (0.56mm/year) than when common iliac artery aneurysm was left untreated (0.16mm/year). The completely excluded aneurysm did not expand.[18]

## Conclusion

Definition of iliac artery aneurysm is varied in the literature as is the proposed repair threshold. There is also not much differentiation between the different iliac vessels, although aneurysms of the internal and common iliac artery are likely to differ somewhat from one another. In the case of asymptomatic aneurysms, follow-up until the diameter of 3.5–4cm seems warranted. Historically, results of rupture of iliac artery aneurysm and of surgical treatment have been poor but more recent data show results comparable or even better than those for abdominal aortic repair. The modern endovascular methods like iliac branched stent grafts are promising in treating common iliac artery aneurysms and enable the preservation This is preferable to occluding it as this can lead to significant complications in some cases, especially when both internal iliac arteries are occluded. In the case of internal iliac artery aneurysm, the preservation on flow in the vessel is usually impossible.

## Summary

- Iliac artery aneurysms are often found in patients with abdominal aortic aneurysms.

- Aneurysm most often involves the common iliac artery, sometimes the internal iliac artery and very rarely the external iliac artery.

- Iliac artery aneurysm repair is indicated in aneurysms with a diameter >3.5–4.0cm and in symptomatic aneurysms.

- Iliac artery aneurysms can be treated by endovascular repair with good results.

- Occluding internal iliac arteries may occasionally lead to serious complication.

- Iliac branched devices show promising results in preserving internal iliac artery patency.

- Treatment of internal iliac aneurysm requires the occlusion of the distal branches of the aneurysm, causing symptoms to many patients.

## References

1. Thompson JE. Early history of aortic surgery. *J Vasc Surg* 1998; **28** (4): 746–52.
2. Cooper AP. Lectures on the principles and practice of surgery (2nd edn). F.C. Westley: London, 1830.
3. Mott V. Successful ligation of the common iliac artery. *Am J Med Sci* 1827; **1**: 156–61.
4. Johnston KW, Rutherford RB, Tilson MD, *et al*. Suggested standards for reporting on arterial aneurysms. subcommittee on reporting standards for arterial aneurysms, ad hoc committee on reporting standards, Society for Vascular Surgery and North American Chapter, International Society for Cardiovascular Surgery. *J Vasc Surg* 1991; **13** (3): 452–58.
5. Richardson JW, Greenfield LJ. Natural history and management of iliac aneurysms. *Journal of Vascular Surgery* 1988; **8** (2): 165–71.
6. Brunkwall J, Hauksson H, Bengtsson H, *et al*. Solitary aneurysms of the iliac arterial system: an estimate of their frequency of occurrence. *J Vasc Surg* 1989; **10** (4): 381–84.
7. Huang Y, Gloviczki P, Duncan AA, *et al*. Common iliac artery aneurysm: expansion rate and results of open surgical and endovascular repair. *J Vasc Surg* 2008; **47** (6): 1203–10.
8. Laine MT, Bjorck M, Beiles CB, *et al*. Few internal iliac artery aneurysms rupture under 4cm. *J Vasc Surg* 2017; **65** (1): 76–81.
9. Santilli SM, Wernsing SE, Lee ES. Expansion rates and outcomes for iliac artery aneurysms. *J Vasc Surg* 2000; **31**(1 Pt 1): 114–21.
10. McCready RA, Pairolero PC, Gilmore JC, *et al*. Isolated iliac artery aneurysms. Surgery 1983; **93** (5): 688–93.
11. Lowry SF, Kraft RO. Isolated aneurysms of the iliac artery. Arch Surg 1978; **113** (11): 1289–93.
12. Wilhelm BJ, Sakharpe A, Ibrahim G, *et al*. The 100-year evolution of the isolated internal iliac artery aneurysm. *Annals of Vascular Surgery* 2014; **28** (4): 1070–77.
13. Krupski WC, Selzman CH, Floridia R, *et al*. Contemporary management of isolated iliac aneurysms. *J Vasc Surg* 1998; **28** (1): 1–11.
14. Jongsma H, Bekken JA, Bekkers WJ, *et al*. Endovascular treatment of common iliac artery aneurysms with an iliac branch device: Multicenter experience of 140 patients. *J Endovasc Ther* 2016. Epub.
15. Mylonas SN, Rumenapf G, Schelzig H, *et al*. A multicenter 12-month experience with a new iliac side-branched device for revascularization of hypogastric arteries. *J Vasc Surg* 2016; **64** (6): 1652—59.
16. van Sterkenburg SM, Heyligers JM, van Bladel M, *et al*. Experience with the GORE EXCLUDER iliac branch endoprosthesis for common iliac artery aneurysms. *J Vasc Surg* 2016; **63** (6): 1451–57.

17. Lobato AC, Camacho-Lobato L. The sandwich technique to treat complex aortoiliac or isolated iliac aneurysms: results of midterm follow-up. *J Vasc Surg* 2013; **57** (2 Suppl): 26S–34S.
18. Krievins DK, Savlovskis J, Holden AH, *et al.* Preservation of hypogastric flow and control of iliac aneurysm size in the treatment of aortoiliac aneurysms using the Nellix EndoVascular Aneurysm Sealing endograft. *J Vasc Surg* 2016; **64** (5): 1262–69.
19. Jean-Baptiste E, Brizzi S, Bartoli MA, *et al.* Pelvic ischemia and quality of life scores after interventional occlusion of the hypogastric artery in patients undergoing endovascular aortic aneurysm repair. *J Vasc Surg* 2014; **60** (1): 40–49.
20. Chitragari G, Schlosser FJ, Ochoa Chaar CI, Sumpio BE. Consequences of hypogastric artery ligation, embolization, or coverage. *J Vasc Surg* 2015; **62** (5): 134–47.

# Abdominal compartment syndrome after abdominal aortic surgery

S Ersryd, K Djavani-Gidlund, A Wanhainen
and M Björck

## Introduction

Abdominal compartment syndrome represents a serious and potentially lethal complication after surgery for abdominal aortic aneurysm.[1] The mortality remains high; without treatment, it is nearly 100% and in the range of 30–70% with treatment.[2–4] The risk of developing abdominal compartment syndrome after both intact and ruptured abdominal aortic aneurysm depends on case mix, the proportion of patients treated prophylactically with open abdomen, and the routines for resuscitation.[5] Although abdominal compartment syndrome is more common after repair of ruptured abdominal aortic aneurysms, affecting 8–20% of the patients,[2, 6] it may also occur after intact abdominal aortic aneurysm repair. The incidence of abdominal compartment syndrome requiring surgical treatment after intact abdominal aortic aneurysm repair is historically low, however, with figures below 1%.[4] In 2004, an international society focused on abdominal compartment syndrome was formed—the World Congress of the Abdominal Compartment Society (WACS). The society published consensus documents on abdominal compartment syndrome in 2006 and 2007 and updated these documents in 2013.[7] The current consensus document used the GRADE technology for a systematic review of current knowledge, and included definitions, consensus statements and a proposed treatment algorithm.[7] In the consensus documents, several medical treatment options to reduce the intra-abdominal hypertension, and prevent abdominal compartment syndrome, are described in detail. Medical treatment may serve as initial and sometimes sufficient treatment. In many cases, however, the treatment of abdominal compartment syndrome will ultimately require surgery through a decompressive laparotomy.[8] The procedure includes leaving the patient with an open abdomen.[9] The open abdomen is preferentially managed with negative pressure wound therapy.[7] Treatment with open abdomen is rather resource intensive and is by itself a cause of morbidity.[7,10] The focus in recent years has, therefore, been on the prevention and early recognition of abdominal compartment syndrome. As a testimony to this, repeated intra-abdominal pressure measurements in the critically ill are now an established routine in many intensive care units.[7]

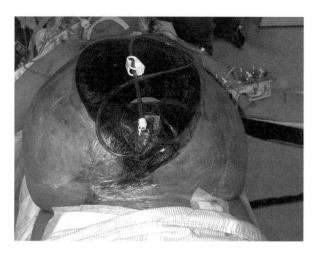

**Figure 1:** A patient treated with open abdomen after a ruptured abdominal aortic aneurysm, using the vacuum-assisted wound closure and mesh-mediated fascial traction method.[12] The patient's abdomen underwent primary delayed fascial closure after four weeks.

## Contemporary data from the Swedish vascular registry, Swedvasc

In Sweden, all vascular repairs are reported to the nationwide vascular registry, Swedvasc. In a recent international validation, the external validity of abdominal aortic aneurysm surgery in Sweden was 100% (no missing cases).[11] Since May 2008, data for abdominal compartment syndrome and decompressive laparotomy have been entered prospectively into the registry, making it possible to identify and further study these complications in a population-based setting. In the studied time-period, May 2008–December 2013, all entries in the aortic module containing infra- and juxta-renal abdominal aortic aneurysm repairs were examined and 6,634 patients were subsequently included.[8] They had a mean age of 72.8 years and 16.6% were women. There were 5,271 repairs for intact abdominal aortic aneurysm, equaling 79.6% of the total, and 1,341 repairs for rupture (20.4%). The proportion of endovascular aneurysm repair (EVAR) procedures among intact aneurysms was 62% and was 28% among ruptured aneurysms.

In the intact aneurysm group, 1.6% and 0.5%, respectively, developed abdominal compartment syndrome after open repair and after EVAR. Among the patients

## Definitions

**Intra-abdominal pressure:** The steady-state pressure concealed within the abdominal cavity.

**Intra-abdominal hypertension:** A sustained or repeated pathological elevation in intra-abdominal pressure ≥12mmHg. Graded as follows:

- Grade I, IAP 12–15mmHg
- Grade II, IAP 16–20mmHg
- Grade III, IAP 21–25mmHg
- Grade IV, IAP >25mmHg.

**Abdominal compartment syndrome:** Sustained intra-abdominal pressure >20mmHg that is associated with new organ dysfunction or failure.

who developed abdominal compartment syndrome, 68.6% were treated with decompressive laparotomy after open repair and 25% after EVAR. In the ruptured abdominal aortic aneurysm group, 6.8% developed abdominal compartment syndrome after open repair and 6.9% after EVAR. Among those who developed abdominal compartment syndrome, 77.3% and 84.6%, respectively, underwent decompressive laparotomy when the primary treatment was open repair or when it was EVAR.

In a separate validation of 300 patients treated with open repair for ruptured abdominal aortic aneurysm, the abdomen was left open prophylactically in 10.7% (95% [confidence interval; CI] 7.2–14.3). In summation, approximately 15% of the patients treated with open repair for ruptured abdominal aortic aneurysm received open abdomen treatment.

## Outcome

After ruptured abdominal aortic aneurysm repair, patients with abdominal compartment syndrome had a mortality rate of 42.4% at 30 days, rising to 60.7% at one year. These rates were significantly worse, and almost doubled, than those for patients with ruptured aneurysms who did not develop abdominal compartment syndrome after repair; the mortality rates for these patients were 23.5% at 30 days and 31.8% at one year. The mortality rates did not differ between open repair and EVAR in the patients treated for rupture.

An even greater increase was seen after intact abdominal aortic aneurysm repair. Patients with abdominal compartment syndrome had a 30-day mortality rate of 11.5%, rising to 27.5% at one year. The corresponding mortality rates for patients

## Medical treatment options

### Improve abdominal wall compliance

- Optimal pain and anxiety relief (consider epidural anaesthesia)
- Neuromuscular blockade (48 hours is safe)

### Evacuation of intraluminal contents

- Nasogastric and/or rectal tube.

### Evacuation of intra-abdominal content (seldom possible after aortic surgery)

- Percutaneous drainage.

### Optimise fluid administration

- Avoid positive cumulative fluid balance
- Enhanced ratio of plasma/packed red cells during resuscitation of massive haemorrhage
- Consider slow albumin infusion together with furosemide or RRT.

### Optimise systemic/regional perfusion

- Goal-directed resuscitation.

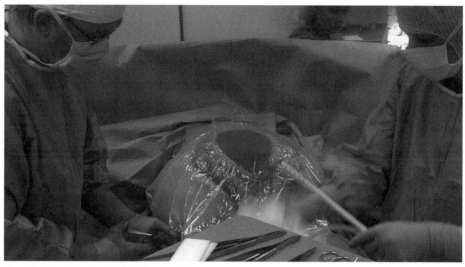

**Figure 2:** Redressing the patient with open abdomen.

with intact abdominal aortic aneurysm repair who did not develop abdominal compartment syndrome were 1.8% at 30 days and 6.3% at one year. Likewise, no difference in mortality between primary open repair and EVAR was found among those treated for intact abdominal aortic aneurysm.

In accordance with the findings on mortality rates, the rates of renal failure, multiorgan failure, intestinal ischaemia, intensive care unit treatment more than five days, were all significantly higher in patients with abdominal compartment syndrome.

## Conclusion

In this first ever and large population-based study, abdominal compartment syndrome and treatment with open abdomen were common after ruptured abdominal aortic aneurysm repair. The outcome associated with abdominal compartment syndrome after both ruptured abdominal aortic aneurysm and intact abdominal aortic aneurysm repair was devastating; with no differences in neither incidence nor outcome depending on if the primary treatment was open or endovascular.

## Summary

- In the first large population-based study on abdominal compartment syndrome after abdominal aortic aneurysm surgery (6,634 patients), the risk was similar if the primary treatment was open or endovascular.

- Open abdomen treatment was more common after open repair of a ruptured abdominal aortic aneurysm; however, since one in 10 had their abdomen left open at the end of the primary operation.

- The risk was much higher after repair of a ruptured abdominal aortic aneurysm, which was expected, but the consequences in terms of increased risks of complications and death were more severe in those operated on for an intact aneurysm.

## References

1. Kron IL, Harman PK, Nolan SP. The measurement of intra-abdominal pressure as a criterion for abdominal re-exploration. *Annals of Surgery* 1984; **199** (1): 28–30.
2. Mayer D, Rancic Z, Meier C, *et al*. Open abdomen treatment following endovascular repair of ruptured abdominal aortic aneurysms. *Journal of Vascular Surgery* 2009; **50** (1) :1–7.
3. Rasmussen TE, Hallett JW Jr, Noel AA, *et al*. Early abdominal closure with mesh reduces multiple organ failure after ruptured abdominal aortic aneurysm repair: guidelines from a 10-year case-control study. *Journal of Vascular Surgery* 2002; **35** (2): 246–53.
4. Sorelius K, Wanhainen A, Acosta S, *et al*. Open abdomen treatment after aortic aneurysm repair with vacuum-assisted wound closure and mesh-mediated fascial traction. *European Journal of Vascular and Endovascular Surgery* 2013; **45** (6): 588–94.
5. Balogh ZJ, Lumsdaine W, Moore EE, Moore FA. Postinjury abdominal compartment syndrome: from recognition to prevention. *Lancet* 2014; **384** (9952): 1466–75.
6. Karkos CD, Menexes GC, Patelis N, *et al*. A systematic review and meta-analysis of abdominal compartment syndrome after endovascular repair of ruptured abdominal aortic aneurysms. *Journal of Vascular Surgery* 2014; **59** (3): 829–42.
7. Kirkpatrick AW, Roberts DJ, De Waele J, *et al*. Intra-abdominal hypertension and the abdominal compartment syndrome: updated consensus definitions and clinical practice guidelines from the World Society of the Abdominal Compartment Syndrome. *Intensive Care Medicine* 2013; **39** (7): 1190–206.
8. Ersryd S, Djavani-Gidlund K, Wanhainen A, Bjorck M. Editor's Choice - Abdominal compartment syndrome after surgery for abdominal aortic aneurysm: A nationwide population-based study. *European Journal of Vascular and Endovascular Surgery* 2016; **52** (2): 158–65.
9. Bjorck M. Management of the tense abdomen or difficult abdominal closure after operation for ruptured abdominal aortic aneurysms. *Seminars in Vascular Surgery* 2012; **25** (1): 35–38.
10. Bjorck M, D'Amours SK, Hamilton AE. Closure of the open abdomen. *The American Surgeon* 2011; **77** Suppl 1: S58–61.
11. Venermo M, Lees T. International Vascunet validation of the Swedvasc registry. *Eur J Vasc Endovasc Surg* 2015; **50** (6): 802–08.
12. Petersson U, Acosta S. Björck M. Vacuum-assisted wound closure and mesh-mediated fascial traction – a novel technique for closure of the open abdomen. *World J Surg* 2007; **31**: 2133–37.

# The consequences of performing fewer open abdominal aortic aneurysm repairs

J Budtz-Lilly, M Venermo and K Mani

## Introduction

Several studies indicate that the prevalence of abdominal aortic aneurysms has decreased over the past decades.[1–3] Despite this, the number of aneurysm repairs is still significant, because of increased opportunistic and screening-related detection of disease as well as increased possibilities to surgically treat elderly comorbid patients who were previously not regarded as candidates for repair.[4] Furthermore, the introduction of endovascular aneurysm repair (EVAR) has dramatically transformed the treatment of aneurysms. The number of EVAR procedures has increased steadily since its introduction in the previous millennium. Data from the Vascunet registry, an international collaboration of vascular surgical registries from 11 countries, demonstrates this trend in Figure 1. These data show that, overall, the percentage of EVAR procedures for intact aneurysms has increased by almost 150% from 2005 to 2013. Endovascular repair is now the preferred treatment modality in most countries.[5] In the USA and in Australia, more than 70% of all intact repairs are performed with EVAR—making open repair a marginalised technique.

The major limitation for EVAR application is aneurysm morphology. However, increasing technical advancements are enabling the treatment of complex iliac involvement and juxtarenal and thoracoabdominal aneurysms.[6–9] Nonetheless, the concern for treatment failure is not unwarranted, as it is well documented that performing EVAR outside device instructions for use leads to increased failures and complications.[10] Additionally, the recent publication of the long-term results of the EVAR-1 trial indicate that the risk of EVAR failure—with catastrophic outcome—continues in the long term.[11]

The increasing use of EVAR has important considerations for open repair. Two questions arise: first, can high-quality training be maintained if fewer, but more technically challenging, open repair cases are being performed? Second, can high-quality surgical outcomes be maintained if experience to open repair (because it is no longer a routine procedure) decreases and the complexity of these procedures increases? The evidence that addresses these questions is of obvious interest, but perhaps the critical aspect lies in how we adjust or deal with the consequences of these considerations.

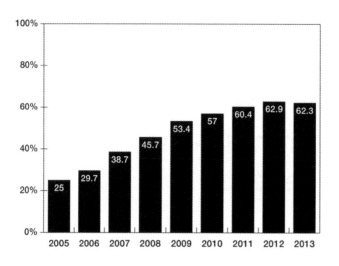

**Figure 1:** The percentage of intact aneurysms treated with EVAR from 2005 to 2013 (for 11 countries from the Vascunet registry).

## Training in open surgery

Worldwide, the demand for vascular surgeons is generally still high. However, the number of aneurysms requiring treatment does not appear to be increasing and, as mentioned, there is quite a clear trend towards EVAR being offered to the majority of patients. The equation is thus simple: there are fewer open procedures assigned to an increasing number of vascular surgery trainees, who may not work at academic or high-volume surgical centres. Data from the USA show that even between 1999 and 2008, the average number of open repairs dropped by 50%.[12] According to one prediction model, a vascular surgeon fellow may be exposed to no more than three open procedures per year by 2020.[13]

The concern about the point at which too few open repair procedures, for fellows to achieve sufficient experience, will be performed is difficult to address. Landry and colleagues suggest that suitable experience will be lacking for operating the complex aneurysm cases and that "regionalisation" of these repairs may be necessary.[14] Although the majority of trainee-specific data come from the USA, similar concerns of reduced open repair are observed in other countries.[15] Data from Australia and New Zealand are somewhat reassuring, however, as they demonstrate that, despite diminishing open repairs, there is no significant worsening of outcomes among those patients treated by surgeons trained in the endovascular era.[16]

A thought-provoking consideration to this discussion is the observation made by McPhee and colleagues regarding procedure volumes. They found that a high surgeon volume was associated with a greater mortality reduction than a high institution volume.[17]

## Outcomes following open repair in the endovascular era

The evolution of EVAR from a so-called "failed experiment" to the preferred aneurysm treatment in many countries in less than a decade has been dramatic.[18] The EVAR-1 and EVAR-2 trials have led to many interpretations.[11,19] In particular, the reduced short-term mortality, despite the cost of increased reinterventions, has an appeal for both patients and surgeons alike. Open repair is now typically reserved for those patients with anatomical constraints (for EVAR), but other considerations such as age, comorbidities, and patient preference may also play a role.

It is fair to state that the growth of EVAR has led to more complicated open repair. Ballotta and colleagues noted more frequent suprarenal aortic cross-clamping, left renal vein division, and longer operating times.[20] Landry *et al* also found increased use of suprarenal cross-clamping and operative time and greater blood loss.[14] Additionally, the incidence of coexisting iliac aneurysmal and occlusive disease is greater among those patients now offered open repair than it was in the past. Open repair patients, in current practice, are older than in previous years—although this trend is seen with EVAR patients as well. It is important to recognise that a significant number of patients are offered open repair because of failed or even infected EVAR grafts, which invariably increases the level of technical complexity.[21]

There are several studies comparing outcomes before and after the implementation of EVAR treatment. Hiromatsu *et al* reported an impressive perioperative mortality of 0% both before and after the introduction of EVAR in their department.[22] The study by Landry *et al* found that the increased need for suprarenal cross-clamping in the more complex open repairs did not lead to significant differences in perioperative mortality, but there was an increase in the occurrence of renal and pulmonary complications.[14] An earlier study, a nationwide analysis by Giles and colleagues, showed unchanged perioperative mortality after the introduction of EVAR.[6]

There is an inherent risk of type II errors in these analyses, but there are other factors that may play a role in maintaining acceptable outcomes. Quality initiative programmes, such as one implemented in the UK in 2008, raise the focus on the quality of care in these patients that cannot be neglected.[23] Muehling *et al* have reported on the results of a fast-track optimal care protocol, which reduced the number of postoperative complications.[24]

It is, therefore, incumbent upon us to follow and update the outcomes of aneurysm treatment and, hence, appreciate the value of large vascular surgery registries. The

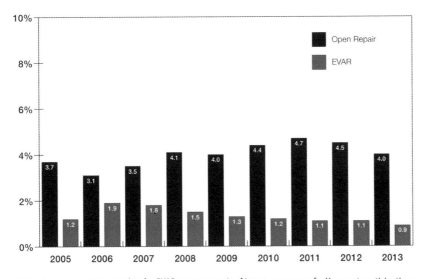

**Figure 2:** Crude perioperative mortality for EVAR or open repair of intact aneurysms for Vascunet participating countries from 2005 to 2013.

above-mentioned Vascunet collaboration collates data from multinational registries and provides benchmarks for standard levels of care. The most recent report includes outcomes from more than 80,000 operations, of which about 37,000 were treated with open repair. Overall, it appears that the perioperative mortality is declining, but this is driven by the two-fold consequence of first, an increasing number of EVAR procedures and, second, a decreasing perioperative mortality of EVAR. As evident in Figure 2, the crude perioperative mortality for open repair has increased over the past years and is mirrored by a decrease in the perioperative mortality for EVAR. After adjusting for age and gender, the perioperative mortality odds ratio for open repair for 2010–13, as compared to 2005–09, was 1.17 (95% confidence interval, 1.03-1.30).

This is the first time a significant increase in short-term mortality after repair has been witnessed in recent years. Previous national analyses of open repair have indicated continued improvement in perioperative outcome, because of improved perioperative care.[4]

## Controversies and solutions

Despite the rapid increase in the use of EVAR for elective repair, one cannot help but notice the much slower increase in the use of EVAR for ruptured aneurysms. The report by Sachs *et al* found that EVAR was used for 78% of the elective aneurysms for Medicare beneficiaries in 2008, whereas for only 31% of the ruptured aneurysms.[12] This is similar to data from the Vascunet participating countries: 60.3% for intact aneurysms and only 23.1% for ruptured aneurysms.

There are many explanations for this difference, including technical constraints and issues of graft availability. One must also speculate, however, as to whether these patients were admitted to centres where open repair was the preferred method of acute treatment. Regardless of the explanations, if the door to open repair is closing, the gap between the number of standard EVAR procedures and those of EVAR for ruptured aneurysms must also close. This may require severe structural, financial, and political decisions.

One of the additional important findings from the Vascunet open repair data was the difference in mortality between high- and low-volume centres. In the international analysis, the mortality after open repair increased over time in low-volume centres while it was stable in high-volume centres. The volume-outcome relationship in complex vascular surgical procedures is well established.[25]

In light of the worsening outcomes for open repair given here, particularly among low-volume centres, it is time to more aggressively consider structural changes in the delivery of open vascular surgery. The establishment of high open-surgical-volume centres could also avail themselves to those trainees who desire exposure to these procedures. Again, this may require difficult decisions in care delivery.

## Conclusion

The increase in EVAR treatment of aneurysms has been dramatic, and there are few signs to suggest a reversal in the near future. Open repair is generally reserved for more complex anatomy, but even here, advancing EVAR technology is making inroads. Moreover, it now appears that perioperative mortality is worsening for patients undergoing open repair, particularly in centres with low volumes. On the other hand, most ruptured aneurysms are still treated with open repair, so clearly the door for open repair is not entirely closed. It may be that technical and anatomical constraints continue to support the need for open repair, but its future will also be impacted by political and administrative decisions—especially in the implementation of centres of high volume.

## Summary

- EVAR has rapidly overtaken open repair and comprises approximately two thirds of procedures for treatment of intact aneurysms.

- Training in aortic open repair is falling dramatically.

- Perioperative mortality following open intact aneurysm repair now appears to be worsening, despite various efforts for improved quality care.

- Open repair still dominates treatment for ruptured aneurysms, presumably due to multiple factor—not least of which include issues of access and the delivery of acute vascular care.

- Establishment of high-volume centres may improve both the teaching and outcomes of open aortic repair.

# References

1. Anjum A, Powell JT. Is the incidence of abdominal aortic aneurysm declining in the 21st century? Mortality and hospital admissions for England & Wales and Scotland. *Eur J Vasc Endovasc Surg* 2012; **43**: 161–66.

2. Björck M, Bown MJ, Choke E, *et al.* International update on screening for abdominal aortic aneurysms: issues and opportunities. *Eur J Vasc Endovasc Surg* 2015; **49**: 113–15.

3. Jacomelli J, Summers L, Stevenson A, *et al.* Impact of the first 5 years of a national abdominal aortic aneurysm screening programme. *Br J Surg* 2016; **103**: 1125–31.

4. Mani K, Björck M, Wanhainen A. Changes in the management of infrarenal abdominal aortic aneurysm disease in Sweden. *Br J Surg* 2013; **100**: 638–44.

5. Beck AW, Sedrakyan A, Mao J, *et al.* Variations in Abdominal Aortic Aneurysm Care: A Report from the International Consortium of Vascular Registries. *Circulation* 2016; **134** (24):1948–58.

6. Giles KA, Pomposelli F, Hamdan A, *et al.* Decrease in total aneurysm-related deaths in the era of endovascular aneurysm repair. *J Vasc Surg* 2009; **49**: 543–50.

7. Wolf YG, Fogarty TJ, Olcott IV C, *et al.* Endovascular repair of abdominal aortic aneurysms: Eligibility rate and impact on the rate of open repair. *J Vasc Surg* 2000; **32**: 519–23.

8. Greenberg RK, Lu Q, Roselli EE, *et al.* Contemporary analysis of descending thoracic and thoracoabdominal aneurysm repair a comparison of endovascular and open techniques. *Circulation* 2008; **118**: 808–17.

9. Bicknell CD, Cheshire NJW, Riga C V, *et al.* Treatment of complex aneurysmal disease with fenestrated and branched stent grafts. *Eur J Vasc Endovasc Surg* 2009; **37**: 175–81.

10. Schanzer A, Greenberg RK, Hevelone N, *et al.* Predictors of abdominal aortic aneurysm sac enlargement after endovascular repair. *Circulation* 2011; **123**: 2848–55.

11. Patel R, Sweeting MJ, Powell JT, Greenhalgh RM. Endovascular *versus* open repair of abdominal aortic aneurysm in 15-years' follow-up of the UK endovascular aneurysm repair trial 1 (EVAR trial 1): a randomised controlled trial. *Lancet* 2016; **388** (10058): 2366–74.

12. Sachs T, Schermerhorn M, Pomposelli, *et al.* Resident and fellow experiences after the introduction of endovascular aneurysm repair for abdominal aortic aneurysm. *J Vasc Surg* 2011; **54:** 881–88.

13. Dua A, Koprowski S, Upchurch G, *et al.* Progressive shortfall in open aneurysm experience for vascular surgery trainees with the impact of fenestrated and branched endovascular technology. *J Vasc Surg* 2016. Epub.

14. Landry G, Lau I, Liem T, *et al.* Open abdominal aortic aneurysm repair in the endovascular era: effect of clamp site on outcomes. Arch Surg 2009; **144:** 811–16.

15. Johnston MJ, Singh P, Pucher PH, *et al.* Systematic review with meta-analysis of the impact of surgical fellowship training on patient outcomes. *Br J Surg* 2015; **102:** 1156–66.

16. Beiles CB, Walker S. Mortality after open aortic aneurysm surgery by Australasian surgeons trained in the endovascular era. ANZ J Surg 2016; **86:** 544–48.

17. McPhee JT, Robinson WP, Eslami MH, *et al. Surgeon* case volume, not institution case volume, is the primary determinant of in-hospital mortality after elective open abdominal aortic aneurysm repair. *J Vasc Surg* 2011; **53:** 591–99.

18. Collin J, Murie JA. Endovascular treatment of abdominal aortic aneurysm: a failed experiment. *Br J Surg* 2001; **88:** 281–82.

19. Greenhalgh RM. Endovascular aneurysm repair and outcome in patients unfit for open repair of abdominal aortic aneurysm (EVAR trial 2): Randomised controlled trial. *Lancet* 2005; **365:** 2187–92.

20. Ballotta E, Giau G Da, Bridda A, *et al.* Open abdominal aortic aneurysm repair in octogenarians before and after the adoption of endovascular grafting procedures. *J Vasc Surg* 2008; **47:** 23–30.

21. Moulakakis KG, Dalainas I, Mylonas S, *et al.* Conversion to open repair after endografting for abdominal aortic aneurysm: a review of causes, incidence, results, and surgical techniques of reconstruction. *J Endovasc Ther* 2010; **17:** 694–702.

22. Hiromatsu S, Sakashita H, Okazaki T, *et al.* Perioperative outcomes for elective open abdominal aortic aneurysm repair since the adoption of endovascular grafting procedures. *Eur J Vasc Endovasc Surg* 2011; **42:** 178–84.

23. Dimick JB, Upchurch GR. Measuring and improving the quality of care for abdominal aortic aneurysm surgery. *Circulation* 2008; **117:** 2534–41.

24. Muehling BM, Ortlieb L, Oberhuber A, Orend KH. Fast track management reduces the systemic inflammatory response and organ failure following elective infrarenal aortic aneurysm repair. Interact Cardiovasc Thorac Surg 2011; **12:** 784–88.

25. Holt PJ, Poloniecki JD, Gerrard D, *et al.* Meta-analysis and systematic review of the relationship between volume and outcome in abdominal aortic aneurysm surgery. *Br J Surg* 2007; **94:** 395–403.

# Reducing errors during minimally invasive procedures for elective AAA repair

AJ Batchelder and CD Bicknell

## Introduction

There is growing recognition that healthcare is a high-risk industry, and that a significant number of patients come to harm while in hospital.[1] The highest rate of adverse events occurs in patients undergoing procedural interventions, especially in patients undergoing vascular procedures.[2] The cost of error is high—in 2008, measureable errors cost approximately US$17.1 billion. A paper by Van Den Bos *et al* suggested that 10 types of errors accounted for more than two-thirds of the total cost of errors.[3] Most errors identified in this study were complications of interventions, including postoperative infection, perioperative haemorrhage or haematoma, inadvertent intraoperative injury and mechanical complications of implants or grafts.

Over the past few decades, vascular surgical care has developed markedly. In 1987, Ukrainian surgeon Nicholas Volodos performed the first endovascular repair of a traumatic thoracic aortic aneurysm. Subsequently, in 1990, Juan Parodi and his team in Buenos Aires, Argentina, successfully undertook the first endovascular repair of an abdominal aortic aneurysm (AAA). It was this work that served to catalyse interest in this area.

In 1999, the first report of use of a fenestrated aortic stent was published. These interventions have been designed and refined to tackle the major surgical complication rate that is inevitable in patients who have high rates of comorbidity. This technology has been rapidly and universally adopted. It continues to evolve, for example, through the use of branched devices, chimney techniques and percutaneous access. However, increasing evolution inevitably brings an increase in complexity. In order to optimise patient outcomes, attention must be focussed not only on patient and technical factors, but also on the role of wider aspects of the surgical system in patient safety.[1,4]

Between 2012 and 2014, a multicentre observational study—the LEAP Study (Landscape of error in aortic procedures)—recruited 20 vascular surgical teams from 10 hospitals in England with the aim of identifying the nature, frequency and determinants of errors and failures in aortic surgery.[5] During the initial phase of this work, the vascular surgical teams were trained to use a validated self-reporting tool.[6] Subsequently, the teams collected data for consecutive aortic procedures. In 185 aortic cases, the teams reported a median of three errors per procedure (interquartile range two to six). The most frequently-reported errors related to equipment (33.9%). The most frequent major or harm-producing errors were communication failures. Critical errors leading to direct patient harm were present in 6.5% of cases, and over 50% of the root cause of these errors was communication-based. Importantly, error frequency directly correlated with clinical outcomes. Increased error frequency was associated with a significantly increased risk of return to theatre, development of major complication and postoperative death. Thus, this study evidenced the importance of systemic and non-technical elements in aortic surgery and highlighted the significant harm that may result from potentially avoidable errors.

An unpublished systematic search of the UK National Reporting and Learning System (NRLS) and subsequent thematic analysis identified 2,698 aortic surgery safety incidents, of which 1,126 were elective; 448 preoperative; 302 intraoperative; and 376 postoperative. Five categories account for 80% of all reports: medical devices, resources/organisational management, clinical process/procedure, medication and documentation. Of the 1,126 incidents, 885 affected the patient (78.6%), 307 caused harm (27.3%); severe harm or death occurred in 7.3%.

NHS England has recently established standards for interventional procedures, stratified at organisational and individual levels.[6] This guidance was introduced due to persisting incidence of "never events"—serious incidents that are wholly preventable because safety recommendations that provide strong systemic protective barriers are available at a national level (and thus, should be implemented by all healthcare providers). The guidance formalises practices that are already common in many surgical departments but emphasises the basic tenets of safe delivery of care.

As a vascular surgical community, therefore, we have proof that the aortic endovascular procedures we provide—designed to reduce the morbidity and mortality of older patients with extensive comorbidity—can be safer and the key determinants error and potential patient harm have been mapped effectively. Communication, effective use of technology, team working and leadership appear to be key targets for improvements in care. This chapter briefly discusses the use of simulation, rehearsal, team training and reporting registries.

## Simulation

The role of simulation in training operators in procedural techniques has gained widespread acceptance. In the context of endovascular surgery, simulation training has been reported to improve overall technical proficiency and to reduce total procedural time, use of contrast media and fluoroscopy time.[7-9] Thus, high-fidelity procedure-based simulators may be a valuable tool for improving the technical skills of individual operators. The technical skill improvements seen with effective training using high-fidelity simulators are well reported in the literature.

## Rehearsal

Mental team rehearsal prior to endovascular cases is, in itself, effective in streamlining procedures and avoiding error. We have found that a simple extension to the WHO checklist, with detailed run-through of procedural steps, can reduce the rate of errors significantly. This is especially the case for communication and equipment error, and staff absence during critical steps and planning.

More recently, patient-specific modelling is being used to practise cases prior to intervention, especially in particularly challenging aortic morphology. A prospective, multicentre trial randomised 100 patients undergoing elective endovascular repair of infrarenal aortic or iliac aneurysms to preoperative patient-specific rehearsal using a virtual reality simulator and a three-dimensional reconstruction based on the patient's aortic anatomy or standard care.[10] This study reported that patient-specific rehearsal yielded a 26% reduction in minor errors, a 76% reduction in major errors and a 27% reduction in errors causing procedural delay. The number of angiograms performed to visualise proximal and distal landing zones reduced in the rehearsal group. Whilst not statistically significant, there were also trends towards decreased contrast use and decreased radiation dose in the rehearsal group. These results highlight the importance of preprocedural preparation and planning in endovascular aneurysm surgery and the implications this has on efficiency and patient safety.

## Team training

Simulation exercises are also beneficial in training all team members involved in interventions in non-technical aspects of safe delivery of care. Crisis resource management is a proactive risk-minimisation strategy historically adopted by high-risk organisations, such as the aviation and nuclear power industries. It recognises human variability and environmental complexities, and is used to train teams in a range of non-technical skills. These include interpersonal skills (e.g. communication, team working, leadership and followership) and cognitive skills (e.g. situational awareness, planning, decision making and task management).[11]

A single-centre before/after study investigating the effects of a three-month crisis resource management teaching programme in general and vascular surgical teams demonstrated significant improvements in non-technical skills and attitudes towards safety.[12] This study also reported a significant reduction in the incidence of technical and non-technical errors. Simulated team training may be particularly helpful in preparing for uncommon emergency scenarios. The feasibility of fully-immersive multidisciplinary training in endovascular repair of ruptured abdominal aortic aneurysm has been demonstrated, and such education serves to provide a useful tool for improving technical and non-technical aspects of perioperative care.[13]

At Imperial College London, we have instituted a programme of team training on a weekly basis to train teams in elective and emergency cases as well as dealing with specific issues that may arise from clinical incident reporting—a reactive training pathway. The success of this programme has been documented through quantitative and qualitative feedback mechanisms.

The practicalities of team training, however, are not insignificant. There needs to be engagement from all staff. Interestingly, the authors of one study noted reluctance amongst some senior medical staff to engage with this type of training and this is likely to represent a challenge for cultural change.[12] Our view is that training should be the responsibility of all and the distinction between trainee and trainer should be fluid in different circumstances. Finance must always be a consideration and further evidence is needed for the cost-effectiveness of a dedicated programme.

## Debriefing

Several of the previously mentioned studies coincidentally identified failures to subsequently respond to problems identified during procedures. In order to continually improve care delivery, it is vital that individuals and organisations learn from errors and take steps to avoid recurrence of these issues. The development of a collective memory was one of the principle recommendations of *To err is human: Building a safer health system*, which highlighted the extent and impact of clinical error.[14] Central to this process is a systematic approach to recognising errors and debriefing can effectively facilitate this. Current reporting systems in the UK are too far removed from the clinical team, and actions arising from "serious incident" investigations are often ineffective.

A number of tools have been developed to aid error identification and recall, including the Imperial Collage Error Capture (ICECAP) tool. This tool was developed from a comprehensive log of vascular procedural errors, which were graded according to their potential to cause delays or harm.[15] The tool has seven distinct error groupings, including those relating to equipment, communication, procedure-independent pressures, safety, patient-related factors and technical factors. The use of ICECAP was shown to significantly improve error recall during debriefing following arterial procedures. Unpublished data from our experience at the 10 centres involved in the LEAP study has demonstrated that using the ICECAP data collection prompts is an effective debriefing tool. Similar mechanisms should be considered by all units to close a loop of feedback and improvement at the grassroots level.

## Radiation safety

The advent of endovascular techniques exposes vascular surgeons and their patients to significant doses of radiation. The issue of radiation exposure has recently received a great deal of attention in the medical press. Long-term outcome data from the EVAR1 trial have identified a significant increase in cancer-related mortality in patients undergoing endovascular repair after eight years.[16] Conventional endovascular repair of infrarenal aortic aneurysms exposes the primary operator to 52.5µSv (area uncovered by lead garment) and 4µSv (area covered by lead garment).[17] Obliquity of the C-arm and repeated digital subtraction angiography increase the exposure. Radiation doses during thoracic, fenestrated and branched cases are significantly higher. These studies and similar demonstrate that with the increasing number of procedures performed by teams each year, the risk of long-term radiation exposure is a real concern. Care must, therefore, be taken to minimise behaviours that increase radiation exposure.

A survey of US vascular trainees reported a lack of formal radiation safety training.[18] Surgeon education has been shown to significantly reduce patient radiation doses through improved operating practices, such as elevation of table height and use of collimation.[19] We believe that team training is key to protecting all team members from radiation and the lead operator is responsible for the entire team.

In addition to the role of education in enhancing radiation safety, there are a number of ergonomic considerations as well. Hybrid theatre suites with flat-panel detectors provide improved imaging resolution and can reduce radiation exposure by up to 30% compared to X-ray image intensifiers. This technology requires major capital investment. However, even in centres where such investment is not available, other strategies may be employed to improve radiation safety. A reduction in operator radiation dose may be achieved through the use of disposable radiation-absorbing surgical drapes. A small, randomised controlled trial demonstrated that these drapes decreased doses to the hand and chest of the primary interventionalist by 49% and 55% respectively.[20]

## Reporting systems and registries

In most healthcare systems the reporting of outcomes is of importance, often stimulated by high-profile failures in care. In the UK, one of the key recommendations of the public inquiry into high mortality rates in children undergoing cardiac surgery at the Bristol Royal Infirmary in the late 1980s and early 1990s was that outcome data should be more widely available.[21] Subsequently, in 2004 the Society of Cardiothoracic Surgeons of Great Britain and Ireland published activity data and mortality rates for all UK cardiac surgeons. In 2013, the National Vascular Registry was established to collect and report surgeon-specific outcome data for vascular surgeons in the UK. This has allowed identification of statistical outliers and provision of additional support for these individuals. However, concerns exist around data quality, risk-adjustment methodologies and case selection. Additionally, clinical outcomes are influenced by the wider hospital team and resource availability, not solely individual surgeon performance. Greater transparency in reporting, with appropriate corresponding support and remedial mechanisms, provides a useful tool in improving patient safety. Device-specific registries provide a further strategy for enhancing patient care. Such registries, in conjunction with regulatory reporting schemes, serve as a collective learning tool and allow identification of device-specific issues.

## Conclusion

We cannot be complacent in "not being an outlier" in large-scale outcome-based registries. Systems must be set up to target all errors that occur to really optimise the outcomes for patients in endovascular surgery of the aorta. Errors occur at a significant rate during all endovascular procedures. Most of these errors are latent failures within a system but a significant number become active errors in vascular surgery leading to patient harm; this is the basis of the Swiss Cheese Model of error propagation.[22] Strategies for enhancing patient safety must therefore be targeted towards the creation of safer systems.

There is a growing understanding of the nature and impact of errors within the context of aortic surgery; nevertheless, further work needs to be done to identify the best ways of sustained improvement. Ultimately, the delivery of safe care mandates a system with multiple protective barriers to error and a culture of transparency with emphasis on learning and continual improvement. The published literature appears to support focused interventions aimed at addressing specific errors. There is, however, no data for comprehensive safety programmes within vascular surgery adopting a multifaceted approach.

## Summary

- Errors occur frequently during endovascular aortic procedures and a significant number of these will result in harm to the patient.

- There is a growing evidence base for strategies targeting individual factors implicated in error propagation.

- Reducing error frequencies in endovascular surgery relies upon the creation of systems incorporating multiple protective mechanisms, including educational, organisational and ergonomic elements.

# References

1. Vincent C. Understanding and responding to adverse events. *N Engl J Med* 2003; **348** (11): 1051–56.
2. Leape LL, Brennan TA, Laird N, Lawthers A, de Leval MR, Barnes BA, *et al.* The nature of adverse events in hospitalized patients: Results of the Harvard Medical Practice Study II. *N Engl J Med* 1991; **324** (6): 377–84.
3. Van Den Bos J, Rustagi K, Gray T, *et al.* The $17.1 billion problem: the annual cost of measurable medical errors. *Health Aff* 2011; **30** (4): 596–603.
4. Weerakkody RA, Cheshire NJ, Riga C, *et al.* Surgical technology and operating-room safety failures: a systematic review of quantitative studies. *BMJ Qual Saf* 2013; **22** (9): 710–18.
5. Lear R, Riga C, Godfrey AD, *et al.* Multicentre observational study of surgical system failures in aortic procedures and their effect on patient outcomes. *Br J Surg* 2016; **103** (11): 1467–75.
6. Mason SL, Kuruvilla S, Riga CV, *et al.* Design and validation of an error capture tool for quality evaluation in the vascular and endovascular surgical theatre. *Eur J Vasc Endovasc Surg* 2013; **45** (3): 248–54.
7. Chaer RA, DeRubertis BG, Lin SC, *et al.* Simulation improves resident performance in catheter-based intervention: results of a randomized, controlled study. *Ann Surg* 2006; **244** (3): 343–52.
8. Dawson DL, Meyer J, Lee ES, Pevec WC. Training with simulation improves residents' endovascular procedure skills. *J Vasc Surg* 2007; **45** (1): 149–54.
9. Aggarwal R, Black SA, Hance JR, *et al.* Virtual reality simulation training can improve inexperienced surgeons' endovascular skills. *Eur J Vasc Endovasc Surg* 2006; **31** (6): 588–93.
10. Desender LM, Van Herzeele I, Lachat ML, *et al.* Patient-specific rehearsal before EVAR: influence on technical and nontechnical operative performance. A randomised controlled trial. *Ann Surg* 2016; **264** (5): 703–09.
11. Rudarakanchana N, Van Herzeele I, Desender L, Cheshire NJW. Virtual reality simulation for the optimization of endovascular procedures: current perspectives. *Vasc Health Risk Manag* 2015; **11**: 195–202.
12. McCulloch P, Mishra A, Handa A, *et al.* The effects of aviation-style non-technical skills training on technical performance and outcome in the operating theatre. *Qual Saf Health Care* 2009; **18** (2): 109–15.
13. Rudarakanchana N, Van Herzeele I, Bicknell CD, *et al.* Endovascular repair of ruptured abdominal aortic aneurym: technical and team training in an immersive virtual reality environment. *Cardiovasc Intervent Radiol* 2014; **37**: 920–27.
14. Committee on Quality of Health Care in America. To err is human: building a safer health system. Washington DC, National Academies Press, 1999.
15. Mason SL, Kuruvilla S, Riga CV, *et al.* Design and validation of an error capture tool for quality evaluation in the vascular and endovascular surgical theatre. *Eur J Vasc Endovasc Surg* 2013; **45** (3): 248–54.
16. Patel R, Sweeting MJ, Powell JT, *et al.* Endovascular *versus* open repair of abdominal aortic aneurysm in 15 years' follow-up of the UK endovascular aneurysm repair trial 1 (EVAR trial 1): a randomised controlled trial. *Lancet* **388** (10058): 2366–74.
17. Patel AP, Gallacher D, Dourado R, *et al.* Occupational radiation exposure during endovascular aortic procedures. *Eur J Vasc Endovasc Surg* 2013; **46** (4): 424–30.
18. Bordoli SJ, Carsten CG 3rd, Cull DL, *et al.* Radiation safety education in vascular surgery training. *J Vasc Surg* 2014; **59** (3): 860–64.

19. Kirkwood ML, Arbique GM, Guild JB, *et al. Surgeon* education decreases radiation dose in complex endovascular procedures and improves patient safety. *J Vasc Surg* 2013; **58** (3): 715–21.
20. Kloeze C, Klompenhouwer EG, Brands PJM, *et al*. Use of disposable radiation-absorbing surgical drapes results in significant dose reduction during EVAR procedures. *Eur J Vasc Endovasc Surg* 2014; **47** (3): 268–72.
21. Kennedy I. Learning from Bristol: the report of the public inquiry into children's heart surgery at the Bristol Royal Infirmary 1984-1995. London, The Stationery Office, 2001.
22. Reason J. Human error. New York, Cambridge University Press, 1990.

# Management of challenging access

E Gallito, C Mascoli, R Pini, G Faggioli, S Ancetti, A Stella and M Gargiulo

## Introduction

Data from randomised controlled trials have shown endovascular aneurysm repair (EVAR) to be associated with lower 30-day morbidity and mortality than the open repair.[1] The feasibility and effectiveness of EVAR depend on specific anatomic aortioiliac features. After proximal neck anatomy, the challenging iliac-femoral access (small diameter, severe angulations/tortuosity, extensive calcification and occlusive disease) represent the second excluding factor for EVAR.[2,3] Patients undergoing EVAR have concomitant iliac-femoral atherosclerosis in up to 40% of cases, and severe femoral-iliac artery disease precludes patients from EVAR in up to 25% of cases in historical published series.[2,4,5] Hostile iliac-femoral anatomy carries the risk of intraoperative vessel injury, such as iliac rupture, dissection, thrombosis and distal ischaemia.[5,6] In the EUROSTAR registry, limitation of access was one of the most common reason for conversion to open repair, and access complications were reported in 13% of patients.[7] Over the last decade, several strategies have been reported to manage EVAR in challenging access. Despite the availability of new abdominal devices (low profile, high pushability/trackability devices), several issues remain unsolved. Moreover, thoracic and fenestrated/branched endovascular aortic repair still involve the use of a large profile delivery system that could be associated with problems in cases of challenging access. The aim of the present paper is to describe pre- and intra-procedural strategy, addressing difficult access in EVAR, and to discuss the advantages and disadvantages of each one.

## Preoperative evaluation

Patients with aortic aneurysms are studied by computer tomography (CT) angiography. Preoperative CT angiography is usually performed following a standard aortic protocol with basal (calcium-burden) and arterial (true lumen, thrombus load) acquisitions.

Post-processing reconstructions (volume rendering, centre lumen line, multi-planar and maximum intensity projection reconstructions) can be performed by dedicated software for the advanced vessel analysis in order to accurately evaluate the femoral and iliac access. Access vessel evaluation consists on definition of common femoral, external/common iliac arteries diameters (intima-intima linear distance), iliac tortuosity, steno-obstructive lesions and/or presence of calcification.

# Challenging access: Definition and grading

Chaikof *et al* reported an accurate description of the challenging aortioiliac anatomy.[8] They described four grades of morphological risk (0: absent; 1: mild; 2: moderate; 3: severe) according to preoperative evaluation of iliac diameters, angulations/tortuosity, presence of calcifications and thrombosis. An iliac access was defined severe in the presence of almost one of the following features: diameter <7mm, stenosis with diameter <7mm and >3cm length, more than one focal stenosis of diameter <7mm, calcification >50% of the vessel length, tortuosity index >1.6 or iliac angles >90 degrees. In their daily practice, physicians use the term "severe" or "challenging" to describe the iliac anatomy grade three of the Chaikof's classification.

# Iliac artery tortuosity

An aneurysm is not only characterised by an enlargement in diameter, but also by artery elongation.[5] As the distal aorta is fixed, the elongation is confined to the iliac artery and cause tortuosity.[5] Tortuosity of the iliac axis could increase the risk of technical failures and iliac injuries in patients undergoing EVAR.[5,6]

Iliac tortuosity can be managed by stiff or extra-stiff guidewires (single or double).[5] The rigidity of the wire stretches the iliac axis, and the resulting alignment of the femoral, iliac and infra-renal aorta, facilitates the advancement and the navigability of the endograft through the iliac axis.[5] Iliac changes are not always feasible/effective in cases of heavy calcifications of the arterial wall.

In the case of abdominal aortic aneurysm with iliac artery tortuosity, the use of a stiff guidewire can be replaced or supported by a "through and through" working-way.[5] The transfemoral guide is snared in the descending aorta or aortic arch from brachial or axillary access. By applying tension to both ends (from brachial/axillary and femoral access), the aortic and iliac axis is straightened; this manoeuvre is mandatory to protect the aortic-subclavian angle with a reinforced sheath to decrease the risk of aortic injury.[5]

In presence of iliac tortuosity, the completion angiography should be always performed in three-projection without stiff guidewires in order to detect stenosis or kinking of the iliac limb or native iliac arteries.[9] In cases of residual stenosis or kinking, percutaneous transluminal angioplasty with stenting is suggested to correct any defects and maintain the limb patency during follow-up.[9]

# Iliac arteries with small diameter or steno-obstructive disease

### Low-profile endografts

In the last few years, industries have refocused their endografts to achieve lower profiles for the treatment of abdominal aortic aneurysm with challenging access. Delivery systems with diameter >20Fr are disappearing, and the majority of introduced sheaths and delivery systems have hydrophilic coating to allow easier insertion and navigability.

Moreover, new devices with ultra-low-profile features are commercially available. These devices, requiring an access of 7mm diameter for the main-body, enlarge the rate of abdominal aortic aneurysm fit for EVAR.

The INNOVATION trial (60 patients at six European centres), reported the safety/effectiveness at two-year follow-up for the Incraft endograft (Cordis).[10] At one-month, the primary endpoint of safety and effectiveness was achieved in 97% of cases. All patients were free from abdominal aortic aneurysm-enlargement, and there were no type I-III endoleaks at two-years. Overall mortality was 11.5% and no deaths were device- or procedure-related. Three patients required re-interventions—two for type-I endoleak and one for limb occlusion. Recently, Sugimoto *et al* reported on their postmarket clinical experience with the Incraft endograft in 24 patients with challenging access routes. Adjunctive interventions for iliac artery disease (percutaneous transluminal angioplasty-stenting) were performed in eight patients (33%).[11] Ninety-two per cent of patients were managed by a percutaneous approach, and technical success was 100%. At a mean follow-up of 12.5 months, there were 4.2% of access-related complications, with one case of bilateral limb thrombosis.

Metha *et al* reported the outcomes of the US regulatory trial for the Ovation abdominal endograft (Trivascular, 161 patients at 36 US centres).[12] Technical success was 100% and the 30-day major adverse event rate was 2.5%. The one-year clinical success was 99.3% with a 0.6% of abdominal aortic aneurysm-related mortality. Abdominal aortic aneurysm-related reinterventions were performed in 10 patients (6.2%) for 12 findings, including endoleak (six), aortic main body stenosis (three), and iliac limb stenosis or occlusion (three). The authors concluded that the one-year results of the Ovation abdominal endograft (Trivascular) demonstrate excellent safety/effectiveness for abdominal aortic aneurysms, particularly in patients with challenging anatomic characteristics, including short aortic necks and narrow iliac arteries.

The Italian multicentre registry for the Zenith abdominal Alfa endograft (unpublished data) enrolled 232 abdominal aortic aneurysm patients, who underwent EVAR in order to report the real-life outcomes of this new device. Technical success, 30-day mortality and 30-day reinterventions were 99%, 2.5% and 0.4%, respectively. At a mean follow up of 4.7 months, iliac limb occlusion rate was 1.9%. Severe anatomical iliac characteristics were not risk factors for technical failure, predischarge complications, 30-day survival, limb occlusion and reinterventions.

It is important to underline that all these devices have become commercially available in the last few years, and no long-term data are available. However, early and mid-term data showed good results in term of technical/clinical success and iliac leg patency during this follow-up.

## Endovascular tips to facilitate device navigation

Several adjunctive endovascular tips can be used to facilitate the device navigation through a challenging iliac axis by transfemoral approach.[5,13] It is always desirable to start from simple strategies and proceed with more complex solutions only in cases of primary failure.

In the presence of small iliac diameters, progressive mechanical dilatations can be performed by dedicated dilatators; this manoeuvre could be therapeutic and diagnostic as a test of device navigability.

In case of focal or multiple stenotic lesions, percutaneous transluminal angioplasty could be sufficient to overcome the iliac problem. If the diameter required is then not achieved, or recoiling is observed, self-expanding or balloon expandable stents or stent grafts can be used.[5,13] However, it is important to underline that it should desirable to stent the iliac axis at the end of the procedure because the presence of stents could cause problems during the endografting manoeuvres.

In cases of very challenge steno-obstructive lesions, when the previous proposals have failed, some authors reported off-label endovascular procedures that allow endovascular aortic repair.

The "*in situ* sheath dilatation" was described by von Segesser et al.[14] It consists of the placement of a sheath in the iliac artery with a diameter smaller than that recommended for the endograft, and the inflation of a balloon catheter inside the sheath, stretching it to a diameter compatible with the introduction of the device. It allows physicians to increase the access vessel diameter by 50% (from six to 9mm) or the luminal circumference from 18Fr to 27Fr.[14] The authors reported five cases successfully treated by this technique. However, in our opinion, the risk of iliac rupture and massive bleeding is not negligible, especially when the sheaths are removed.

Hinchliffe *et al* reported the feasibility of the "paving and cracking" technique.[15] It consists of the deployment of covered stents or iliac limb endograft in the stenotic iliac artery (paving), that are dilated until a controlled rupture of the vessel occurs (cracking).[5,15] After deployment of the stent graft, the device is ballooned at its proximal and distal ends in order to seal. Only after this manoeuvre, the central stent graft segment is aggressively ballooned with a noncompliant balloon, creating the controlled rupture of the native iliac artery. The authors suggested that angioplasty with a non-compliant 10mm balloon allows passage of delivery sheaths up to 22Fr, while a 12mm balloon is required for 24Fr.[5,15] It is important to underline that at the completion angiography, iliac access requires a meticulous control in order to detect any remaining bleeding or stenosis needing further treatment.

Van Bogerijen *et al* reported a comparison between iliac artery endoconduits (16 cases) and retroperitoneal open iliac conduits (ROIC; 23 cases) in patients who underwent thoracic endovascular aortic repair (TEVAR) with challenging access.[16] The technical success was reported in all cases and at a median follow-up of 10.1 months, the incidence of iliac-femoral complications was less for iliac artery endoconduits compared with the ROIC (12.5% *vs.* 26.1%; p=0.301). No patients sustained limb loss. Lower extremity claudication occurred in one patient after iliac artery endoconduits. Early mortality occurred in one patient in the iliac artery endoconduit group. Two-year Kaplan-Meier survival for the entire cohort was 74.4%, and did not differ between groups (ROIC, 78.3% *vs.* iliac artery endoconduit, 68.8%; p=0.35). Two-year Kaplan-Meier freedom from limb loss, claudication, or revascularisation did not differ between the two approaches (ROIC, 91.3% *vs.* iliac artery endoconduit, 93.8%; p=0.961). The authors suggested that the iliac artery endoconduit approach can be considered safe and effective. It was also associated with low rates of early mortality and late iliac-femoral complications. The approach avoids complications associated with the retroperitoneal approach, and allows transfemoral TEVAR. Coverage of hypogastric artery during endoconduit technique could be associated with potential risk of back bleeding from patent hypogastric and the low pelvic perfusion. In the small reported experiences, these complications were not found.[5,13] If it is possible, a coil embolisation of the hypogastric artery before placement of the endoconduit should theoretically be performed. This cautious approach has not been necessary in the most of these cases, where the iliac arteries are too small and diseased (preoperative hypogastric occlusion).[5,13] Ideally, perfusion through the contralateral hypogastric artery should be maintained. If possible, the internal iliac artery should be preserved in order to avoid pelvic ischaemia complications, especially in setting of contralateral hypogastric artery occlusion.[5,13]

It is important to underline that these off-label techniques are described in few case reports or small clinical series without evidences and follow-up data. Larger series needs to be examined before any conclusions can be made about the safety of this technique.

## Aorto-uni-iliac endograft.

In patients with unilateral iliac artery occlusion, it is indicated to perform aortic uni-iliac endografting associated with extra-anatomic cross femoral-femoral bypass.

Yilmaz et al reported the use of aorto-uni-iliac endografts associated with a cross-over femoro-femoral bypass as an effective and durable solution with acceptable rate of complications (5.4% over a mean follow-up of 23.6 months) in patients with unfit anatomy for a standard EVAR. However, potential complications such as graft infection (inguinal wounds) or crossover occlusion are not negligible and are dangerous.[17]

Jean-Baptiste et al compared mid-term results of bifurcated and aorto-uni-iliac endograft in the treatment of abdominal aortic aneurysm unfit for open repair.[18] Technical success was 94% and 99% in bifurcated and aorto-uni-iliac endograft, respectively (p=0.002). Major perioperative complications occurred in 13 aorto-uni-iliac endograft patients (10%) vs. 12 bifurcated endograft patients (4%, p=0.005). The 30-day mortality rate was 3.2% vs. 1.5% (p=0.2). During the follow-up period (median 24 months), secondary procedures were required in 11% and 5% of aorto-uni-iliac and bifurcated endograft patients, respectively (p=0.01). Freedom from reintervention at 12, 24 and 36 months was 98%, 90%, and 85% in bifurcated endograft vs. 96%, 92%, and 92% in aortic uni-iliac endograft patients (p<0.005). In the aorto-uni-iliac endograft group, the cross femoral-femoral bypass was responsible for three major complications (2.4%). Upon uni- and multivariate analysis, concomitant iliac arterial occlusive disease was a significant predictor of clinical failure (open repair 3.996; 95% CI: 1.996 to 7.921; p<0.0001). Although this paper concludes that bifurcated graft was associated with better results than was aorto-uni-iliac endograft, the aortic uni-iliac endograft is the technique of choice in patients with abdominal aortic aneurysm and unilateral iliac artery occlusion.

## Iliac artery recanalisation before EVAR

Endovascular iliac recanalisation is safe and effective for peripheral arterial occlusive disease with clinical success at mid/long-term follow-up. According with these results and with development of endovascular experience, bifurcated endografts could become an option for abdominal aortic aneurysm and concomitant iliac artery occlusion. Vallabhaneni et al reported short/mid-term outcomes of bifurcated EVAR in patients with abdominal aortic aneurysm and concomitant chronic iliac occlusions requiring recanalisation.[19] Fifteen occluded iliac arteries (14 patients) were treated (unilateral common iliac artery occlusion: seven; unilateral external iliac artery occlusion: four; unilateral combined common iliac artery and external iliac artery occlusion: three; bilateral common iliac artery occlusion: one). Successful recanalisation was achieved in 14 of the 15 vessels (93%). One external iliac artery ruptured occurred during recanalisation but was controlled by covered-stent. Overall, 13 bifurcated devices were successfully implanted. During a mean follow-up of 28.2 months (range, one–86 months), there was 100% primary patency of successfully recanalised iliac arteries. The authors concluded that the use of bifurcated endovascular devices after recanalisation of an occluded iliac system is technically feasible and durable at midterm follow-up. This technique allows to re-establish aorto-iliac inflow to both lower extremities, and to obviate the need for extra-anatomic bypass. It may preserve hypogastric perfusion in some patients.[19]

## Iliac surgical conduit

Surgical conduit is an available therapeutic option to guarantee the endovascular treatment of abdominal aortic aneurysm in patients with external iliac arteries unfit for the device navigation.[5,13] The level of the anastomosis should be carefully evaluated and particular attention is required for the vessel diameter, the grade of calcification and the quality of the proximal common iliac artery and the distal aorta.

After retroperitoneal exposure, the conduit is performed by suturing a synthetic graft (10mm diameter) to the common iliac artery (generally in the distal segment) in an end-to-side fashion.[5,13] The graft is tunnelled to the femoral region to  work in a straight line, the distal end is closed (clip, suture or clamp) to avoid blood loss during component exchanges. The endovascular procedure can be performed by introducing the device through this bridging vessel. At the end of the procedure, the surgical conduit can be removed in patients with iliac arteries with small diameter, or used as an iliac-femoral bypass in those with ipsilateral iliac artery occlusion or residual steno-obstructive disease.

Lee *et al* found the use of surgical conduits to be associated with a significantly higher morbidity rate compared to the standard femoral access (1.8 higher complications; 2.6 greater blood loss; 1.5 day longer length of stay and 82% longer procedure time when retroperitoneal exposure rather than femoral access was used in conjunction with EVAR).[20] However, in experienced hands, the construction of a surgical conduit represents a fast, direct and controlled EVAR approach.

In an effort to avoid the use of a prosthetic conduit, Carpenter *et al* described a direct aortic or iliac access through a limited retroperitoneal exposure.[21] With this approach, a purse-string suture is placed in the access vessel, the artery is punctured in the middle of this purse-string, and the device is delivered without the need for a prosthetic conduit.[5,21] At the end of procedure, the adventitial purse-string suture is cinched down to close the entry site. This method avoids leaving prosthetic material behind as a potential nidus of infection or confusion in follow-up imaging.[5,21]

## Summary

- Challenging iliac access reduces EVAR suitability and could increase the intra/ post-operative morbidity and mortality.

- Accurate preoperative planning (CT angiography and post-processing process) should be used to identify potential anatomical critical issues at the level of iliac arteries.

- Severe aortio-iliac tortuosity can be successfully managed by stiff guidewires. If this maneuvre does not guarantee the device navigation, the "through and through" subclavian-femoral technique can be useful. At the completion angiography, it is crucial to pay attention to the iliac limb/external iliac artery residual stenosis. Three-projection angiography without stiff guidewires and aggressive use of stents are suggested in order to guarantee the iliac leg patency during follow-up.

- Progressive mechanical dilatations can be used in cases of small iliac diameter using dedicated dilatators (16–22Fr) as therapeutic manoeuvre or test of device navigability.

- In cases of focal or multiple stenosis, conventional percutaneous transluminal angioplasty could allow the navigation of the device

- According with aortic-iliac anatomy and instructions-for-use of the endograft, it is desirable to approach patients with challenging iliac access with ultra-low profile devices.

- Aortic-uni-iliac endograft and extra-anatomic cross femoral-femoral bypass is indicated in cases of chronic and long, iliac occlusion.

- In cases of external iliac arteries unfit for the device navigation (i.e. small diameter, occlusion) a surgical iliac conduit is a safe and effective surgical solution.

- Off-label adjunctive endovascular procedures, (i.e. paving-cracking technique) were described as feasible and effective, but they are not supported by large clinical data. For these reason, they should be used only in cases where previous reported approaches are not feasible.

## References

1. United Kigndom EVAR Trial Investigators, Greenhalgh RM, Brown LC, *et al*. Endovascular *versus* open repair of abdominal aortic aneurysm. *N Engl J Med* 2010; **362**: 1863–71.
2. Arko FR, Filis KA, Seidel SA, *et al*. How many patients with infrarenal aneurysms are candidates for endovascular repair? *J Endovasc Ther* 2004; **11:** 33–40.
3. Carpenter JP, Baum RA, Barker CF, *et al*. Impact of exclusion criteria on patient selection for endovascular abdominal aortic aneurysm repair. *J Vasc Surg* 2001; **34** (6): 1050–54.
4. Murray D, Ghosh J, Khwaja N, *et al*. Access for endovascular aneurysm repair. *J Endovasc Ther* 2006; **13 (6):** 754–61.
5. Bischoff MS, Peters AS, Meisenbacher K, Böckler D. Challenging access in endovascular repair of infrarenal aortic aneurysms. *J Cardiovasc Surg* (Torino) 2014; **55** (2 Suppl 1): 75–83.
6. Tillich M, Bell RE, Paik DS, Fleischmann D, *et al*. Iliac arterial injuries after endovascular repair of abdominal aortic aneurysms: correlation with iliac curvature and diameter. *Radiology* 2001; **219 (1):** 129–36.

7. Cuypers PW, Laheij RJ, Buth J. Which factors increase the risk of conversion to open surgery following endovascular abdominal aortic aneurysm repair? The EUROSTAR collaborators. *Eur J Vasc Endovasc Surg* 2000; **20** (2): 183–89.

8. Chaikof EL, Fillinger MF, Matsumura JS, *et al.* Identifying and grading factors that modify the outcome of endovascular aortic aneurysm repair. *J Vasc Surg* 2002; **35** (5): 1061–66.

9. Bianchini Massoni C, Gargiulo M, Giovanetti F, *et al.* Adjunctive stenting of endograft limbs during endovascular treatment of infrarenal aortic and iliac aneurysms according to 3-projection completion angiography. *J Endovasc Ther* 2011; **18** (4): 585–90.

10. Torsello G, Scheinert D, Brunkwall JS, *et al.* Safety and effectiveness of the INCRAFT AAA Stent Graft for endovascular repair of abdominal aortic aneurysms. *J Vasc Surg* 2015; **61** (1): 1–8.

11. Sugimoto M, Torsello GF, Torsello GB, *et al.* Postmarket Clinical Experience with the INCRAFT AAA Stent Graft System for Challenging Access Routes. *Ann Vasc Surg*. 2016; [Article in press] DOI: http://dx.doi.org/10.1016/j.avsg.2016.07.073.

12. Mehta M, Valdés FE, Nolte T, *et al.* One-year outcomes from an international study of the Ovation Abdominal Stent Graft System for endovascular aneurysm repair. *J Vasc Surg* 2014 Jan; **59 (1):** 65–73.

13. Peterson BG, Matsumura JS. Tips and tricks for avoiding access problems when using large sheath endografts. *J Vasc Surg* 2009; **49** (2): 524–27.

14. Von Segesser LK, Marty B, Tozzi PG, Corno A. *In situ* introducer sheath dilatation for complex aortic access. *Eur J Cardiothorac Surg* 2002; **22** (2): 316–18.

15. Hinchliffe RJ, Ivancev K, Sonesson B, Malina M. "Paving and cracking": an endovascular technique to facilitate the introduction of aortic stent-grafts through stenosed iliac arteries. *J Endovasc Ther 2007*; **14** (5): 630–33.

16. Van Bogerijen GH, Williams D, Eliason J, *et al.* Alternative access techniques with thoracic endovascular aortic repair, open iliac conduit *versus* endoconduit technique. *J Vasc Surg* 2014; **60:** 1168–76.

17. Yilmaz LP, Abraham CZ, Reilly LM, *et al.* Is cross-femoral bypass grafting a disadvantage of aortomonoiliac endovascular aortic aneurysm repair? *J Vasc Surg* 2003; **38** (4): 753–57.

18. Jean-Baptiste E, Batt M, Azzaoui R, *et al.* A comparison of the mid-term results following the use of bifurcated and aorto-uni-iliac devices in the treatment of abdominal aortic aneurysms. *Eur J Vasc Endovasc Surg* 2009; **38** (3): 298–304.

19. Vallabhaneni R, Sorial EE, Jordan WD Jr, *et al.* Iliac artery recanalization of chronic occlusions to facilitate endovascular aneurysm repair. *J Vasc Surg* 2012; **56** (6): 1549–54.

20. Lee WA1, Berceli SA, Huber TS, *et al.* Morbidity with retroperitoneal procedures during endovascular abdominal aortic aneurysm repair. *J Vasc Surg* 2003; **38** (3): 459–63.

21. Parmer S, Carpenter J. Techniques for large sheath insertion during endovascular thoracic aortic aneurysm repair. *J Vasc Surg* 2006; **43 Suppl A:** 62A-68A.

# Outcomes & follow-up

# Embolisation for type I endoleaks after EVAR— patient selection, technical tips and outcomes

S Ameli-Renani, V Pavlidis and RA Morgan

## Introduction

Type I endoleaks are seen in up to 10% of patients following endovascular aneurysm repair (EVAR), and they are one of the leading factors necessitating secondary intervention.[1] They can be defined as a failure to create or maintain an adequate seal at the proximal (type Ia) or distal attachment site (type Ib), allowing direct of flow into the aneurysm sac. They result from adverse aortic anatomy, including short, wide or excessively calcified proximal necks, type and size of stent graft used, stent migration and aortic degeneration with time.[2] The resultant communication between the high pressure aortic lumen and the perigraft space can result in increased sac pressurisation, sac expansion and rupture. There is general consensus on the need for early treatment of type I endoleaks.

Standard endovascular treatment options include placement of an aortic cuff to extend coverage proximally, or insertion of a large-calibre stent inside the proximal endograft to improve the seal. The treatment of type Ib endoleaks typically entails extension of distal endograft coverage to increase the sealing zone.[3]

Transcatheter embolisation offers an alternative percutaneous approach for management in cases unsuitable or refractory to conventional treatments. Mainly used for proximal endoleaks, the procedure can be undertaken by most operators familiar with catheter embolisation techniques and can be performed as a day case under conscious sedation with a relatively short procedure time. The procedure needs to be performed methodically in view of the risk of non-target embolisation into the aorta and renal arteries. Herein, we will outline technical tips and suggestions on patient selection to optimise outcome in these cases and provide a brief review of the literature and our institutional outcomes.

## Patient selection

The main indications for type I endoleak embolisation are cases in which conventional methods of endoleak management are not possible due to adverse aortic anatomy or severe comorbidities prohibiting general anaesthesia or open repair. The former applies in cases where there is inadequate length or diameter of landing zone for an aortic cuff or where this zone is heavily diseased.

Ideal type I endoleak characteristics for embolisation include a long, narrow entrance (communicating neck space between aorta and endoleak cavity) and an endoleak cavity that is not too small or too large. Where the endoleak cavity is very small, embolisation may be best deferred whilst the patient has regular surveillance, as the chances of successful engagement of the endoleak cavity and achieving complete occlusion of the cavity are limited. Conversely, very large endoleak cavities and those with a wide endoleak entrance are similarly difficult to embolise with a durable outcome. Occlusion of the endoleak entrance is important to avoid a recurrent endoleak. Large endoleaks require a large volume of embolic material, and it is difficult to completely occlude the endoleak entrance whilst avoiding non target embolisation, which is more likely with a wide endoleak neck. In our experience, this risk can be reduced by filling the endoleaks with coils prior to liquid embolisation. We have not yet analysed endoleak morphology in detail to determine an "unfavourable" endoleak cavity and neck threshold for embolisation. However, we consider an endoleak cavity volume of more than 30ml and an endoleak entrance of more than 15mm as unfavourable predictors of success.[4]

There are, however, patients unsuitable for standard therapy or surgery, in whom embolisation is the only possible option to avoid imminent sac rupture. These cases may benefit from embolisation as a "palliative step" to prevent sac growth and rupture for as long as possible with the understanding that complete occlusion of the endoleak entrance may not be feasible. We have performed two cases of embolisation in patients with impending abdominal aortic aneurysm rupture, both whom survived for four and five months, and believe that palliative embolisation can be considered in patients without any other alternative.

In type I endoleak cases following EndoVascular Aneurysm Sealing (EVAS) with the Nellix device (Endologix), standard management options are not usually feasible and transcatheter embolisation may be offered as the first-line treatment option for managing proximal endoleaks with these endografts at our centre.

Embolising a distal type I endoleak is usually only required in cases were the distal landing zone cannot be extended. Examples from our experience include endoleaks at the distal end of a thoracic aortic endograft and a case of aortic uni-ilac endograft with a bypass graft originating close to the end of the endograft.

## Technical tips and considerations

The embolisation technique has been previously fully described.[5] In brief, embolisation is performed via a microcatheter advanced co-axially through a parent catheter into the endoleak sac and embolic material injected until the endoleak cavity is completely occluded (Figure 1). Technical considerations and some "tips and tricks", which in our experience help optimise the procedure, are as follows:

- Use a long access sheath (e.g. a 45cm 6Fr) sheath advanced into the aorta with the sheath tip a few centimetres below the top of the endograft in order to maximise support when attempting to engage the endoleak cavity and during embolisation
- Use a reverse shape curved catheter (e.g. 5Fr) to engage the endoleak cavity. The endoleak cavity is the space between the endograft and aortic wall. The tip of a reverse shaped catheter is likely to "drop" into the endoleak cavity as the catheter is pulled down from above the tip of the endograft

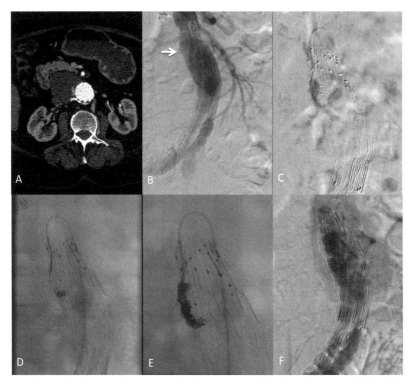

**Figure 1:** Eighty-four year-old male presenting with proximal type 1 endoleak. (A) Axial CT angiography image shows endoleak adjacent to the proximal end of the endograft. (B) Oblique aortic angiogram confirms proximal endoleak (white arrow). Endoleak cavity catheterised with reverse shaped catheter and microcatheter. (C) Endoleakogram more accurately confirms size and morphology of endoleak cavity. (D) Embolisation performed first with detachable micro-coils and then with (E) Onyx. (F) Completion angiography confirms occlusion and isolation of the endoleak.

- Perform an "enoleakogram" after advancing a microcatheter co-axially through the reverse shaped catheter into the endoleak cavity. This helps to better define the size and morphology of the endoleak and to evaluate for the occasional presence of any exit vessels. The endoleakogram can also act as a road map for the embolisation procedure.

Consider embolising the endoleak cavity with coils prior to liquid embolisation. Following earlier experience, we now initially deploy detachable coils in the endoleak cavity to form a "scaffold" prior to occlusion of the endoleak by liquid embolics. In our experience, this approach helps to deliver better sealing of the endoleak in the long term and has also minimised the risk of non-target embolisation. We favour the use of detachable coils because of the potential for coil misplacement and migration out of the endoleak cavity.

Use a liquid embolic to occlude the endoleak cavity. The authors prefer to use Onyx (Medtronic) as the embolic agent, although other liquid embolics may be used. In general, use of a liquid embolic is essential to achieve complete filling of the endoleak sac. Advantages of Onyx in this context include non-adhesive properties and gradual precipitation with a long solidification time in a dependent fashion forming a spongy cast; allowing for a controlled delivery and enabling the polymer to conform to the variable shape of the endoleak cavity. The authors use Onyx-34 for EL1 embolisation. The higher viscosity of this formulation compared with Onyx 18 may produce a better seal of the endoleak cavity and reduce risk of reflux.

For EL1b embolisation, the procedure and steps are similar, apart from the use of a short regular sheath at the access site and the use of an angled-tip catheter to engage the endoleak cavity.

In cases where embolisation is being performed following the use of the Nellix system, one must consider the location of the endoleak in relation to the orientation of the endograft limbs and choose the side of access most favourable for engaging the endoleak. For example, an endoleak on the right of the aortic sac is best accessed from a left common femoral artery approach, because the Nellix endografts cross over at the aortic bifurcation and the limb on the right of the proximal aorta extends distally to the left iliac artery.

## Outcomes

Transarterial embolisation of type I endoleaks was first described by Golzarian and colleagues in 1997,[6] who later described results in a cohort of 32 cases of type Ia endoleak embolised with coils with or without gelatine sponge and thrombin with two cases of endoleak recurrence amongst 22 followed-up patients.[7] Amesur et al used coils only in five patients, with two requiring repeat embolisation.[8] Maldonado and colleagues embolised 13 proximal and four distal type-I endoleaks using n-butyl cyanoacrylate (NBCA) adhesive, or coils and thrombin with clinical success in 12 and three patients respectively.[9] Choi et al used NBCA with or without coils in seven cases, with three requiring repeat embolisation.[10] More recently, two groups have reported outcomes of embolisation of type I endoleaks using Onyx, with or without coils, in a total of 14 patients with technical success achieved in all cases and one case of endoleak recurrence.[11,12]

We have previously reported our initial experience in six type I endoleak cases following conventional EVAR[13] and seven cases following Nellix EVAS.[5] More recently we published our cohort of 27 embolisation cases to date performed in 25 patients with mid-term outcome data.[4] This comprised 25 cases with proximal and two distal endoleaks. The average aneurysm sac size prior to embolisation was 8.2cm and the average time between endoleak diagnosis and EVAR was 685 days and was 27 days between endoleak diagnosis and embolisation. Onyx and coils were used in 11 cases and Onyx as sole embolisation agent was used in 16 cases. Complete isolation of the endoleak on completion angiography was achieved in all procedures.

During the average follow-up time of 311 days, seven patients developed endoleak recurrence. Two of these patients underwent a second embolisation procedure, one had no further endoleak, and the other developed a recurrent endoleak and died from sac rupture. Amongst the other five cases of endoleak recurrence, two were successfully managed by other procedures, one had a persistent endoleak despite aortic cuff placement and the other two were deemed unsuitable for further intervention. Three of the four patients with persistent endoleaks have died from sac rupture. The freedom from endoleak recurrence at the mean follow-up of 311 days was 80% and freedom from sac growth was 85%.

There were two interesting observations amongst our patient cohort. Endoleak recurrence was more common in patients undergoing embolisation with Onyx only compared with Onyx and coils. Six of seven patients with endoleak recurrence were embolised with Onyx only and only one patient had Onyx and coils. We have also observed a trend for a reduced risk of non-target embolisation with the latter approach. Secondly, post-embolisation outcomes were better in patients with the Nellix device compared with conventional endografts with only one of 11 Nellix patients developing endoleak recurrence, which was subsequently managed successfully with a second embolisation procedure. This compared with six of 14 patients with conventional endografts who developed recurrent endoleaks. One reason for this may be that the endoleaks were generally smaller in Nellix patients, possibly because of being constrained by the endobag in the perigraft space.

There were six procedural complications, none of which had long-term sequela. Three patients developed puncture site haematomas with two requiring surgical revision. There were three cases of Onyx reflux at the end of the embolisation procedure. Two of these occurred in patients with Nellix grafts within one of the two Nellix limbs and were both treated successfully by deployment of an additional stent within the Nellix endograft to affix the Onyx between the outside wall of the newly placed stent and the inside wall of the Nellix endograft. In another patient with a conventional aorto-uni-iliac endograft, a small amount of Onyx reflux into the endograft was identified, but was not thought to be significant and was not treated. The patient remained asymptomatic with no adverse findings on the follow-up computed tomography imaging.

## Conclusion

Transcatheter embolisation provides a safe treatment option for patients unsuitable or refractory to conventional type I endoleak treatment options with a high technical success and low endoleak recurrence rate. In our experience Onyx embolisation following deployment of coils within the endoleak cavity produces a more durable outcome, with a lower risk of non-target embolisation particularly with larger endoleaks.

## Summary

- Transcatheter embolisation offers a safe and feasible treatment option for type I endoleak cases unsuitable or refractory to conventional treatments.

- Endoleak cavities that are too small or too big are more difficult to treat using this option.

- Even with large endoleaks, in which all other options are exhausted, there is a role for emobolisation as a palliative measure.

- We suggest placement of coils within the endoleak cavity to form a "scaffold" prior to embolising the endoleak cavity with a liquid embolic, particularly with larger endoleaks.

# References

1. Van Marrewijk C, Buth J, Harris PL, *et al.* Significance of endoleaks after endovascular repair of abdominal aortic aneurysms: The EUROSTAR experience. *J Vasc Surg* 2002; **35** (3): 461–73.

2. Green N, Sidloff D, Stather PW, *et al.* Endoleak after endovascular aneurysm repair: Current status. *Rev Vasc Med* 2014; **2** (2): 43–47.

3. Rosen RJ, Green RM. Endoleak management following endovascular aneurysm repair. *J Vasc Interv Radiol* 2008; **19** (6 Suppl): S37–43.

4. Ameli-renani S, Pavlidis V, Morgan RA. Early and midterm outcomes after transcatheter embolization of type I endoleaks in 25 patients. *J Vasc Surg* 2017; **65** (2): 346–55.

5. Ameli-Renani S, Morgan RA. Transcatheter Embolisation of Proximal Type 1 Endoleaks Following Endovascular Aneurysm Sealing (EVAS) Using the Nellix Device: Technique and Outcomes. *Cardiovasc Intervent Radiol* 2015; **38** (5): 1137–42.

6. Golzarian J, Struyven J, Abada HT, *et al.* Endovascular aortic stent-grafts: transcatheter embolization of persistent perigraft leaks. *Radiology* 1997; **202** (3): 731–34.

7. Golzarian J, Maes EB, Sun S. Endoleak: Treatment options. *Tech Vasc Interv Radiol* 2005; **8** *(1 Special Issue):* 41–49.

8. Amesur NB, Zajko AB, Orons PD, Makaroun MS. Embolotherapy of persistent endoleaks after endovascular repair of abdominal aortic aneurysm with the ancure-endovascular technologies endograft system. *J Vasc Interv Radiol* 1999; **10** (9): 1175–82.

9. Maldonado TS, Rosen RJ, Rockman CB, *et al.* Initial successful management of type I endoleak after endovascular aortic aneurysm repair with n-butyl cyanoacrylate adhesive. *J Vasc Surg* 2003; **38** (4): 664–70.

10. Choi SY, Lee DY, Lee KH, *et al.* Treatment of type i endoleaks after endovascular aneurysm repair of infrarenal abdominal aortic aneurysm: Usefulness of N-butyl cyanoacrylate embolization in cases of failed secondary endovascular intervention. *J Vasc Interv Radiol* 2011; **22** (2): 155–62.

11. Henrikson O, Roos H, Falkenberg M. Ethylene vinyl alcohol copolymer (Onyx) to seal type 1 endoleak. A new technique. *Vascular* 2011; **19** (2): 77–81.

12. Eberhardt KM, Sadeghi-Azandaryani M, Worlicek S, *et al.* Treatment of type I endoleaks using transcatheter embolization with onyx. *J Endovasc Ther* 2014; **21** (1):1 62–71.

13. Chun J-Y, Morgan R. Transcatheter embolisation of type 1 endoleaks after endovascular aortic aneurysm repair with Onyx: when no other treatment option is feasible. *Eur J Vasc Endovasc Surg* 2013; **45** (2): 141–44.

# Fabric degeneration and type IIIb endoleaks remain a problem

## A England and R McWilliams

## Introduction

Over the past two decades, endovascular aneurysm repair (EVAR) has become the dominant treatment option for asymptomatic abdominal aortic aneurysms. More than half of all patients are these days treated with EVAR, and in many instances, elective open abdominal aortic aneurysm repair is reserved only for those who are anatomically unsuitable for EVAR.[1] Despite the success of EVAR and its widespread acceptance, there are still concerns regarding its durability.

Endoleak is the presence of blood flow outside the lumen of the stent graft but within the aneurysm.[2–5] Five categories of endoleak exist and classification is based on the origin of flow in the aneurysm.[2–4,6.] Type III endoleaks generally occur late during follow-up and are caused by modular disconnection (IIIa) or a fabric defect (IIIb).[7] Evidence suggests that type III endoleaks are associated with aneurysm rupture[8] and consequently urgent treatment is recommended.[2,9–11]

Endoleaks are present in between 15% and 52% of patients following EVAR.[12–20] Data from a recent conference paper reported a 7% incidence of type III endoleaks in first and second generation EVAR devices, and a lower (3%) rate for third-generation devices.[21] Jones and colleagues argue that limited data currently exist for the true incidence of type III endoleaks due to complexities in diagnosis and the convention of reporting types I and III endoleaks together.[22] Even when these endoleaks are reported separately, there is often a lack of distinction between types IIIa and IIIb. The EVAR trials contained a total of 21 type III endoleaks, but even in the in-depth analysis of 27 post-EVAR ruptures, type III endoleaks were not subdivided.[23]

## Structural disintegration and type III endoleaks

Structural disintegration is known to occur with stent grafts used in the repair of abdominal aortic aneurysms.[22] In a systematic review of late ruptures following EVAR, graft material failure was the cause of rupture in 97 out of 270 cases.[8] A limitation of this work is that only 40 of these cases included a description of the type of stent graft implanted. Fabric tears leading to type IIIb endoleaks can lead to pressurisation of the aneurysm with consequences such as aneurysm expansion and late rupture.[22]

Fabric tears commonly result from the apex of a stent rubbing against the fabric. The current configurations of stent grafts allow for micromotion of the individual metal stents against the fabric leading to graft wear.[24] Contact between the stent and the fabric can be further exacerbated as a result of stent graft distortion and suture breakage.[22] Stent fractures provide a further mechanism for direct trauma to the graft fabric.[25] In a study of 60 patients with stent graft fatigue, 43 had metallic stent fractures, 14 had suture stent disruptions and three had graft holes.[24] This report identified stent fractures in nitinol, stainless steel and cobalt-chromium/nickel based stents. Stress fatigue was identified as one of the possible causes of stent fracture together with metal corrosion.[24] This work also identified a relationship between the severity of the corrosive irregularity and the implantation time. The aetiology of type IIIb endoleaks suggests that this complication should be late occurring; however, there are emerging reports of early type IIIb endoleaks within the literature.[26]

Abouliatim and colleagues reported an intraoperative type IIIb endoleak in a patient with an Endurant stent graft (Medtronic).[26] They speculated that the cause of the fabric defect was due to one of four reasons: (i) excessive endovascular manipulation; (ii) excessive pressure of ballooning; (iii) damage to the fabric by the acute tip of a stent displaced by severe neck angulations; and (iv) a manufacturing defect. Van der Vliet and colleagues also described an early type IIIb endoleak which was caused by a fabric tear from low-pressure balloon modeling of a Zenith stent graft (Cook Medical).[27]

Reports regarding late type IIIb endoleaks are more frequent. Lee and colleagues[28] reported on a late type IIIb endoleak from graft erosion of an Excluder (Gore) stent graft. In this case, the patient presented symptomatically 12 months post-repair with a new pulsatile abdominal mass. Urgent CT demonstrated an intact aneurysm with a large endoleak. Catheter angiography demonstrated a large type IIIb endoleak originating from the proximal aspect of the ipsilateral limb. Review of prior surveillance imaging demonstrated no evidence of stent fractures. The authors concluded that both ePTFE and Dacron-based graft materials may be subject to tears or erosions resulting in a type IIIb endoleak and as such patients must be diligently followed for late device failure.

Banno and colleagues[29] reported on a late type IIIb endoleak leak from a fabric tear in the main body of a Zenith bifurcated stent graft approximately 19 months after implantation. More recently, Barburoglu and colleagues[30] reported a case of a type IIIb endoleak 14 months after successful EVAR with an Endurant device.

## Diagnosing type III endoleaks

Type IIIb endoleaks are notoriously difficult to diagnose and may be more common in second- and third-generation stent grafts than reports suggest.[22] Type IIIb endoleaks may be intermittent and multimodality imaging is often required for confident diagnosis. Diagnosis at catheter angiography may be difficult but definitive diagnosis is made if a selective catheter engages the defect (Figure 1). The visualisation difficulties at CT and catheter angiography have been further considered by Wanhainen and colleagues.[31] They postulated that pressure inside the intact aneurysm can prevent sufficient extravasation of iodinated contrast medium for detection.

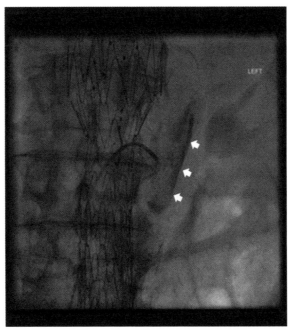

**Figure 1:** A type IIIb endoleak visualised during catheter angiography. The image presented in an unsubstracted angiogram where the catheter can be seen protruding through a hole in the stent graft fabric. Iodinated contrast media injected through the catheter can be visualised in the aneurysm (white arrows).

There has been significant discussion within the literature regarding difficulties in separating type II and III endoleaks and also identifying combined type II/III endoleaks. In the report by Turney *et al,* several patients presented with type III endoleaks combined with either type I or II endoleaks.[32] In problematic cases of aneurysm growth, type II endoleaks should not be accepted as the sole cause of aneurysm expansion until multimodality investigations with temporal information regarding perigraft flow have been completed.[22] The pattern of aneurysm growth with time may be a possible indicator of a graft-related endoleak. Sudden aneurysm growth late in follow-up is not typical of isolated type II endoleak. A rapid change in the aneurysm expansion rate should also be considered as potentially indicative of a graft-related endoleak. For example, in our experience, we have seen gradual expansion of an aneurysm during follow-up and then a sudden rapid increase in size. This patient was assessed using both CT and catheter-based angiography, and a type IIIb endoleak was confirmed.

There are accepted challenges when imaging suspected type IIIb endoleaks using CT, ultrasound and magnetic resonance (MR) imaging. In many instances, a definitive diagnosis can only be possible by positioning a catheter either close or directly through a fabric hole. In some patients, this will not be possible and diagnosis can only be confirmed at open conversion/graft explantation.

## Management of type IIIb endoleaks

Type IIIb endoleaks can be treated endovascularly or surgically. Endovascular options include repairing the defect with an aortic cuff extension or placement of a new stent graft, either bifurcated or aorto-uni-iliac with a femoro-femoral crossover graft.[30] If a diagnosis of a type IIIb endoleak can be made in a timely manner, then relining of the stent graft may be possible and would carry less risk than open surgical solution. A further treatment option is graft explanation with conversion to open repair. Up to 73% of explanations are performed for types I, II, or III endoleak.[33,34] Electively, explanation may be performed with between 0 and  3.3% mortality but in the presence of rupture this can be considerably higher.[34]

In more advanced EVAR procedures the treatment of type IIIb endoleaks can be more complex. McWilliams and colleagues presented a case of a type IIIb endoleak in a patient with a fenestrated EVAR device, and noted that treatment of such cases by relining would require incorporation of the target vessels in the repair.[35] In this scenario, the authors described a successful repair of the type IIIb endoleak using an Amplatzer septal occluder (Abbott). This case illustrates the operator's choice between focal repair of a fabric defect and relining of the entire graft. There are also reports of focal treatment at open repair where fabric holes have been repaired using a Teflon pledget or tissue glue.[22]

There are emerging reports of treating type IIIb endoleaks with endovascular sealing using the Nellix graft (Endologix).[36] It is, therefore, reassuring that a number of treatment options are available for managing type IIIb endoleaks and worldwide experience of these cases is growing.

## Summary

- No device is immune from structural failure leading to type IIIb endoleaks.

- Type IIIb endoleaks were originally thought to be late occurring but evidence now suggests that these can occur at any time point.

- Diagnosis can be difficult and is likely to require multimodality imaging together with a thorough review of the aneurysm history.

- Successful treatment is possible and in many instances this can be via an endovascular approach. Recent *in vitro* experiments have suggested that the shape of supporting stents should be revisited in order to further reduce the incidence of type IIIb endoleaks.[37]

- Greater understanding of the causes and incidence of fabric degradation would be achieved if explanted stent grafts were routinely subjected to structural analysis.[38,39]

## References

1. Chaikof EL, Brewster DC, Dalman RL, *et al*. The care of patients with an abdominal aortic aneurysm: the Society for Vascular Surgery practice guidelines. *Journal of Vascular Surgery* 2009; **50** (4 Suppl): S2–49.
2. Heikkinen MA, Arko FR, Zarins CK. What is the significance of endoleaks and endotension. *The Surgical Clinics of North America* 2004; **84** (5):1337–52.
3. White GH, May J, Waugh RC, *et al*. Type III and type IV endoleak: toward a complete definition of blood flow in the sac after endoluminal AAA repair. *Journal of Endovascular Surgery* 1998; **5** (4): 305–09.
4. White GH, May J, Waugh RC, Yu W. Type I and Type II endoleaks: a more useful classification for reporting results of endoluminal AAA repair. *Journal of Endovascular Surgery* 1998; **5** (2): 189–91.
5. White GH, Yu W, May J. Endoleak—a proposed new terminology to describe incomplete aneurysm exclusion by an endoluminal graft. *Journal of Endovascular Surgery* 1996; **3** (1): 124–25.

6. White SB, Stavropoulos SW. Management of endoleaks following endovascular aneurysm repair. *Seminars in Interventional Radiology* 2009; **26** (1): 33–38.

7. Teruya TH, Ayerdi J, Solis MM, *et al.* Treatment of type III endoleak with an aortouniiliac stent graft. *Annals of Vascular Surgery* 2003; **17 (2):** 123–8.

8. Schlosser FJ, Gusberg RJ, Dardik A, *et al.* Aneurysm rupture after EVAR: can the ultimate failure be predicted? *European Journal of Vascular and Endovascular Surgery* 2009; **37** (1): 15–22.

9. Politz JK, Newman VS, Stewart MT. Late abdominal aortic aneurysm rupture after AneuRx repair: a report of three cases. *Journal of Vascular Surgery* 2000; **31 (3):** 599–606.

10. Teutelink A, Van der Laan MJ, Milner R, Blankensteijn JD. Fabric tears as a new cause of type III endoleak with Ancure endograft. *Journal of Vascular Surgery* 2003; **38** (4): 843–46.

11. Zarins CK, White RA, Fogarty TJ. Aneurysm rupture after endovascular repair using the AneuRx stent graft. *Journal of Vascular Surgery*. 2000; **31** (5): 960–70.

12. May J, White GH, Waugh R, *et al.* Life-table analysis of primary and assisted success following endoluminal repair of abdominal aortic aneurysms: the role of supplementary endovascular intervention in improving outcome. *European Journal of Vascular and Endovascular Surgery* 2000; **19 (6):** 648–55.

13. Schurink GW, Aarts NJ, van Bockel JH. Endoleak after stent-graft treatment of abdominal aortic aneurysm: a meta-analysis of clinical studies. *The British Journal of Surgery* 1999; **86** (5): 581–87.

14. White GH, Yu W, May J, *et al.* Endoleak as a complication of endoluminal grafting of abdominal aortic aneurysms: classification, incidence, diagnosis, and management. *Journal of Endovascular Surgery* 1997; **4** (2): 152–68.

15. Buth J, Laheij RJ. Early complications and endoleaks after endovascular abdominal aortic aneurysm repair: report of a multicenter study. *Journal of Vascular Surgery* 2000; **31** (1 Pt 1) : 134–46.

16. Chuter TA, Faruqi RM, Sawhney R, *et al.* Endoleak after endovascular repair of abdominal aortic aneurysm. *Journal of Vascular Surgery* 2001; **34** (1): 98–105.

17. Zarins CK, White RA, Hodgson KJ, *et al.* Endoleak as a predictor of outcome after endovascular aneurysm repair: AneuRx multicenter clinical trial. *Journal of Vascular Surgery* 2000; **32** (1): 90–107.

18. Greenberg RK, Lawrence-Brown M, Bhandari G, *et al.* An update of the Zenith endovascular graft for abdominal aortic aneurysms: initial implantation and mid-term follow-up data. *Journal of Vascular Surgery* 2001; **33** (2 Suppl): S157–64.

19. Moore WS, Kashyap VS, Vescera CL, Quinones-Baldrich WJ. Abdominal aortic aneurysm: a 6-year comparison of endovascular *versus* transabdominal repair. *Annals of Surgery* 1999; **230 (3):** 298–308.

20. Arko FR, Hill BB, Olcott C, *et al.* Endovascular repair reduces early and late morbidity compared to open surgery for abdominal aortic aneurysm. *Journal of Endovascular Therapy* 2002; **9** (6): 711–18.

21. Poorteman L, Saint-Lebes B, Heye S, *et al.* Type III endoleak after endovascular aortic repair: incidence, etiology and management. European Congress of Radiology; Vienna, Austria 2015.

22. Jones SM, Vallabhaneni SR, McWilliams RG, Naik J, Nicholas T, Fisher RK. Type IIIb endoleak is an important cause of failure following endovascular aneurysm repair. *Journal of Endovascular Therapy* 2014; **21** (5): 723–27.

23. Wyss TR, Brown LC, Powell JT, Greenhalgh RM. Rate and predictability of graft rupture after endovascular and open abdominal aortic aneurysm repair: data from the EVAR Trials. *Annals of Surgery* 2010; **252** (5): 805–12.

24. Jacobs TS, Won J, Gravereaux EC, *et al.* Mechanical failure of prosthetic human implants: a 10-year experience with aortic stent graft devices. *Journal of Vascular Surgery* 2003; **37** (1): 16–26.

25. Chuter TA. Durability of endovascular infrarenal aneurysm repair: when does late failure occur and why? *Seminars in Vascular Surgery* 2009; **22** (2): 102–10.

26. Abouliatim I, Gouicem D, Kobeiter H, *et al.* Early type III endoleak with an Endurant endograft. *Journal of Vascular Surgery* 2010; **52** (6): 1665–67.

27. Van der Vliet JA, Blankensteijn JD, Kool LJ. Type III endoleak caused by fabric tear of a Zenith endograft after low-pressure balloon modeling. *Journal of Vascular and Interventional Radiology* 2005; **16** (7): 1042–44.

28. Lee WA, Huber TS, Seeger JM. Late type III endoleak from graft erosion of an Excluder stent graft: a case report. *Journal of Vascular Surgery* 2006; **44** (1): 183–5.

29. Banno H, Morimae H, Ihara T, *et al.* Late type III endoleak from fabric tears of a zenith stent graft: report of a case. Surgery Today 2012; **42** (12): 1206–09.

30. Barburoglu M, Acunas B, Onal Y, *et al.* Late Type 3b Endoleak with an Endurant Endograft. *Case Reports in Radiology* 2015: 783468.

31. Wanhainen A, Nyman R, Eriksson MO, Bjorck M. First report of a late type III endoleak from fabric tears of a Zenith stent graft. *Journal of Vascular Surgery* 2008; **48 (3):** 723–26.

32. Turney EJ, Steenberge SP, Lyden SP, *et al.* Late graft explants in endovascular aneurysm repair. *Journal of Vascular Surgery* 2014; **59** (4): 886–93.

33. Brinster CJ, Fairman RM, Woo EY, *et al*. Late open conversion and explantation of abdominal aortic stent grafts. *Journal of Vascular Surgery* 2011; **54** (1): 42–46.

34. Kelso RL, Lyden SP, Butler B, *et al*. Late conversion of aortic stent grafts. *Journal of Vascular Surgery* 2009; **49 (3):** 589–95.

35. McWilliams RG, Chan TY, Smout J, *et al*. Endovascular repair of type IIIb endoleak with the Amplatzer Septal Occluder. *Journal of Endovascular Therapy* 2016.

36. Swaelens C, Poole RJ, Torella F, *et al*. Type IIIb Endoleak and Relining: A mathematical model of distraction forces. *Journal of Endovascular Therapy* 2016; **23** (2): 297–301.

37. Lin J, Wang L, Guidoin R, *et al*. Stent fabric fatigue of grafts supported by Z-stents *versus* ringed stents: an in vitro buckling test. Journal of Biomaterials Applications 2014; **28**(7): 965–77.

38. Lin J, Guidoin R, Wang L, *et al*. Fatigue and/or failure phenomena observed in the fabric of stent-grafts explanted after adverse events. Journal of Long-Term Effects of Medical Implants 2013; **23 (1):** 67–86.

39. Riepe G, Heintz C, Kaiser E, *et al*. What can we learn from explanted endovascular devices? *European Journal of Vascular and Endovascular Surgery* 2002; **24** (2): 117–22.

# Influence of on-off instructions for use adherence on outcomes following EVAS

S Zerwes, S Bachhuber, Y Gosslau, R Jakob and
L Schnitzler

## Introduction

When Parodi first described a successful endovascular aneurysm repair (EVAR) in 1991 and hence enabled the birth of EVAR, he caused both a clinical and industrial revolution[1]—a "clinical revolution" because, following the introduction of EVAR, open aortic repair slowly but surely lost its status as the number one treatment option for abdominal aortic aneurysms, and an "industrial" one because this completely new platform generated innovation and development.[2,3] As with any revolution though, after the initial blast, some order and rules were needed. Again, this was both clinically and industrially: instructions for use (IFU) entered the scene and became indivisibly associated with any new EVAR device that came on to the market. Consequently, each endovascular device manufacturer published an IFU guideline that specified anatomic features for "proper" use of the EVAR device, exactly defining the indications and limitations of each stent graft.[4] What all the devices had in common was the fact that they depended on proximal and distal fixation to exclude the aneurysm.[5]

Close to 20 years after EVAR was developed, a new concept was introduced to vascular surgery: EndoVascular Aneurysm Sealing (EVAS).[6] This new system was different from all previous EVAR stent grafts because it abandoned the EVAR principles of proximal and distal fixation. Instead, polymer filled endobags achieved both the fixation of the stent grafts within the aorta and the exclusion of the aneurysm by completely filling the aneurysm sac with polymer.[7,8]

At our institution, we began using EVAS in 2013 and have since performed well over 200 procedures.[9] While plenty of data exist regarding the effects of the adherence to the IFUs on clinical outcomes for EVAR devices, there is only limited knowledge regarding the same effect for EVAS procedures.[4,10–12] We present our experience for 200 EVAS cases and pursue the question of how "on-off" IFU adherence influences outcomes following EVAS.

## Description of the IFU and patient cohort

When our institution performed the first EVAS implantation in July 2013, the IFU were similar to those for EVAR devices: an infrarenal aortic neck diameter that ranged from 16mm to 32mm, a minimum non-aneurysmal aortic proximal neck length ≥10mm, a proximal aortic neck angulation ≤60 degrees, and a diameter of the iliac arteries ranging from 8mm to 35mm.[7,9,13] However, a new requirement with EVAS was for a blood lumen diameter of ≤60mm. Taking the blood lumen into consideration, given the different types of aneurysm exclusion created by the endobags, seemed to be logical.

Between July 2013 and September 2016, at our institution, 200 consecutive patients were treated with EVAS. The term "consecutive" is important in this context because it meant no patient who underwent EVAS was later excluded from the retrospective study. Therefore, our cohort truly represents "real-world" patients and indeed comprised of patients with a large variety of pathologies and anatomies undergoing EVAS. This included 142 infrarenal aneurysms, 39 of which extended to the iliac arteries; 38 juxtarenal pathologies, eight of which also involved the iliac arteries; seven isolated iliac artery aneurysms; and lastly, 13 repair procedures for patients who had previously undergone EVAR. Not surprisingly, considering these pathologies, nearly 50% (i.e. 98 cases) of the EVAS procedures in our study were performed outside of the IFU.

However, the reasons why we classified a case as being outside of the IFU varied: the first reason, and most obvious of all, was that anatomic prerequisites for EVAS were not met; the second was that the procedure involved EVAS being combined with chimneys/snorkels for the treatment of juxtarenal or iliac artery aneurysms; third was that EVAS was being used to treat an acute rupture; and fourth was that the procedure was to repair an aneurysm that had been previously treated with EVAR. Naturally when we first started performing EVAS, we did not treat the more advanced cases—only feeling comfortable to use EVAS in these more complex anatomies when we had gained more experience.

## Outcomes within and outside IFU

Of 200 patients, 195 were successfully treated with EVAS—resulting in a primary technical success rate of 97.5%. Two of the five technical failures were intraoperative aneurysm ruptures caused by the endobags, two related to EVAS being unable to stop the bleeding after an acute rupture, and one involved the endobag itself rupturing and causing intra-arterial polymer leakage. Overall, four were cases that were classified as being outside of the IFU.

Thirty-day mortality was 3% (i.e. six out of 200 patients died). Of the patients who died, four were treated outside of the IFU for EVAS and were also considered to have had device-related deaths—all were affected by the technical failures previously described. Hence, performing EVAS outside of the IFU is clearly associated with higher rates of technical failure and 30-day mortality. That nearly 50% of patients in our study were treated outside of the IFU might explain why the outcomes in our study were not as good as those seen in previous experiences of EVAS.[8,12]

During a mean follow-up of 325 days (median 272, range 2–1,128), 10.5% of patients had an endoleak. However, more than twice as many patients who were treated outside of the IFU had an endoleak than had patients who were treated inside the IFU: 14.3% vs. 6.9%, respectively. While this difference was statistically not significant, it did call for a closer analysis of patients' initial diagnosis. This revealed

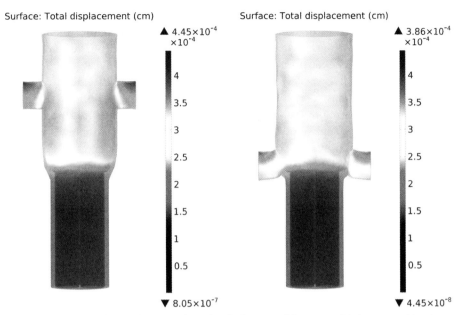

Surface: Total displacement (cm)     Surface: Total displacement (cm)

▲ 4.45×10⁻⁴     ▲ 3.86×10⁻⁴

**Figures 1 and 2:** Total surface displacements. The surface displacement of the aortic wall is demonstrated in colours ranging from black (minor displacement) to white/light grey (major displacement). Figure 1 shows a rather low proximal landing of the EVAS stent grafts and consequently a considerable (white/light grey) surface displacement, i.e. movement of the aortic segment above the stent grafts. Figure 2 shows a juxtarenal landing of the EVAS stent grafts, resulting in less movement of the aortic segment above the stent grafts and potentially explaining the lower endoleak rate in patients treated with EVAS in combination with chimney grafts.

a surprising finding; while one might expect patients with infrarenal aneurysms to have had the lowest rate of endoleaks, it was actually the patients with juxtarenal pathologies—treated with a combination of chimney grafts and EVAS—who did (3.2%).

We hypothesised that different flow dynamics might have played a role in why this anatomically challenging juxtarenal cohort treated with chimney grafts, and thus clearly outside of the IFU, came "out on top". Therefore, we asked our physics department to simulate two different scenarios: one, a very low (infrarenal) landing; two, a relatively high (juxtarenal) landing of the proximal ends of the EVAS stent grafts (Figures 1 and 2). The simulation showed that in the setting of a relatively low landing, there was considerably more total surface displacement, and hence movement of the aortic segment, compared with a relatively high landing.

Although it is important to note the limited follow-up time in our study, these preliminary findings might explain the low endoleak rate found in the subgroup treated with EVAS and chimney grafts. Additionally, they are in line with the suggestions of Matt Thomson *et al,* who argued that the majority of endoleaks were due to technical aspects of the implantation procedure (resulting in low landing of the device).[12]

## Conclusion

Endovascular repair is still in a phase of constant evolution—as such, EVAS is a new concept that differs from previous stent grafts mainly because of its use of polymer

Influence of on-off instructions for use adherence on outcomes following EVAS    ·    S Zerwes, S Bachhuber, Y Gosslau, R Jakob and L Schnitzler

technology. This means that the procedure not only departs from the traditional concept of proximal and distal fixation, but also involves the whole aneurysm sac being filled with polymer. In our experience, the cases treated outside of the IFU were associated with lower primary technical success, higher 30-day mortality, and higher rates of endoleaks. Nevertheless, it was a subgroup of the outside of IFU cases that had the lowest persisting endoleaks rate—patients who underwent EVAS in combination with chimney grafts for the treatment of juxtarenal pathologies. While one potential explanation might lie in the different set of flow dynamics, resulting in less total surface displacement and hence movement of the aortic segment, further studies and longer follow-up are needed to define the role of EVAS in the armamentarium for treatment of abdominal aortic aneurysms.

## Summary

- 20 years into EVAR evolution, EVAS is a new concept for treating abdominal aortic aneurysms by using a polymer technology that abandons the traditional principals of proximal and distal fixation.

- While plenty of data exist regarding the effects of the adherence to the IFUs on clinical outcomes for EVAR devices, there is only limited knowledge regarding the same effect for EVAS procedures.

- In our experience of 200 patients treated with EVAS, the cases carried out outside of the IFUs were associated with lower primary technical success, higher 30-day mortality and higher rates of endoleaks.

- Surprisingly, patients that received an EVAS implantation in combination with chimney grafts for treatment of juxtarenal pathologies, hence clearly being outside of the IFUs, had the lowest persisting endoleak rates.

- We believe that flow dynamics resulting in less aortic movement at the proximal neck, might be a potential explanation of the low endoleak rate of patients treated with EVAS and chimney grafts in juxtarenal pathologies.

## References

1. Parodi JC, Palmaz JC, Barone HD. Transfemoral intraluminal graft implantation for abdominal aortic aneurysms. *Ann Vasc Surg* 1991; **5**: 491–99.
2. Greenhalgh RM, Brown LC, Powell JT, *et al.* Endovascular *versus* open repair of abdominal aortic aneurysm. *N Engl J Med* 2010: **362** (20): 1863–71.
3. Schwarze ML, Shen Y, Hemmerich J, *et al.* Age-related trends in utilization and outcome of open and endovascular repair for abdominal aortic aneurysm in the United States, 2001–2006. *J Vasc Surg* 2009; **50**: 722–29.
4. Walker J, Tucker LY, Goodney P, *et al.* Adherence to endovascular aortic aneurysm repair device instructions for use guidelines has no impact on outcomes. *J Vasc Surg* 2015; **61** (5): 1151–59.
5. Leurs LJ, Kievit J, Dagnelie PC, *et al.* Influence of infrarenal neck length on outcome of endovascular abdominal aortic aneurysm repair. *J Endovasc Ther* 2006: **13** (5): 640–48.
6. Donayre CE, Zarins CK, Krievins DK, *et al.* Initial clinical experience with a sac-anchoring endoprosthesis for aortic aneurysm repair. *J Vasc Surg* 2011; **53** (3): 574–82.
7. Krievins DK, Holden A, Savlovskis J, et al., EVAR using the Nellix Sac-anchoring endoprosthesis: treatment of favourable and adverse anatomy. *Eur J Vasc Endovasc Surg* 2011; **42** (1): 38–46.
8. Bockler D, Holden A, Thompson M, *et al.* Multicenter Nellix endovascular aneurysm sealing system experience in aneurysm sac sealing. *J Vasc Surg* 2015; **401** (2):249–54.

9. Zerwes S, Nurzai Z, Leissner G, *et al*. Early experience with the new endovascular aneurysm sealing system Nellix: First clinical results after 50 implantations. Vascular 2016; **24** (4): 339–47.
10. Lee JT, Ullery BW, Zarins CK, *et al*. EVAR deployment in anatomically challenging necks outside the IFU. *Eur J Vasc Endovasc Surg* 2013; **46** (1): 65–73.
11. Zerwes S. Seduction and Its Impact on Instructions for Use. *J Endovasc Ther* 2016; **23** (5): 693–94.
12. Thompson MM, Heyligers JM, Hayes PD, *et al*. Endovascular aneurysm sealing: early and midterm results from the EVAS FORWARD Global Registry. *J Endovasc Ther* 2016; **23** (5): 685–92.
13. Chaikof EL, Brewster DC, Dalman RL, *et al*. The care of patients with an abdominal aortic aneurysm: the Society for Vascular Surgery practice guidelines. *J Vasc Surg* 2009; **50** (4 Suppl): S2–49.

# Classification of endoleak after EndoVascular Aneurysm Sealing

LH van den Ham, EJ Donselaar and MMPJ Reijnen

## Introduction

After its commercial release in 2013, the Nellix EndoVascular Aneurysm Sealing system (EVAS, Endologix) has been used to treat abdominal aortic aneurysms in over 7,000 cases, both within and outside the instructions for use (IFU).[1] The device's concept of sealing the aneurysmal sac is aimed at reducing the incidence of endoleaks and the subsequent reinterventions. The sealing concept using two polymer-filled endobags also acts as intraluminal fixation of the two individual stent grafts. The published literature so far has shown promising short-term results with ongoing research for long-term efficacy. However with more common usage and widespread application of EVAS, the first occurrences of different types of endoleaks have been reported, with type Ia endoleak being the most prevalent. Type II endoleaks are very rare with a small volume, usually detected by a core lab only, while type III endoleak could only occur in case of distal extensions. Because of the different concept of EVAS, when compared to standard endovascular aortic aneurysm repair (EVAR), a different approach is needed to diagnose and treat these endoleaks. In this chapter, we will review the occurrence of endoleak after EVAS and introduce a novel classification system with its clinical relevance.

## Reported endoleak incidence after EVAS

Clinical studies of patients treated with EVAS have shown a low incidence of early endoleaks (30 days) varying from 4% in a single-centre study to 4.7–6% in large multicentre registries.[2–4] The majority of endoleaks in all of these studies were type Ia endoleaks with type Ib, II and III being far less frequent. The EVAS FORWARD Global Registry was a postmarket, multicentre, open-label, single-arm registry that enrolled 277 patients without preoperative screening. Consequently, patients were treated both inside and outside of the IFU. Anatomical measurements and judgement of the presence of endoleak were performed by a core lab. Within 30 days, a type Ia endoleak was seen in eight cases, a type Ib endoleak in one case and a type II endoleak in five cases. Four of the reported type Ia endoleaks were treated with coils, and one resolved spontaneously. Four reported type II endoleaks resolved spontaneously and one remained patent without signs of aneurysm growth. Root cause analysis of the type Ia endoleaks by the core lab suggested the majority was caused by inadequate use of the proximal seal zone (low stent positioning) and underfilling of the endobags. Between 30 days and one year four new type Ia endoleaks developed and all were treated. There was also one type III endoleak between the Nellix device and a distal extension limb. At one year, the persistent endoleak rate was 0.7%, with one type Ia and one type II endoleak. The Kaplan-Meier estimates of freedom from types I and II endoleak at 12-month follow-up were 96% and 98%, respectively.

The Nellix system investigational device exemption (IDE) pivotal trial, as published by Carpenter *et al*, which enrolled 142 patients within IFU, reported a total endoleak rate at 30 days of 6.3% (type I, 0.7%; type II, 5.6%).[3] All of the type II endoleaks were less than 1ml in volume and involved only lumbar arteries. At one year the overall endoleak rate was 3.1% (type I, 0.8%; type II, 2.3%). There was no type III or IV endoleak at any time. In one case, a type Ia endoleak caused a contained rupture and was converted to open repair. All the type II endoleaks were left untreated. A type II endoleak after EVAS means there is an underfilled space inside the aneurysm sac with direct connection to a side branch with retrograde flow, or it is an open flow channel through the thrombus that was not filled by the endobags.

## Appearance on imaging and classification system

The most commonly used imaging modality for the detection of endoleaks is computed tomography (CT) angiography. In an evaluation of type Ia endoleaks after EVAS in 14 EVAS-experienced centres, CT angiography was predominantly used for the annual follow-up (unpublished data). Additionally duplex ultrasound was often used at a six-month interval to monitor aneurysm growth and endoleaks. Because of EVAS' unique appearance on CT angiography follow-up of EVAS patients requires knowledge of both the normal appearance as well as of early signs for endoleaks. The normal appearance after EVAS has been previously described and changes over time; for example, there is a normal change in the endobag density during the first months and also the intensity of the thrombus changes during the first year.[5,6]

Signs for a proximal endoleak can include one or more of the following:

1) The presence of contrast between the endobag and the aneurysmal wall or mural thrombus (at neck level or inside the aneurysmal sac)
2) The presence of contrast in between the endobags (at neck level or inside the aneurysmal sac)
3) Distal stent migration over time compared to previous imaging
4) Endobag separation. The distance between the two endobags should remain stable over time. Any displacement without visible contrast leak is associated with the presence of a proximal type endoleak. As such the space between the endobags is usually filled with fresh thrombus[7]
5) Aneurysm sac growth without presence of one of the above factors. Sac growth is suggestive for pressurisation of the aneurysm and is, therefore, indicative of inadequate seal either proximally or distally

When there is a suspicion of an endoleak without proof, for instance in aneurysm growth, without a visible contrast leak other imaging modalities should be considered. In the past both magnetic resonance (MR) angiography and ECG-gated CT angiogram have been proven viable in the detection of endoleaks.[8,9]

At the conception of the classification system for endoleaks after EVAR, the flow routing was used to define where the leak was present, what could have caused it and what the best way to treat it was. However, after EVAS, the routes are predominantly from the cranial part of the aneurysm (hence a type Ia), but the aethiology and clinical consequences of each are different and, consequently, a new classification suitable for Nellix EVAS is required. This new classification should be based on the device's (inadequate) sealing mechanism and can, therefore, be referred to as a type "Is(eal)" endoleak.

A type Is1 endoleak is defined as the appearance of contrast between the endobag and the wall of the proximal neck but not reaching the aneurysm sac itself. Per definition this would not be considered as being an endoleak but in EVAS they require consideration. When they do not disappear spontaneously in the early phase or progresses over time these endoleaks should be treated, as they seem to be prone for progression into a more severe type of endoleak. Type Is2 endoleaks are defined as those where there is contrast between the endobag and the aneurysmal wall or thrombus inside the aneurysm sac. This situation should be considered as a repressurisation of the aneurysmal sac that may lead to rupture. There have been anecdotal cases in which these endoleaks present with an outflow vessel, either a lumbar artery or the inferior mesenteric artery. A type 1s2 endoleak usually requires treatment. A type Is3 endoleak differs from the two endoleaks mentioned before as they show contrast or fresh thrombus between the endobags inside the aneurysm sac. This type of endoleak is mostly seen in combination with migration of stent grafts and has a late presentation due to their nature. These endoleaks do require urgent reintervention as they can lead to rupture due to the increase in sac pressure. This endoleak should be considered as the most unstable situation. Lastly, a type Is4 endoleak is the presence of sac pressurisation without proof or with the presence of secondary signs. If there is, for instance, an increase in aneurysm diameter or an increase in the distance from the proximal part of the stent to the lowest renal artery further investigation for an endoleak is required. ECG-gated CT angiography is a viable option for further imaging in these types of endoleak. Especially in the earlier generation devices special attention should be given to the distal seal as in this generation the endobag did not have a distal fixation and as such might not have been positioned well in the common iliac artery.

## Prevention and treatment of endoleaks

Current data suggest that endoleaks after EVAS can be prevented in multiple ways. Firstly, patient selection and subsequent aneurysmal morphology are vital to a successful outcome. Ongoing studies include both patient groups within and outside of the IFU. Strict adherence to the IFU is associated with lower reintervention rates. The EVAS FORWARD Global Registry reported a 98% freedom from reintervention within the IFU patients compared to 86% freedom from reintervention in the non-IFU group after 12 months. Recently, the IFU have been refined in an attempt to further minimise late complications and reinterventions.

Another key factor in endoleak prevention is proper stent placement. Nellix EVAS is suitable for necks with a minimal length of 10mm, but one should use these lengths to its full extent in order to gain adequate seal. Placement of the endobags flush below the renal arteries will maximise the sealing zone. Preliminary data from an upcoming multicentre study in which type Ia endoleaks were analysed showed that the majority of endoleaks might have been prevented if there was a full use of the neck's entire sealing length. In cases with short necks the use of renal and/or visceral chimneys is advised to prevent endoleak and migration. Furthermore, the stent grafts should be aligned as much as possible during placement. Any apposition or offset of either stent graft can lead to failure in sealing on one side of the sac and therefore lead to an endoleak. Particular anatomies may complicate procedural placement. Asymmetrical "stomach shaped" aneurysms are particularly difficult to treat as competition of the endobags may lead to an offset position of the stents. Small common iliac arteries may reduce the options for repositioning as the stents are balloon-expandable with a diameter of 10mm.

Procedural type Ia endoleaks may occur after primary fill and are sometimes hard to detect. A secondary fill can be performed to gain extra seal from the device's endobags and possibly exclude the endoleak. It is advised to perform high-quality angiography in at least two directions using a pigtail catheter with one device still in place to perform a secondary fill if required. A lateral view is important to detect possible ventral or dorsal endoleaks that can be missed on anteroposterior view and can be present at the attachment zones of the two endobags. If the endoleak is still persisting after secondary fill direct embolisation is advised.

Individual cases have been described in which an early endoleak disappeared on later imaging without reintervention. A prolonged wait-and-see policy regarding these endoleaks is, however, not advised as they tend to increase over time. If there is a type Is1 endoleak in early follow-up a transcatheter embolisation using coils with Onyx (Medtronic) or glue is an effective treatment option.[10,11] This method of embolisation prevents the endoleak from progressing towards the aneurysm sac and becoming a type Is2 or Is3 endoleak. The same treatment strategy could be applied in Is2 endoleaks when the endoleak occurs with a proper position of the stents (Figure 1).

If the endoleak is related to malpositioning of the stents, distal migration or when a more extensive type Is2 or type Is3 endoleak is present the sealing length

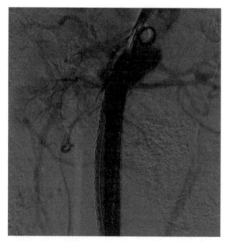

**Figure 1A:** Procedural type Is2 endoleak on lateral view.

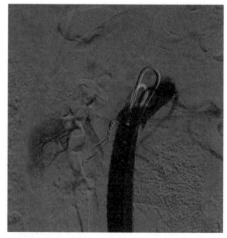

**Figure 1B:** Successful selective coiling of the endoleak.

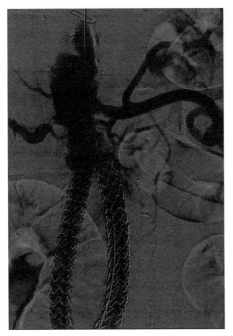 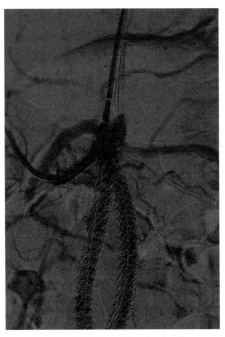

**Figure 2A:** Procedural angiography before Nellix-in-Nelix with chimney placement, webbing of the stent grafts can be seen caused by migration.

**Figure 2B:** Two Nellix devices placed with a chimney in the right renal artery.

should be improved. Proximalisation using two extra Nellix stents (Nellix-in-Nellix) is a feasible method in cases where there is inadequate seal and/or device migration, but obviously outside of the IFU for the device.[12] Careful planning is paramount in the success of Nellix-in-Nellix proximalisation (Figure 2). To gain adequate neck seal length a protrusion of at least 3cm to 4cm, depending on the neck diameter, is needed above the original stents. The use of chimneys should not be withheld to reach adequate sealing length. Obviously, open conversion should always be considered if the patient is fit. In type Is4 the treatment will depend on the most likely cause of growth. Close surveillance could be a first strategy but careful judgement of all sealing zones is essential.

## Conclusion

Endoleaks after EVAS do occur but are not frequent, with type Ia being the most predominant type. Patient selection and technique seem to play an important role in their prevention. A new classification method is helpful to correctly diagnose and treat these endoleaks and standardise reporting.

## Summary

- Endoleaks after EVAS are uncommon and differ from endoleaks after EVAR.

- Type Ia endoleaks after EVAS are often related to case selection and technique.

- Different appearances in type Ia endoleaks require a different classification system.

- Transcatheter embolisation and proximal extensions can both be applied successfully, depending on the cause of the endoleak.

## References

1. van den Ham LH *et al*. Abdominal aortic aneurysm repair using Nellix endovascular aneurysm sealing. *Surg Technol Int* 2015; **26**: 226–31.
2. Brownrigg JR *et al*. Endovascular aneurysm sealing for infrarenal abdominal aortic aneurysms: 30-day outcomes of 105 patients in a single centre. *Eur J Vasc Endovasc Surg* 2015; **50** (2): 157–64.
3. Carpenter JP *et al*. Results of the Nellix system investigational device exemption pivotal trial for endovascular aneurysm sealing. *J Vasc Surg* 2016; **63** (1): 23–31 e1.
4. Thompson MM *et al*. Endovascular Aneurysm Sealing: Early and midterm results from the EVAS FORWARD Global Registry. *J Endovasc Ther* 2016; **23** (5): 685–92.
5. Holden A *et al*. Imaging after Nellix Endovascular Aneurysm Sealing: A consensus document. *J Endovasc Ther*, 2016; **23** (1): 7–20.
6. Van den Ham LH *et al*. Evolution of computed tomography imaging the first year after endovascular sealing of infrarenal aortic aneurysms using the Nellix device. Submitted for publication, 2016.
7. Cheng LF *et al*. Early enlargement of aneurysmal sac and separation of endobags of Nellix Endovascular Aneurysm Sealing System as signs of increased risk of later aneurysm rupture. *Cardiovasc Intervent Radiol* 2016; **39** (11): 1654–57.
8. Koike Y *et al*. Dynamic volumetric CT angiography for the detection and classification of endoleaks: application of cine imaging using a 320-row CT scanner with 16-cm detectors. *J Vasc Interv Radiol* 2014; **25** (8): 1172–80.
9. Wieners G *et al*. Detection of type II endoleak after endovascular aortic repair: comparison between magnetic resonance angiography and blood-pool contrast agent and dual-phase computed tomography angiography. Cardiovasc Intervent Radiol 2010; **33** (6): 1135–42.
10. Ameli-Renani S and RA Morgan. Transcatheter embolisation of proximal type 1 dndoleaks following Endovascular Aneurysm Sealing (EVAS) using the Nellix device: Technique and outcomes. *Cardiovasc Intervent Radiol* 2015; **38** (5): 1137–42.
11. Ameli-Renani S *et al*. Embolisation of a proximal type I endoleak post-Nellix aortic aneurysm repair complicated by reflux of Onyx into the Nellix endograft limb. *Cardiovasc Intervent Radiol* 2015; **38** (3): 747–51.
12. Donselaar EJ *et al*. Feasibility and technical aspects of proximal Nellix-in-Nellix extension for late caudal endograft migration. *J Endovasc Ther* 2016. Epub.

# Type II endoleak

# The transiliac route for the embolisation of type II endoleaks after EVAR: Technique, when to attempt it and efficacy

S Ameli-Renani, V Pavlidis, L Mailli and RA Morgan

## Introduction

Type II endoleaks are the most common type of endoleak following EVAR and result from retrograde flow of blood from aortic or iliac collaterals into the aneurysm sac.

Whilst there is consensus on prompt treatment of type I and III endoleaks, which tend to be high-pressure leaks, the management of type II endoleaks is a subject of debate. This reflects the low pressure, and often transient, nature of type II endoleaks, which are usually fed by low flow vessels. Hence, their natural progression and clinical significance are poorly understood and as such, indications for treatment are controversial. Whilst several studies have shown conservative management to be safe, others have shown risk of sac expansion and rupture with these.[1-4] However, most would advocate intervention for patients with a persistent endoleak associated with a significant increasing aneurysm sac size of more than 5mm.[5-9]

The transiliac approach is a novel technique for transarterial embolisation of type II endoleaks by accessing the endoleak sac via a paraendograft approach through the distal landing zone, termed the transiliac paraendograft embolisation (TAPE) approach by the authors.[10]

## Technique—how we do it

The computed tomography (CT) angiogram images are reviewed prior to the procedure specifically to assess the degree of apposition between the distal aspect of each iliac endograft limb and the wall of the native common iliac artery. On close inspection, it is not uncommon for there to be complete apposition of the entire circumference of the endograft limb to the artery wall, usually due to angulation of the native iliac artery. The side with the least apposition between the iliac limb and iliac artery wall is selected for access. If there is complete apposition between the limb and artery wall on both sides, the technique may still be feasible, and the side with the shortest extent of the iliac limb in the common iliac iliac artery is chosen.

A short 6Fr sheath is advanced following retrograde femoral artery access. A combination of an angled 4/5Fr catheter (e.g. cobra or vertebral) and a hydrophilic guidewire (usually straight) is used to find a path into the paraendograft space between the iliac endograft and the vessel wall. The guidewire and subsequently the catheter are advanced upwards between the limb and the artery wall until they access the aneurysm sac.

Entry into the endoleak nidus is confirmed by the retrograde flow of blood from the proximal end of the catheter. If, at this point, the guidewire and catheter are found to be located in the sac thrombus, it is usually possible to access the nidus using standard catheter/guidewire manipulations. In cases where this is difficult because of the narrow space between the endograft limb and the iliac arterial wall, it may be helpful to place a longer supporting sheath (6Fr or larger) over the guidewire into the paraendograft space.

After engaging the endoleak with the catheter, a microcatheter is advanced coaxially into the endoleak cavity and an "endoleakogram" is performed to outline the size and anatomy of the endoleak nidus prior to performing embolisation.

The authors prefer to use ethylene vinyl alcohol copolymer (Onyx, Medtronic) for embolisation. However, other embolic agents such as glue may be used according to operator preference. The use of a liquid embolic is thought to be important, however, in order to achieve complete filling of the endoleak nidus including the origins of the inflow and outflow vessels, without selective catheterisation of each vessel.[9]

Embolisation is performed until there is complete filling of the nidus (Figure 1). Onyx (Medtronic) may also pass into the feeding arteries although this is not invariably observed using the Onyx 34 formulation. After occlusion of the endoleak nidus, the catheter is removed.

A road map to define the location of the nidus obtained by selective angiography of the artery supplying the endoleak, e.g. the ipsilateral internal iliac artery or the superior mesenteric artery, may be helpful in targeting the nidus.

As with other interventions in patients with endografts, we administer intravenous antibiotic prophylaxis to avoid subsequent graft infection.

## The rationale for parailiac embolisation

The treatment of type II endoleaks aims to halt sac expansion and prevent aneurysm rupture by occluding the endoleak. The mainstay of type II endoleak embolisation is transarterial embolisation using a coaxial technique to catheterise the nidus of the endoleak selectively via its feeding vessels.[9,11,12] This technique is often feasible when treating endoleaks arising from the inferior mesenteric artery and if there is a clear path from the superior mesenteric artery via the marginal artery to the inferior mesenteric artery. However, it is frequently difficult when a lumbar artery is the source due to inability to cannulate the responsible vessel or failure to navigating the catheter through small arteries into the endoleak nidus owing to the tortuosity of the small communicating vessels feeding the endoleak.[13] Failure to embolise the endoleak nidus has been shown to be associated with an increased risk of recurrence due to the nidus recruiting additional flow from adjacent vessels.[14]

In recent years new techniques for occluding type II endoleaks have been developed to access the endoleak nidus directly. These include a translumbar

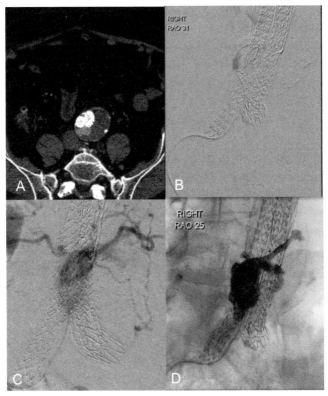

**Figure 1:** Paraendograft transiliac embolisation of type II endoleak. (A) Axial CT angiogram image shows persistent type II endoleak arising from lumbar arteries associated with a 6mm increase in sac size over six months. (B) 6Fr 45cm sheath placed with the tip adjacent to the distal end of the right iliac limb of the Nellix endograft and 5Fr Cobra catheter advanced into the space between the endograft and arterial wall and negotiated into the endoleak cavity over a hydrophilic wire. (C) "Endoleakogram" via injection of contrast through a microcatheter advanced coaxially into the endoleak cavity demonstrates size of endoleak and reflux of contrast into the lumbar arteries. (D) Single image exposure showing filling of the endoleak following Onyx embolisation.

approach, whereby a needle is advanced directly into the nidus under CT or fluoroscopic guidance and transcaval embolisation.[15–17]

Transiliac embolisation is a new technique for accessing and embolising the endoleak nidus. Although the individual lumbar or inferior mesenteric artery vessels responsible for the endoleak are not themselves embolised, the nidus forming the communication between these and the other feeding arteries is abolished, which is similar to embolisation of the central nidus in arteriovenous malformations.

In this regard, the result of this technique is similar to translumbar and transcaval embolisation. However, this technique offers the advantage of avoiding a general anaesthetic and may be attempted at the same time as an attempt at embolisation using the conventional transarterial route, more familiar to operators trained in catheter angiography techniques.

## Feasibility and application

The technique can be applied in all cases where the conventional endovascular embolisation through the feeding vessels in not feasible or unsuccessful. Alternatively, it can be used before other methods are attempted. The procedure is less likely to be successful if the iliac endograft limbs have been extended to the external iliac arteries, and particularly if a bare stent has been used to extend stent coverage distally.

Apart from a technical note on this approach authored by ourselves, there has been only one other publication on this technique.[10] Coppi and colleagues (2014) described a similar approach to obtain access to the endoleak sac in 16 of 17 attempts.[18] They used a combination of a 9Fr access site sheath and a 5/6Fr introducer sheath advanced into the aneurysm sac along the iliac paragraft space and used coils, cyanoacrylate, or fibrin glue for embolisation. They reported one case of intraoperative secondary type Ib endoleak despite routine ballooning of the iliac graft used to access the sac at the end of the procedure. In our experience, the use of a 6Fr sheath at the access site into the paraendograft space and a 4/5Fr catheter rather than a sheath to access the endoleaks sac is technically sufficient and minimises the risk of a procedural distal type I endoleak.

## Summary

- Transiliac paraendograft embolisation enables a transarterial direct access to a type II endoleak nidus at the distal landing zone via the space between the iliac limb and the native artery wall.

- It is particularly useful where the artery feeding the type II endoleak has tortuous branches which are not amenable to direct catheter access.

- A 5Fr catheter is usually sufficient to access the aneurysm sac and endoleak nidus, and minimises the risk of a procedural distal type I endoleak.

## References

1. Rayt HS, Sandford RM, Salem M, *et al*. Conservative management of type II endoleaks is not associated with increased risk of aneurysm rupture. *Eur J Vasc Endovasc Surg* 2009; **38** (6): 718–23.
2. Sidloff D, Gokani V, Stather PW, Choke E, *et al*. Type II endoleak: conservative management is a safe strategy. *Eur J Vasc Endovasc Surg* 2014; **48 (4):** 391–99.
3. Batti S El, Cochennec F, Roudot-thoraval F. Type II endoleaks after endovascular repair of abdominal aortic aneurysm are not always a benign condition. YMVA 2010; **57** (5): 1291–97.
4. Jones JE, Atkins MD, Brewster DC, *et al*. Persistent type II endoleak after endovascular repair of abdominal aortic aneurysm is associated with adverse late outcomes. *J Vasc Surg* 2007; 46: 1–8.
5. Ozdemir BA, Chung R, Benson RA, *et al*. Embolisation of type II endoleaks after endovascular aneurysm repair. *J Cardiovasc Surg* (Torino) 2013; **54** (4): 485–90.
6. Chung R, Morgan R. Type II endoleaks post-EVAR: Current evidence for rupture risk, intervention and outcomes of treatment. Cardiovasc Intervent Radiol 2014; **38** (3): 507–22
7. Moll FL, Powell JT, Fraedrich G, *et al*. Management of abdominal aortic aneurysms clinical practice guidelines of the European society for vascular surgery. *Eur J Vasc Endovasc Surg* 2011; **41** Suppl 1: S1–S58.
8. Gallagher KA, Ravin RA, Meltzer AJ, *et al*. Midterm outcomes after treatment of type II endoleaks associated with aneurysm sac expansion. *J Endovasc Ther* 2012; **19** (2): 182–92.
9. Aziz A, Menias CO, Sanchez L a, *et al*. Outcomes of percutaneous endovascular intervention for type II endoleak with aneurysm expansion. *J Vasc Surg* 2012; **55** (5): 1263–67.
10. Ameli-Renani S, Pavlidis V, Mailli L, *et al*. Transiliac paraendograft embolisation of type 2 endoleak: An alternative approach for endoleak management. *Cardiovasc Intervent Radiol* 2016; **39** (2): 279–83. Transiliac Paraendograft Embolisation of Type 2 Endoleak: An Alternative Approach for Endoleak Management.
11. Hongo N, Kiyosue H, Shuto R, *et al*. Double coaxial microcatheter technique for transarterial aneurysm sac embolization of type II endoleaks after endovascular abdominal aortic repair. *J Vasc Interv Radiol* 2014; **25** (5): 709–16.

12. Abularrage CJ, Patel VI, Conrad MF, Schneider EB, *et al.* Improved results using Onyx glue for the treatment of persistent type II endoleak after endovascular aneurysm repair. *J Vasc Surg* 2012; **56** (3): 630–36.
13. Chung R, Morgan R. Technical Note: "Remote" transarterial embolisation technique of lumbar artery type II endoleaks with Onyx. *EJVES Extra* 2014; **27** (4): e32–33.
14. Massis K, Carson WG, Rozas A, Patel V, *et al.* Treatment of type II endoleaks with ethylene-vinyl-alcohol copolymer (Onyx). *Vasc Endovascular Surg* 2012; **46** (3): 251–57.
15. Sidloff D a, Stather PW, Choke E, Bown MJ, *et al.* Type II endoleak after endovascular aneurysm repair. *Br J Surg* 2013; **100** (10): 1262–70.
16. Baum R, Carpenter JP, Golden M, *et al.* Treatment of type II endoleaks after endovascular repair of abdominal aortic aneurysms: Comparison of transarterial and translumbar techniques. *J Vasc Surg* 2002; **35** (1): 23–29.
17. Mansueto G, Cenzi D, Scuro A, *et al.* Treatment of type II endoleak with a transcatheter transcaval approach: results at 1-year follow-up. *J Vasc Surg* 2007; **45** (6): 1120–27.
18. Coppi G, Saitta G, Gennai S, Lauricella a, *et al.* Transealing: a novel and simple technique for embolization of type II endoleaks through direct sac access from the distal stent-graft landing zone. *Eur J Vasc Endovasc Surg* 2014; **47** (4): 394–401.

**Ruptured aneurysm**

# EVAR simulation for ruptured aortic aneurysm saves lives

M Venermo, L Vikatmaa and P Aho

## Introduction

Open surgery for the treatment of ruptured abdominal aortic aneurysms (AAA) has been available for more than 60 years and is associated with a mortality rate of 30–40%.[1,2] Due to long traditions, the time from patient presentation to the start of the procedure is one of the shortest in operating rooms. In a large operating room—such as ours at the Helsinki University Hospital, treating some 50 emergency aneurysms annually—personnel frequently face medical emergencies in which a short door-to-procedure time is life-saving.

The treatment of an aneurysm changed dramatically after the introduction of endovascular aneurysm repair (EVAR) 25 years ago; today, most of the elective cases are managed by endovascular means.[2,4]

EVAR has also established a place in the treatment of ruptured aneurysms. Although randomised trials have failed to show lower mortality with ruptured EVAR, an increasing number of experts acknowledge the benefits of endovascular treatment and prefer it—at least for anatomically suitable patients.[5–8] One of the major benefits of ruptured EVAR is the haemodynamic stability that can be achieved by using local anaesthesia. General anaesthesia is mainly used for open abdomen treatment in patients who develop or who are at risk of developing abdominal compartment syndrome.[9]

While the treatment process of ruptured aneurysm patients undergoing open surgery in our hospital is rapid, this was initially not the case for such patients undergoing EVAR. The elective EVAR procedures that are performed at our hospital are usually performed by the same team; therefore, when such a procedure is performed, all members of the team are familiar with the endovascular approach. However, most ruptured aneurysm patients present during "off hours"—i.e. during the evenings, nights or weekends—when there is a high probability that the operating team on duty (given in our operating department, there is more than 200 staff) is not familiar with EVAR.

Compared to open surgery, the ruptured EVAR team includes a radiology nurse as an "extra player". Furthermore, the anaesthesia personnel in the team have to be familiar with the benefits of using local anaesthesia for ruptured EVAR. While the vascular surgeons who perform elective EVAR will also be the ones who perform ruptured EVAR, they do need to change their mindset to ensure that they achieve the fastest possible haemodynamic control with an aortic occlusion balloon. Preparation time and time from door-to-aortic closure were unacceptably long at our hospital. To shorten this timeframe, from August 2015, we began to perform ruptured EVAR simulations once a month. The aim of the simulations is to practise the pathway of the ruptured aneurysm patient from the operating room door to the point at which the occlusion balloon is in place. The ultimate goal is to perform this in five minutes. We plan to continue with the monthly simulations until the entire operating room staff is trained and, thereafter, proceed with a less frequent but still regular simulation schedule to keep up the awareness and train new personnel.

## Simulation sessions and development of the performance

The simulations take place in the same hybrid suite where all the real-life procedures for ruptured aneurysms are performed. The room is equipped with a Artis zeego interventional angiography system (Siemens Healthineers). A patient simulator (Resusci Anne Simulator, Laerdal), designed for the training of emergency care staff in both pre-hospital and in-hospital environments, is used. It is anatomically realistic with functionalities for airway management, live defibrillation and synchronised ECG, blood pressure and heart rate monitoring, voice, lung and heart sounds, and cardiopulmonary resuscitation (CPR) feedback. Each simulation session is video recorded.

All participants receive electronic material on the simulation a week before the actual session. Furthermore, they fill out an electronic questionnaire beforehand, which they repeat after the simulation. The simulation session includes three parts:

1. The briefing. Participants are informed on the course of the simulation and receive their duty cards. There are six different types of duty cards (Figure 1), one for each player in the team—the scrub nurse, anaesthesiology nurse, radiology nurse, second scrub nurse (assisting), anaesthesiologist, and vascular surgeon. During briefing, the duties of each participant are reviewed based on the cards.

2. The simulation. It starts when the vascular surgeon receives a "telephone call" about a ruptured aneurysm patient who has arrived in computed tomography (CT) room at the emergency department and ends when the occlusion balloon is in place. The "patient" arrives in the operating room five

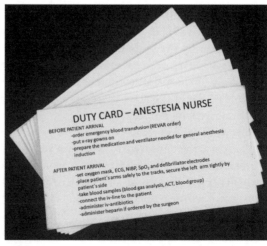

**Figure 1:** The duty card of the anaesthesia nurse. At the beginning of the simulation, each participant receives a duty card that lists his/her duties during the preparation of the patient for ruptured EVAR. There are six different duty cards.

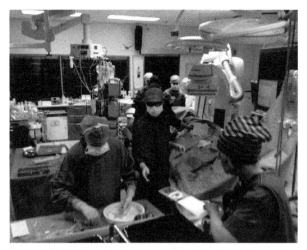

**Figure 3:** Simulation session in progress. The patient is ready for a groin puncture but the scrub nurse is not yet ready with the equipment. The radiological nurse is offering the introducer.

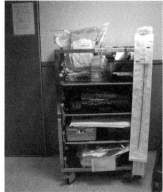

**Figure 4:** All of the equipment needed for the placement of occlusion balloon in local anaesthesia is in one corridor outside the hybrid room. The equipment includes instrument kit for open conversion and aortic clamping.

to 10 minutes after the telephone call. All of the equipment that is needed to insert the occlusion balloon is normally outside the hybrid operating room (Figure 2) and during the simulation the same equipment is used.

3. The debriefing. During the debriefing, a video recording of the simulation session is shown and the participants are free to discuss their views on the simulation as well as provide suggestions as to how to improve future simulations and real-life ruptured EVAR procedures. After each debriefing, the coaches meet to evaluate the session and discuss possible future improvements.

Overall, nine to 10 people participate in each simulation: two scrub nurses, two anaesthesiology nurses, one radiological nurse, one to two anaesthesiologists, and two vascular surgeons. During each session, the time between the patient's arrival in the operating room and when the occlusion balloon is in place is recorded (door-to-occlusion time).

In addition to evaluating the team's performance during the simulation, we analysed the changes in the treatment of real-life ruptured aneurysm patients. All CT-verified patients treated by endovascular means between January 2013 and August 2016 were evaluated retrospectively from hospital and patient records. The time from the patient arriving at the operating room to the start of the procedure (the patient is ready for puncture) was evaluated.

Since August 2015, 20 monthly simulation sessions had been arranged (up to August 2016) (Figure 3). In the first simulations, the door-to-occlusion time was 32 minutes. After modifying the simulation so that the "patient" collapses and requires CPR soon after the beginning of the simulation, the time decreased to 10–13 minutes in the most recent simulations (including a five-minute resuscitation period). Another change was made to the briefing: we highlighted that the main goal of the session is to insert the occlusion balloon into the aorta as soon as possible and focus should be kept on preparation of the occlusion balloon, ultrasound, C-arm and the patient´s groin.

In the electronic questionnaire on the confidence and knowledge of the operating staff regarding the treatment of ruptured EVAR patients before and after simulations, there was improvement in all except one of the questions. The greatest improvement was seen with answer to the question "how I feel about my skills during ruptured EVAR", with the median answer changing from "uncertain" before the simulations to "confident" after the simulations. In only one question, the answer remained at the same before and after the simulations. Responding to the question—on a scale of one to seven (with one representing "not at all" and seven "I totally agree")—I have already enough experience from ruptured EVAR cases in real life", participants, on average, answered with "two" both before and afterwards.

The simulations seemed to have had a significant impact on the treatment of real-life patients. Of 36 ruptured EVAR patients treated at our centre since January 2013, the median door-to-needle time was 68 minutes for 20 aneurysms treated before August 2015 (i.e. before the beginning of the simulations) and 16 minutes for those treated afterwards ($p<0.01$).

## Conclusion

The treatment of ruptured aneurysm patients has shifted from open surgery to EVAR because of the less-invasive nature of the endovascular approach. In a large hospital with a multidisciplinary operating room, building a ruptured EVAR service is challenging as most ruptured EVAR cases do not present during office hours but rather in the evenings and weekends. Therefore, those working during "off hours" have to take responsibility for performing ruptured EVAR and are not, necessarily, the same team members who perform elective EVAR.

To improve the understanding and knowledge of the ruptured EVAR process among operating room staff at our hospital, we started providing regular simulation sessions. This has decreased the door-to-needle time in ruptured aneurysm patients to a quarter of that before the simulations. Not all ruptured aneurysm patients can be treated with EVAR. Therefore, the probable "best-case" scenario for a patient would be to present at a hospital where both surgical and endovascular skills are available and offered at an experienced level. This is the attitude in our hospital.

We do not choose EVAR in cases where it would require clear compromises such as a high risk of later complications—we tend to perform open surgery in cases (e.g. juxtarenal ruptured aneurysms) in which no clear contraindications to surgery exist. As all patients are treated in the same operating room, those who eventually undergo surgery may also benefit from their operating staff having undergone the simulations—the occlusion balloon is a respectable alternative to blind clamping at the beginning of the open procedure.

## Summary

- The successful treatment of a ruptured aneurysm patient with EVAR leads to more rapid recovery, shorter or no stay in the intensive care unit, and a shorter stay at the hospital compared with open surgery. Patients who undergo EVAR under local anaesthesia and do not sustain abdominal compartment syndrome recover particularly well.

- Building a ruptured EVAR service in a large operating room is challenging as all nurses and anaesthesiologists need to master performing ruptured EVAR outside of office hours.

- With ruptured EVAR simulations, the preparation of the patient can be practised safely and effectively. In the simulation, the co-operation between different professional groups in the operating room is practised, with everyone having the same goal—to insert the occlusion balloon in the aorta.

- Ruptured EVAR simulations seem to lead to significant improvement in in real life in terms of shorter aortic occlusion time and maybe also to lesser bleeding, a lower abdominal compartment syndrome incidence as well as a higher survival.

# References

1. Powell JT, Sweeting MJ, Thompson MM, *et al*. Endovascular or open repair strategy for ruptured abdominal aortic aneurysm: 30 day outcomes from IMPROVE randomised trial. *BMJ* 2014; **348**: f7661

2. Mani K, Lees T, Beiles B, Jensen LP, *et al*. Treatment of abdominal aortic aneurysm in nine countries 2005–2009: a vascunet report. *Eur J Vasc Endovasc Surg* 2011; **42**: 598–607.

3. Parodi JC, Palmaz JC, Barone HD. Transfemoral intraluminal graft implantation for abdominal aortic aneurysms. *Ann Vasc Surg* 1991; **5**(6): 491–99.

4. Beck AW, Sedrakyan A, Mao J, Venermo M, *et al*. International Consortium of Vascular Registries. Variations in Abdominal Aortic Aneurysm Care: A report from the international consortium of vascular registries. *Circulation* 2016; **134** (24): 1948–58.

5. Powell JT, Hinchliffe RJ. Emerging strategies to treat ruptured abdominal aortic aneurysms. *Expert Rev Cardiovasc Ther* 2015; **13** (12): 1411–18.

6. Veith FJ, Lachat M, Mayer D, Malina M, *et al*. Collected world and single center experience with endovascular treatment of ruptured abdominal aortic aneurysms. *Ann Surg* 2009; **250** (5): 818–24.

7. Sweeting MJ, Balm R, Desgranges P, *et al*. Individual-patient meta-analysis of three randomized trials comparing endovascular *versus* open repair for ruptured abdominal aortic aneurysm. *Br J Surg* 2015; **102** (10): 1229–39.

8. Powell JT, Hinchliffe RJ, Thompson MM, *et al*. Observations from the IMPROVE trial concerning the clinical care of patients with ruptured abdominal aortic aneurysm. *Br J Surg* 2014; **101** (3): 216–24.

# Challenging anatomy predicts short- and long-term mortality and complications after ruptured EVAR

H Baderkhan, A Wanhainen and K Mani

## Introduction

The introduction of endovascular aneurysm repair (EVAR) at the end of the 80s and beginning of the 1990s by Volodos[1] and Parodi[2] was a milestone in the treatment of aortic aneurysms. This minimally invasive surgical technique is now the primary method for repair of elective aneurysms in many countries.[3] Several randomised trials reported significant improvement in short-term outcome of EVAR compared to open repair in the elective setting.[4–6] In cases of ruptured aneurysms, overall, the use of EVAR is less prevalent, and rate of endovascular repair for treatment of ruptures varies significantly between centres.[7] While some centres almost ubiquitously perform endovascular repair for ruptured abdominal aortic aneurysm (ruptured EVAR),[8] others perform open repair in this setting. This variation is influenced by logistics, tradition and experience. Additionally, ruptured abdominal aortic aneurysms are often larger in size compared with elective aneurysms and have a more challenging anatomy.

The most important limitation with EVAR is the aortic anatomy. This has been extensively studied in the elective setting, and studies show that outcome is affected when EVAR is performed in patients with hostile anatomy or outside device specific instructions for use. In patients with hostile neck anatomy, EVAR is associated with longer fluoroscopy time, more blood loss and higher mortality as well as type I endoleak in up to 18% of the patients.[9] Furthermore, the reintervention rate is increased after elective EVAR outside instructions for use, and continued sac expansion is more common.[10] The outcome of EVAR in ruptured cases with challenging anatomy is scarcely studied.

## Evidence base for performing ruptured EVAR

The outcome of EVAR has been compared with that of open repair in three recent randomised controlled trials.[11–13] A meta-analysis[14] of these trials concluded that there is no early survival benefit with EVAR. Perioperative mortality in these studies was 31% for those undergoing EVAR compared with 34% for open repair. Subgroup analyses indicate that women may have improved early survival with EVAR, and overall analyses show that patients undergoing EVAR treatment have shorter hospital stays and are more likely to be discharged to independent living. The procedure also requires less blood transfusion.

As these trials assessed outcome in patients suitable for both open repair and EVAR, patients with an aortic anatomy that was unsuitable for EVAR were generally not included in the studies. Only a subset of ruptured aneurysms in these trials was deemed suitable for EVAR treatment. The proportion of ruptured aneurysms regarded as suitable for EVAR treatment or randomisation was 39–63%.

Interestingly, an analysis of the IMPROVE (Immediate management of patients with rupture: open vs. endovascular repair) trial showed that aneurysm neck length was a predictor of 30-day mortality after open repair.[12] Other smaller studies report similar findings, with a trend towards lower mortality following open repair of ruptured aortic abdominal aneurysm in patients with friendly morphology.[15,16]

## Ruptured EVAR in patients with hostile anatomy

To assess the outcomes of patients undergoing endovascular repair of a ruptured aneurysm based on aortic anatomy, a multicentre retrospective study was performed that reviewed outcomes for all patients undergoing ruptured EVAR at three European centres (Rotterdam, Holland; Uppsala and Gävle, Sweden).[17] This study enrolled 112 patients, including 43 with aortic anatomy outside EVAR instructions for use. In the short term, there was an increased mortality for patients with hostile aortic anatomy, defined as anatomy outside instructions for use, compared to patients with EVAR "friendly" anatomy (37.2% vs. 14.8% at 90-days; p=0.011). This difference in mortality was sustained throughout the study follow-up, and reached 73.6% at five years for patients with hostile anatomy, compared with 47.8% for friendly anatomy. The rate of graft-related complications for those surviving 30 days were 6% among those treated inside the instructions for use vs. 27% outside the instructions for use (p=0.015). Graft-related secondary intervention rates were 17% inside instructions for use vs. 42% outside (p=0.06); Figure 1.

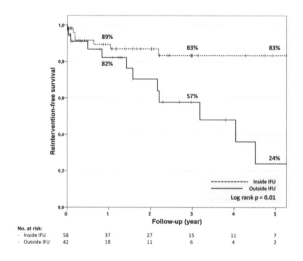

**Figure 1:** Kaplan-Meier plot for reintervention-free survival after EVAR for ruptured abdominal aortic aneurysm repair. The results of patients repaired with EVAR within instructions for use is compared to patients treated outside of instructions for use.

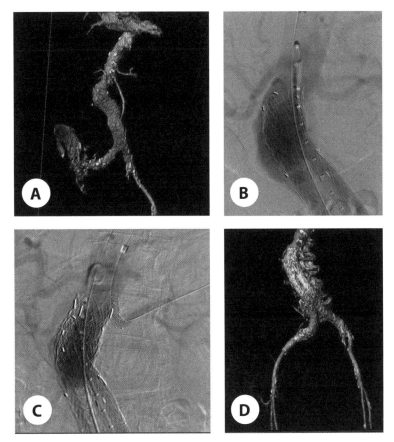

**Figure 2:** (A) CT angiogram of a ruptured abdominal aortic aneurysm with a short and angulated neck; (B) the patient was treated with EVAR, with a Gore excluder stent graft. There was a type I endoleak at the final angiogram; (C) this was corrected with a cuff and left renal artery stent; and D) the one-month postoperative CT angiogram shows a sealed aneurysm.

In a study with 39 patients (44% of them with hostile anatomy), Broos et al[18] reported a comparable one-year outcome in ruptured EVAR between patients with friendly and those with hostile anatomy. However, patients with hostile anatomy more frequently required intraoperative adjunctive procedures. Also, the small number of cases in this study may have affected the outcome; Figure 2.

Although mortality after EVAR is higher in patients with hostile anatomy undergoing ruptured repair, it is important to note that a hostile neck anatomy also negatively affects mortality after open repair. Therefore, it is not certain that an open repair approach would have resulted in improved outcome in these patients. The role of adjunct endovascular procedures for treatment of ruptured aneurysms with hostile anatomy remains of interest. The aforementioned multicentre analysis focused on patients treated with standard EVAR. Available techniques for management of hostile anatomy include use of parallel grafts[19] or fenestrated and branched stent grafts that may either be custom-made, physician-modified, or off -the-shelf.[20] No extensive case series exist that can be used to inform the outcome of EVAR for ruptures with adjunct techniques in the longer term. Centre-based studies, however, indicate that expanded use of EVAR with adjuncts may reach acceptable outcomes when compared to historical open cohorts.[8]

# Conclusion

EVAR for ruptured aneurysms results in shorter hospital stay, less blood transfusion, and higher chance of discharge to independent living when compared with open repair. The use of endovascular repair for ruptured aneurysms is, therefore, likely to increase. However, using EVAR outside instructions for use is associated with significantly more graft-related complications and reinterventions and higher mortality. Ruptured EVAR in patients with hostile anatomy should thus be followed by a meticulous surveillance programme for timely detection of any complications.

## Summary

- The use of EVAR for treatment of ruptures varies significantly between centres.

- Approximately half of the patients with ruptured abdominal aortic aneurysms fulfil the anatomical criteria for EVAR inside instructions for use.

- EVAR provides good short-term outcomes in patients with "friendly" anatomy.

- Using EVAR for treatment of ruptures outside instructions for use is associated with increased graft-related complications and overall mortality.

- The role of adjunct endovascular procedures in treatment of ruptures with EVAR requires further evaluation.

# References

1. Volodos NL. The 30th Anniversary of the First Clinical Application of Endovascular Stent-grafting. *Eur J Vasc Endovasc Surg* 2015; **49** (5): 495–97.
2. Veith FJ, Marin ML, Cynamon J, *et al.* 1992: Parodi, Montefiore, and the first abdominal aortic aneurysm stent graft in the United States. *Ann Vasc Surg* 2005; **19** (5): 749–51.
3. Beck AW, Sedrakyan A, Mao J, *et al.* Variations in abdominal aortic aneurysm care: A report from the International Consortium of Vascular Registries. *Circulation* 2016; **134** (24): 1948–58.
4. Patel R, Sweeting MJ, Powell JT, Greenhalgh RM. Endovascular *versus* open repair of abdominal aortic aneurysm in 15-years' follow-up of the UK endovascular aneurysm repair trial 1 (EVAR trial 1): a randomised controlled trial. *Lancet* 2016; **388** (10058): 2366–74.
5. Lal BK, Zhou W, Li Z, Kyriakides T, *et al.* Predictors and outcomes of endoleaks in the Veterans affairs open *versus* endovascular repair (OVER) trial of abdominal aortic aneurysms. *J Vasc Surg* 2015; **62** (6): 1394–404.
6. Prinssen M, Verhoeven EL, Buth J, *et al.* A randomized trial comparing conventional and endovascular repair of abdominal aortic aneurysms. *N Eng J Med* 2004; **351** (16): 1607–18.
7. Gunnarsson K, Wanhainen A, Djavani Gidlund K, *et al.* Endovascular Versus Open Repair as Primary Strategy for Ruptured Abdominal Aortic Aneurysm: A National Population-based Study. *Eur J Vasc Endovasc Surg* 2016; **51** (1): 22–28.
8. Mayer D, Aeschbacher S, Pfammatter T, *et al.* Complete replacement of open repair for ruptured abdominal aortic aneurysms by endovascular aneurysm repair: a two-center 14-year experience. *Ann Vasc Surg* 2012; **256** (5): 688–95.
9. AbuRahma AF, Yacoub M, Mousa AY, *et al.* Aortic neck anatomic features and predictors of outcomes in endovascular repair of abdominal aortic aneurysms following vs not following instructions for use. J Am Coll Surg 2016; **222** (4): 579–89.
10. Schanzer A, Greenberg RK, Hevelone N, *et al.* Predictors of abdominal aortic aneurysm sac enlargement after endovascular repair. *Circulation* 2011; **123** (24): 284–55.
11. Desgranges P, Kobeiter H, Katsahian S, *et al.* ECAR (Endovasculaire ou *Chirurgie* dans les Anevrysmes aorto-iliaques Rompus): A French randomized controlled trial of endovascular *versus* open surgical repair of ruptured aorto-iliac aneurysms. *Eur J Vasc Endovasc Surg* 2015; **50** (3): 303–10.

12. Powell JT, Sweeting MJ, Thompson MM, *et al*. Endovascular or open repair strategy for ruptured abdominal aortic aneurysm: 30 day outcomes from IMPROVE randomised trial. *BMJ* 2014; 348: f7661.
13. Reimerink JJ, Hoornweg LL, Vahl AC, *et al*. Endovascular repair *versus* open repair of ruptured abdominal aortic aneurysms: a multicenter randomized controlled trial. *Ann Vasc Surg* 2013; **258** (2): 248–56.
14. Sweeting MJ, Balm R, Desgranges P, *et al*. Individual-patient meta-analysis of three randomized trials comparing endovascular *versus* open repair for ruptured abdominal aortic aneurysm. *Br J Surg* 2015; **102** (10): 1229–39.
15. Slater BJ, Harris EJ, Lee JT. Anatomic suitability of ruptured abdominal aortic aneurysms for endovascular repair *Ann Vasc Surg* 2008; **22** (6): 716–22.
16. Perrott S, Puckridge PJ, Foreman RK, *et al*. Anatomical suitability for endovascular AAA repair may affect outcomes following rupture. *Eur J Vasc Endovasc Surg* 2010; **40** (2): 186–90.
17. Baderkhan H, Goncalves FM, Oliveira NG, *et al*. Challenging anatomy predicts mortality and complications after endovascular treatment of ruptured abdominal aortic aneurysm. *Eur J Vasc Endovasc Surg* 2016; **23** (6): 919–27.
18. Broos PP, t Mannetje YW, Cuypers PW, *et al*. Endovascular treatment of ruptured abdominal aortic aneurysms with hostile aortic neck anatomy. *Eur J Vasc Endovasc Surg* 2015; **50** (3): 313–19.

# Internal iliac artery consensus update including aneurysms

# When to deploy an iliac branched device

## KP Donas and G Torsello

## Introduction

Repair of aneurysms extending to the iliac bifurcation remains a challenge. Endovascular therapy mainly includes the use of iliac branched devices, coil embolisation of the hypogastric artery and the bell-bottom technique. A therapeutic algorithm presenting standard indications and use of each technique has been recently published by our group.[1]

The use of iliac branched devices is growing in acceptance. A review analysis of the reported experience with inclusion of 188 patients highlighted the safety and feasibility of iliac branched devices preserving antegrade flow to the hypogastric artery.[2] In agreement with this, profound evaluation of the use of iliac branched devices, regarding the strengths but also limitations and especially the identification of the recommended indications, remains of high scientific interest.

## Indications for use of iliac branched devices

### Young patients with unlimited life expectancy
Jeopardising the hypogastric circulation during endovascular aneurysm repair may be associated with several risks. Generally, lifestyle-limiting buttock claudication and sexual dysfunction have been described as potential complications following occlusion of the hypogastric artery.[1] Buttock claudication and impotence were significantly more frequent in patients treated with hypogastric artery occlusion (19%), compared with those treated with iliac branched devices (4%), as reported by Verzini *et al* in 2009.[3] The infrequent onset of buttock claudication or colonic and pelvic ischaemia represents a strong argument for the use of iliac branched devices, especially in younger, active patients. Additionally, due to the fact that erectile dysfunction is multifaceted, there is no doubt that preservation of hypogastric artery perfusion is important and recommended in patients with an active sexual life.

### Aneurysms with more than 25mm in diameter not suitable for treatment with the bell-bottom technique or contralateral occlusion of the hypogastric artery
The bell-bottom technique with the placement of a maximum 28mm iliac limb has been mainly used for older patients with aortoiliac aneurysms and common iliac diameters up to 25mm. Our group published long-term results of the

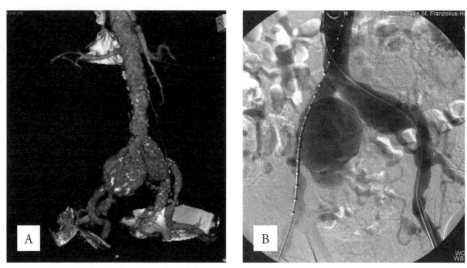

**Figures 1A and 1B:** Preoperative imaging of a bilateral common iliac aneurysm.

Endurant iliac legs (Medtronic) and extensions of 28mm for iliac aneurysms of maximum 25mm in diameter.[4] Consequently, limitation of the technique remains aneurysms extending to the iliac bifurcation with more than 25mm in diameter or further degeneration of the common iliac artery after endovascular treatment and consequently occurrence of Ib endoleak.

For these cases, the use of iliac branched devices is beneficial, allowing better distal fixation in the external iliac artery independent of the diameter of the aneurysms.

### Coexisting hypogastric aneurysm

In 2010, Karthikesalingam *et al* conducted the first systematic review analysis of iliac branched devices including 196 patients. In the same year, the same group published a morphological score to identify patients with aortoiliac aneurysms suitable for endovascular treatment with iliac branched devices.[5,6] The score was based on the recommendations of manufacturers' instructions for use and publications by expert vascular surgeons until 2010. The most common limitation to iliac branched device use was the presence of a hypogastric artery aneurysm.

In our first published work regarding iliac branched devices for 64 patients with aortoiliac aneurysms who were treated with iliac branched devices, the issue of coexistence of a hypogastric artery aneurysm was described *in extenso*.[7] One patient presented with a ruptured 6cm internal iliac artery aneurysm two years after the first placement of an iliac branched device. The cause for the ruptured aneurysm was dislocation of the two balloon-expandable covered stents in the hypogastric artery leading to a type III endoleak and consequent rupture. The patient was treated in the urgent setting with the placement of an Endurant limb at the origin of the internal iliac artery. A recannulation of the dislocated covered stents was not possible. It seems crucial to create a connection between the deployed covered stents and for this reason the use of a flexible self-expanding stent may be beneficial.

In 2013, our group published a novel technique performed in 16 consecutive patients with aneurysms extending to the iliac bifurcation and coexisting

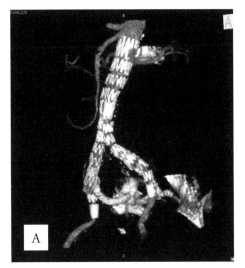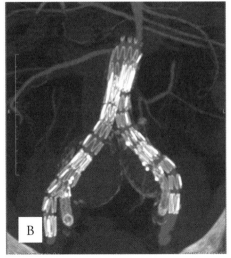

**Figures 2A and 2B:** Postoperative imaging of successful treatment by bilateral placement of an iliac branched device. Please note the recommemded technique in the hypogastric artery of balloon-expandable and self-expanding covered stents.

hypogastric artery aneurysms.[8] The novel approach consisted of placement of a balloon-expandable covered stent in the hypogastric artery branch followed by additional placement of a self-expanding covered stent in the gluteal branch in order to achieve a sufficient landing zone. Finally, additional placement of a long self-expanding bare metal stent in the stented hypogastric artery aims to better fixate the covered stents. Figures 1A, 1B, 2A and 2B present this alternative approach pre- and postoperatively. The overall primary patency of the internal branch was 95.3% and assisted patency was 100%. This approach can be used in aneurysms extending to the iliac bifurcation with aneurysmal involvement of the hypogastric artery. There is no doubt that additional evidence is needed to prove if this approach can be standardised and recommended in cases of coexisting aneurysmal hypogastric arteries.

## Summary

**The main anatomical and clinical indications for the use of iliac branched devices are:**

- Aneurysms of more than 25mm extending to the iliac bifurcation.

- Coexisting aneurysmal involvement of the hypogastric artery.

- Contralateral occlusion of the hypogastric artery.

- Young patients with an active life stand to benefit from techniques maintaining the perfusion of the hypogastric artery.

# References

1.  Panuccio G, Torsello GF, Torsello GB, Donas KP. Therapeutic algorithm to treat common iliac artery aneurysms by endovascular means. *J Cardiovasc Surg* (Torino); **57** (5): 7129–25.
2.  Donas KP, Bisdas T, Torsello G, Austermann M. Technical considerations and performance of bridging stent-grafts for iliac side branched devices based on a pooled analysis of single-center experiences. *J Endovasc Ther*. 2012; **19** (5): 667–71.
3.  Verzini F, Parlani G, Romano L, De Rango P, *et al*. Endovascular treatment of iliac aneurysm: concurrent comparison of side branch endograft *versus* hypogastric exclusion. *J Vasc Surg* 2009; **49**: 1154–61.
4.  Torsello G, Schönefeld E, Osada N, Austermann M, *et al*. Endovascular treatment of common iliac artery aneurysms using the bell-bottom technique: long-term results. *J Endovasc Ther* 2010; **17** (4): 504–09.
5.  Karthikesalingam A, Hinchliffe RJ, Holt PJ, Boyle JR, *et al*. Endovascular aneurysm repair with preservation of the internal iliac artery using the iliac branch graft device. *Eur J Vasc Endovasc Surg* 2010; **39** (3): 285–94.
6.  Karthikesalingam A, Hinchliffe RJ, Malkawi AH, Holt PJ, *et al*. Morphological suitability of patients with aortoiliac aneurysms for endovascular preservation of the internal iliac artery using commercially available iliac branch graft devices. *J Endovasc Ther* 2010; **17**: 163–71.
7.  Donas KP, Torsello G, Pitoulias GA, Austermann M, *et al*. Surgical *versus* endovascular repair by iliac branch device of aneurysms involving the iliac bifurcation. *J Vasc Surg*. 2011; **53** (5): 1223–29.
8.  Austermann M, Bisdas T, Torsello G, Bosiers MJ, *et al*. Outcomes of a novel technique of endovascular repair of aneurysmal internal iliac arteries using iliac branch devices. 2013; **58** (5): 1186–91.

# Patient selection criteria for the internal iliac artery branched device

## DE Cafasso, C Agrusa and DB Schneider

## Introduction

Tremendous advances have been made in the endovascular treatment of abdominal aortic aneurysms. Yet, until recently, the endovascular options for the management of iliac artery aneurysms have been limited. The recent arrival of the first FDA-approved off-the-shelf iliac branch device addresses many of these limitations by providing a dedicated endovascular option for treatment of iliac artery aneurysms.

Isolated iliac artery aneurysms are relatively uncommon, representing less than 2% of all cases of aneurysmal disease and afflicting only 0.03% of the general population. Isolated aneurysms of the internal iliac artery occur even less frequently, representing only 0.4% of all aneurysmal disease.[1,2] However, aneurysms of the iliac arteries are commonly found in patients who have abdominal aortic aneurysms; common iliac artery aneurysms can be seen in 25% to 40% of patients and are often bilateral.[3] Risk factors associated with common iliac artery aneurysms include male gender, age greater than 72 years, hypertension, and a family history of aortic aneurysms.[4] While common iliac arteries are considered aneurysmal once they reach a diameter of 1.5cm, very few are at risk of rupture until they exceed 4cm in diameter. For this reason, it is generally accepted that asymptomatic iliac artery aneurysms can be observed until they reach 3.5cm in diameter.[5] Compressive symptoms, rapid growth, or concomitant endovascular aneurysm repair (EVAR) for an aortic aneurysm are other indications for repair.

## Classic approach to endovascular management of iliac artery aneurysms

Many endovascular treatment options have been used for the management of iliac artery aneurysms. Coil embolisation of the internal iliac artery with covered stent extension to the external iliac artery during EVAR is commonly used to treat aneurysms of both the common and internal iliac arteries. Flared iliac limbs are now available for common iliac artery aneurysms that have adequate distal landing zones proximal to the origin of the internal iliac artery. For patients with common iliac artery morphology unsuitable for flared limbs, a "sandwich technique" has been described where parallel stent grafts are extended from an iliac limb into the external and internal iliac arteries. Hybrid procedures have also been described combining both open and endovascular techniques. Hybrid variations include

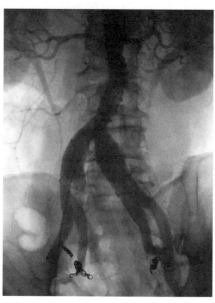

**Figure 1:** Bilateral iliac branch repair in patient with common and internal iliac artery aneurysms. Internal iliac artery branches have been extended into gluteal arteries with embolisation of other internal iliac branches.

EVAR with limb extension into the ipsilateral internal iliac artery and femoral-to-femoral bypass, or exclusion of a common iliac artery aneurysm with an aorto-uni-iliac endograft plus a femoral-to-femoral bypass and contralateral external to internal iliac artery covered stent.

Despite the variety of described treatment options, several limitations remain that affect short- and long-term outcomes of patients with iliac artery aneurysms. Several studies show that patients with abdominal aortic aneurysms are more likely to have failure of their EVAR if they have concomitant iliac artery aneurysms. Hobo *et al* found that EVAR patients with iliac artery aneurysms had higher five-year cumulative rates of distal type Ib endoleaks, iliac limb occlusions, secondary interventions, and aneurysm rupture.[6] Schanzer *et al* found that 44% of EVAR patients are treated outside of device instructions for use (IFU) and consequently, 41% develop aneurysm sac enlargement at five years. Common iliac artery diameter >20mm was found to be an independent predictor of aneurysm sac enlargement.[7] The introduction of flared iliac limbs has improved the management of common iliac artery aneurysms in patients with suitable anatomy. Kirkwood *et al* found no difference in rates of iliac aneurysm sac expansion, secondary interventions, type I endoleaks, or aneurysmal morbidity and mortality in patients with common iliac artery aneurysms treated with flared iliac limbs within the device instructions for use compared to patients without iliac aneurysms.[8] However, a large number of patients with iliac aneurysms do not have adequate vessel morphology for flared iliac limbs and Erben *et al* found that 70% of patients with common iliac artery aneurysms treated with flared iliac limbs were used outside of the endograft IFU. These patients with iliac aneurysms treated with flared limbs outside of IFU guidelines had higher rates of distal type I endoleaks, iliac events, and iliac reinterventions.[9]

Techniques that involve internal iliac artery sacrifice with ligation, embolisation, or coverage of the internal iliac artery are themselves not benign procedures and can lead to a host of ischaemic complications. Immediate buttock claudication has been reported in up to 55% of cases. While some of these patients have resolution of their symptoms, up to 35% will have persistent claudication beyond six months. Sexual dysfunction has been reported in 3% to 46% of patients with very few having symptom improvement over time.[10,11] Spinal cord ischaemia is one of the most feared complications of complex aortic aneurysm repair. In a study of various complex aortic aneurysm repairs by Eagleton *et al,* spinal cord ischaemia occurred in 2.8% of all patients undergoing repair and in 4.6% and 4.8% of patients undergoing repair of thoracic and thoracoabdominal aortic aneurysm repairs, respectively. Fifty per cent of patients that incurred spinal cord ischaemia had occlusion of at least one internal iliac artery.[12] Bilateral embolisation of the internal iliac arteries has been shown to result in higher complication rates among vascular patients.[13] Other devastating complications including colonic and pelvic ischaemia and buttock necrosis, though rare, can also occur.

## Iliac branch devices

The Gore Excluder Iliac Branch Endoprosthesis (IBE) is the only currently FDA-approved off-the-shelf device for treatment of common iliac artery or aortoiliac aneurysms in the US. The Cook Medical Zenith Branch Endovascular Graft-Iliac Bifurcation is not yet FDA-approved and remains in trial. Both the Gore and Cook iliac branch devices are bifurcated stent grafts that are implanted within a common iliac artery aneurysm. One limb extends into the external iliac artery and the other is extended into the internal iliac artery with a covered stent extension that is usually delivered from a contralateral femoral artery approach.

These two iliac branch devices were recently used in prospective pivotal US trials. The Gore Excluder IBE pivotal trial included 63 patients treated at 28 centres from 2013 to 2015. Patients with common iliac artery or aortoiliac aneurysms were treated with the Gore Excluder IBE and Gore Excluder AAA Endoprosthesis. Primary effectiveness endpoints included freedom from patency and/or endoleak-related reinterventions and freedom from occlusion of device branches up to six months. Secondary effectiveness endpoint included freedom from new onset buttock claudication. There was 0% aneurysm-related mortality, 95.2% technical success, 95.2% IBE patency, 100% freedom from new onset buttock claudication, and no type I or III endoleaks at six months.[14] The Cook Medical Zenith Branch Endovascular Graft-Iliac Bifurcation device remains investigational in the USA. This device has a similar delivery platform to the Gore Excluder IBE; however, it uses an Atrium iCAST balloon-expandable covered stent instead of a self-expanding covered stent for the internal iliac component. Results reported from many centres are also promising with a 90% freedom from reintervention rate at one year and 81.3% at five years, a 91.4% patency rate at one and five years, and 95% technical success rate with up to five-year follow-up.[15]

## Anatomical suitability for iliac branch devices

Anatomical requirements for iliac branch devices vary by device according to device specific instructions for use (Table 1). Based upon strict IFU guidelines less

| IFU criteria | Cook Zenith branch endovascular graft-iliac bifurcation | GORE Exclude iliac branch endoprothesis |
|---|---|---|
| Iliofemoral access vessel size/morphology | 20 Fr delivery profile<br>Minimal thrombus, calcification, tortuosity | 16 Fr delivery profile<br>Thrombus <2mm thick and/or <25% of vessel circumference in intended seal zone |
| CIA morphology | Length >50mm<br>Flow lumen diameter >6mm | Flow lumen diameter >17mm |
| EIA landing zone | Length > 20 mm<br>Outer wall diameter 8 mm - 11 mm | Length > 30mm (at least 10mm non-aneurysmal)<br>Diameter 6.5–25mm |
| IIA landing zone | Length >10mm (20–30 mm preferred)<br>Diameter 7–10mm | Length >30mm (at least 10mm non-aneuyrsmal)<br>Diamter 6.5–13.5mm |

**Freedom from significant femoral/iliac artery occlusive disease that would impede flow or outflow of stent-grafts

**Chart: Patient criteria.**

than 50% of patients with aortoiliac aneurysms may be morphologically suitable for treatment with an iliac branch device.[16,17] The most common encountered morphological feature limiting applicability is absence of a suitable internal iliac artery landing zone due to presence of an internal iliac artery aneurysm. Other frequently encountered adverse morphological features include: inadequate common iliac artery lumen diameter, inadequate common iliac artery length, or small internal iliac artery diameter. In the Gore Excluder IBE US pivotal trial, 58.3% of patients screened for enrolment were excluded for anatomical reasons; 58.4% of those excluded were due to inadequate common iliac artery lumen (minimum diameter ≥17mm within the implantation zone of the IBE device and diameter ≥14mm at the iliac bifurcation). Presence of an internal iliac artery aneurysm or aortic anatomy not suitable to receive the Gore Excluder AAA Endoprosthesis was responsible for exclusion of an additional 34.6% of patients not enrolled in the trial.

Applicability may be expanded, specifically in patients with internal iliac artery aneurysms, by using a landing zone in a distal internal iliac artery branch, preferably a gluteal branch.[18] Other internal iliac artery branches are embolised to prevent endoleaks (Figure 1). Wong and colleagues reported that 45% of the patients treated with iliac branch devices in their series had a distal landing zone in an internal iliac artery branch and that there was no adverse impact on patency or incidence of endoleaks.[19]

Patients who develop iliac artery aneurysms and type Ib endoleaks after prior EVAR represent a unique subset of patients with specific anatomical challenges. We have used iliac branch devices to successfully treat several patients with aneurysmal degeneration of the iliac arteries after prior EVAR. While the iliac branch device is delivered from a femoral approach, axillary or brachial artery access is typically needed for delivery of the internal iliac component.

## Which patients should be treated with iliac branch devices?

Based on the previously discussed risks of sacrificing the internal iliac artery, we believe that iliac preservation should be the standard of care in patients with suitable anatomy. Of course, patient selection is paramount for technical success and cost-effectiveness must be considered. Preservation of internal iliac arteries with an iliac branch device should be offered to patients with iliac artery aneurysms who are active to prevent buttock claudication and to preserve sexual function. In patients with multifocal or complex aneurysmal disease, internal iliac artery preservation carries additional importance to minimise risks of spinal cord ischaemia. Patients with advanced age and poor mobility are less ideal candidates for the iliac branch device and may be more appropriately treated with internal iliac embolisation and coverage from a risk and cost-effectiveness perspective. In patients with bilateral iliac artery aneurysm, both internal iliac arteries should be preserved in patients with an active lifestyle or patients with complex aortic disease to prevent ischaemic complications. While bilateral preservation with iliac branch devices is technically feasible and has shown good results, the benefits must also be weighed against the increased associated device costs, radiation dose, and procedure time.

## Conclusion

Iliac artery aneurysms are common in patients undergoing EVAR and prior to the availability of iliac branch devices, sacrifice of internal iliac arteries was routine. Sacrifice of the internal iliac artery is associated with claudication, sexual impotence, spinal cord ischaemia, and even pelvic ischaemia. Iliac preservation using iliac branch devices has been shown to be safe and effective. The iliac branch devices are durable with low branch occlusion rates and reintervention rates comparable to standard EVAR. Furthermore, data from clinical trials have shown a high technical success rate combined with low morbidity and mortality rates. Iliac artery preservation should be standard of care and iliac branch devices should be the preferred approach for management of iliac artery aneurysms in patients with suitable anatomy.

## Summary

- Common iliac artery aneurysms can be seen in 25–40% of patients and are often bilateral. Indications for repair include size >3.5cm, compressive symptoms, rapid growth, or concomitant EVAR for an aortic aneurysm.

- Current techniques to treat iliac artery aneurysms have associated risk of failure or ischaemic complications.

- The Gore Excluder Iliac Branch Endoprosthesis and Cook Medical Zenith Branch Endovascular Graft-Iliac Bifurcation are bifurcated stent grafts for iliac artery aneurysms. Both have been used in prospective pivotal US trials with promising results.

- Anatomical requirements for iliac branch devices vary by device. Key components are suitable internal iliac artery landing zone, adequate common iliac artery length and lumen diameter.

- Iliac preservation should be the standard of care in active patients with suitable anatomy or in patients with multifocal or complex aneurysmal disease. Patients with advanced age and poor mobility are less ideal candidates for the iliac branch device. The benefits of bilateral preservation must be weighed against increased costs, radiation dose, and procedure time.

# References

1. Horejs D, Gilbert PM, Burstein S, Vogelzang RL. Normal aortoiliac diameters by CT. J *Comput Assist Tomogr* 1988; **12** (4): 602–03.
2. Brunkwall J, Hauksson H, Bengtsson H, *et al.* Solitary aneurysms of the iliac arterial system: an estimate of their frequency of occurrence. *J Vasc Surg* 1989; **10** (4): 381–84.
3. Brown CR, Greenberg RK, Wong S, *et al.* Family history of aortic disease predicts disease patterns and progression and is a significant influence on management strategies for patients and their relatives. *J Vasc Surg* 2013; **58** (3): 573–81.
4. Huang Y, Gloviczki P, Duncan AA, *et al.* Common iliac artery aneurysm: expansion rate and results of open surgical and endovascular repair. *J Vasc Surg* 2008; **47** (6): 1203–10.
5. Kasirajan V, Hertzer NR, Beven EG, *et al.* Management of isolated common iliac artery aneurysms. *Cardiovasc Surg* 1998; **6** (2): 171–77.
6. Hobo R, Sybrandy JE, Harris PL, Buth J, EUROSTAR Collaborators. Endovascular repair of abdominal aortic aneurysms with concomitant common iliac artery aneurysm: outcome analysis of the EUROSTAR Experience. *J Endovasc Ther* 2008; **15** (1): 12–22.
7. Schanzer A, Greenberg RK, Hevelone N, *et al.* Predictors of abdominal aortic aneurysm sac enlargement after endovascular repair. *Circulation* 2011; **123** (24): 2848–55.
8. Kirkwood ML, Saunders A, Jackson BM, *et al.* Aneurysmal iliac arteries do not portend future iliac aneurysmal enlargement after endovascular aneurysm repair for abdominal aortic aneurysm. *J Vasc Surg* 2011; **53** (2): 269–73.
9. Erben Y, Oderich G, Duncan A, *et al.* Impact of compliance with anatomic guidelines on sac enlargement and outcomes of "bell-bottom" iliac stent grafts for ectatic or aneurysmal iliac arteries. Society for Vascular Surgery Annual Meeting; May 2013; San Francisco, CA.
10. Farahmand P, Becquemin JP, Desgranges P, *et al.* Is hypogastric artery embolization during endovascular aortoiliac aneurysm repair (EVAR) innocuous and useful? *Eur J Vasc Endovasc Surg* 2008; **35** (4): 429–35.
11. Rayt HS, Bown MJ, Lambert KV, *et al.* Buttock claudication and erectile dysfunction after internal iliac artery embolization in patients prior to endovascular aortic aneurysm repair. *Cardiovasc Intervent Radiol* 2008; **31** (4): 728–34.
12. Eagleton MJ, Shah S, Petkosevek D, *et al.* Hypogastric and subclavian artery patency affects onset and recovery of spinal cord ischemia associated with aortic endografting. *J Vasc Surg* 2014; **59** (1): 89–94.
13. Chitragari G, Schlosser FJ, Ochoa Chaar CI, Sumpio BE. Consequences of hypogastric artery ligation, embolization, or coverage. *J Vasc Surg* 2015; **62** (5): 1340–47.
14. Schneider D, Matsumura J, Oderich GS, *et al.* Pivotal results for the Gore Excluder Iliac Branch Endoprosthesis for treatment of aortoiliac aneurysms in the IBE 12-04 prospective, multicenter study. *J Vasc Surg* 2016; **63** (6): 226–7S.
15. Parlani G, Verzini F, De Rango P, *et al.* Long-term results of iliac aneurysm repair with iliac branched endograft: a 5-year experience on 100 consecutive cases. *Eur J Vasc Endovasc Surg* 2012; **43** (3): 287–92.
16. Karthikesalingam A, Hinchliffe RJ, Holt PJ, *et al.* Endovascular aneurysm repair with preservation of the internal iliac artery using the iliac branch graft device. *Eur J Vasc Endovasc Surg* 2010; **39** (3): 285–94.
17. Gray D, Shahverdyan R, Jakobs C, *et al.* Endovascular aneurysm repair of aortoiliac aneurysms with an iliac side-branched stent graft: studying the morphological applicability of the Cook device. *Eur J Vasc Endovasc Surg* 2015; **49** (3): 283–88.
18. Austermann M, Bisdas T, Torsello G, *et al.* Outcomes of a novel technique of endovascular repair of aneurysmal internal iliac arteries using iliac branch devices. *J Vasc Surg* 2013; **58** (5): 1186–91.
19. Wong S, Greenberg RK, Brown CR, *et al.* Endovascular repair of aortoiliac aneurysmal disease with the helical iliac bifurcation device and the bifurcated-bifurcated iliac bifurcation device. *J Vasc Surg* 2013; **58** (4): 861–69.

# Multicentre experience with one-year results on treatment of isolated concomitant common iliac aneurysms with sac anchor

## JT Boersen and JPPM de Vries

## Introduction

Infrarenal abdominal aortic aneurysm with a concomitant common iliac artery aneurysm occurs in approximately 20% of the aneurysm population.[1,2] Endovascular aneurysm repair (EVAR) in those patients may lead to a significant risk of endoleak and need for associated reinterventions.[1] Treatment of the hypogastric artery in patients with a common iliac artery aneurysm may add time and costs to the procedure, either by embolisation with coils or plugs or by preservation with an iliac branch device or parallel grafting.

EndoVascular Aneurysm Sealing (EVAS) with the Nellix endosystem (Endologix) seals the aneurysm with use of endobags that surround stent frames to provide a flow lumen to both legs.[3,4] The current Nellix generation allows on-label treatment of large concomitant common iliac artery aneurysms with a flow lumen diameter up to 35mm,[5] as long as there is a proper and non-diseased distal landing zone either in the external iliac artery or the distal common iliac artery. The instructions for use include a distal seal zone of at least 10mm with a maximum diameter of 25mm (20mm for the first generation Nellix SQ3+) to properly exclude the aneurysm. EVAS in isolated common iliac artery aneurysm has been demonstrated to be feasible, but this use of the device is strictly considered as off-label.[6]

One of the most important lessons learned regarding the treatment of concomitant common iliac artery aneurysm with EVAS is the need to exclude the entire aneurysm with the endobags. In early clinical experience, it was found that EVAS in common iliac artery aneurysm could be performed without adequate distal sealing zone. Krievins and colleagues showed that partial exclusion (maximum outer diameter >20mm) post-EVAS was associated with continued aneurysm (common iliac artery aneurysm or aortic aneurysm) growth during follow-up (median 24.7 months) and requires reinterventions.[7] They hypothesised that intraluminal thrombus plays an important role in pressurising the common iliac artery or aortic aneurysm, either by disappearance as a consequence of complex flow patterns distal to the stent or by transmitting pressure. These results suggest that landing of the Nellix stent in common iliac artery aneurysm with extensive intraluminal thrombus should be avoided.

Recently, a multicentre registry was initiated to evaluate the use of the Nellix endosystem for treatment of aortic aneurysm patients with concomitant common iliac artery aneurysm and for treatment of patients with an isolated common iliac artery aneurysm. The inclusion criteria for concomitant and isolated common iliac artery aneurysms were based on a minimum diameter of 24mm or 35mm, respectively. The analysis included procedural data and imaging outcomes (computed tomography [CT] angiography or duplex), and indications for reinterventions during one year of follow-up. The primary endpoints were the occurrence of graft migration, stent occlusion and endoleak, and the need for reinterventions.

## Nellix EVAS in common iliac artery aneurysms

In total, 72 patients (median age: 74.9 years [interquartile range: 68.5–80.5 years]; male: 71) were enrolled in this study. Ninety-six common iliac artery aneurysms were treated between April 2013 and May 2015, which included 21 isolated common iliac artery aneurysms and 24 bilateral common iliac artery aneurysms. The median diameter of the right and left aneurysms was, respectively, 36mm [IQR: 29–44mm] vs. 33.5mm [IQR: 28—40mm]. The majority (38) of patients had an American Society for Anesthesiologists score of >2.

Figure 1A depicts the preoperative plan for a male patient (75 years) with cerebrovascular accident, hypertension, and chronic obstructive pulmonary disease (COPD) global initiative on obstructive lung disease (GOLD) IV in history. The patient had a large aneurysm present in the left common iliac artery with a maximum outer diameter of 64mm and occlusion of the internal iliac artery at baseline. The maximum common iliac artery flow lumen diameter was 29mm with adequate sealing zones proximal and distal from the aneurysm. Implantation of a 120mm Nellix stent was performed under local anaesthesia (Figure 1B). The polymer fill volume was 35mL with a fill pressure of 190mmHg. The completion angiogram (Figure 1C) revealed proper exclusion of the common iliac artery aneurysm with a good position of the endosystem. This treatment is off-label use of the Nellix endosystem.

Overall, 98.6% (71 patients) of cases had successful deployment of the Nellix endosystems without the occurrence of type Ia or Ib endoleak. Failure occurred in one patient (1.4%), which was because of a residual type Ib endoleak. In this patient, a parallel graft was used to preserve internal iliac artery flow. An aneurysmal internal iliac artery was treated in 10 patients by pre- or periprocedural hypogastric artery embolisation, including one patient with bilateral internal iliac artery aneurysms. In 15 patients, a distal bare metal stent extension was deemed necessary to better align the distal end of the Nellix stent frame in the common or external iliac artery to improve distal outflow. In eight other patients, the Nellix stent frame had to be extended to the external iliac artery to treat a stenosis (n=5) or a dissection (n=3).

The incidence of stent occlusion during one-year follow-up was 4.2% (n=3), with two early occlusions (<30 days) and one later occlusion (<1 year). In all three patients stent lumen patency was restored by either a thrombectomy and realigning with Viabahn (Gore) (n=2) or thrombolysis (n=1); reocclusion did

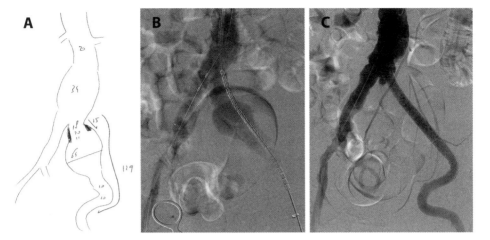

**Figure 1:** (A) Preoperative plan male patient with a large left common iliac artery aneurysm and preexistent left internal iliac artery occlusion; (B) unilateral Nellix endosystem deployment in the common iliac artery; and (C) completion angiography.

not occur. Endoleak was observed in five patients (6.9%) (one type Ia, two type Ib, and two type II endoleaks from a back bleeding hypogastric artery) during one-year follow-up. The type Ia endoleak resolved spontaneously. The two type Ib and two type II endoleaks from the hypogastric arteries persisted but without sac enlargement (so far). Aneurysm-related reinterventions had to be performed in five patients (6.9%) during one year of follow-up, and included treatment of the three stent occlusions. One patient presented with calf claudication three months postprocedure, and this was successfully resolved by percutaneous transluminal angioplasty of a Nellix stent and popliteal stenosis. Additionally, surgical evacuation of a haematoma had to be performed in one patient postprocedure.

The overall mortality was 4.2% (n=3). One procedure-associated death occurred in a patient with fatal haemorrhagic stroke seven days postprocedure. The other two causes of death were not associated to the procedure, or with the abdominal aortic aneurysm.

## Discussion

EVAS can be used to treat large concomitant and isolated common iliac artery aneurysms with a flow lumen diameter up to 35mm, as long as the endobag seals the entire common iliac artery aneurysm in a non-diseased distal landing zone.

The maximum common iliac artery diameter that can be treated with a regular EVAR device is around 24mm.[5] To treat a larger common iliac artery aneurysm, two options are possible. The first option is embolisation of the hypogastric artery and extension of the EVAR device in the external iliac artery, but this may cause erectile dysfunction, buttock claudication or bowel ischaemia.[8] The second is the use of iliac branch devices to preserve the flow into the hypogastric artery—iliac branch device side-branch occlusion has been reported in 7–14% of cases.[9,10] This percentage may be considered acceptable, but the use of an iliac branch device in combination with EVAR leads to a substantial increase in procedure costs.

Furthermore, anatomical restrictions allow treatment within the instructions for use in less than 40% of patients with common iliac artery aneurysmal disease.[11]

With EVAS, it is known that the hypogastric artery can be left untreated if extension to the external iliac artery is deemed necessary, as the seal of the endobag will prevent back bleeding from the hypogastric artery. However, hypogastric treatment is still required in patients with an internal iliac artery aneurysm. These types of aneurysm can be managed by embolisation, or a chimney/periscope in the internal iliac artery to preserve branch patency, although, probably with a higher risk of endoleak.

The stent occlusion rate after one year was low (4.2%) and comparable to previous reported experience on EVAS (5%).[12] The occlusion rate in the current series is comparable to stent occlusion in EVAR (4%).[13] Most of the occlusions still occur within 90 days postprocedure and are associated to technical failure or landing in the external iliac artery.

A high demand for distal stent alignment may be dedicated to variability in (distal) positioning of the stent due to a variable amount of straightening of the aortoiliac anatomy after withdrawal of the delivery system and stiff guidewire.[14] This variability in positioning should be considered mainly in patients with tortuous iliac anatomy. The relative stiffness of the Nellix is considered a limitation of the current stent design. Additionally, positioning variability may be caused by no distal attachment of the endobag to the distal 1cm of the Nellix stent that may result in non-apposition and an inadequate sealing of the common iliac artery aneuyrsm. Therefore, the current generation Nellix includes a distal attachment of the endobag to the stent frame

The incidence of endoleak was comparable to previous experience with EVAS, which has been reported in a range of 2.8–7% type I and type II endoleaks.[2,12] Angiographies in multiple angulations can help to improve endoleak detection at the primary procedure. Endoleak at the follow-up CT can be enhanced by merging of a non-contrast and contrast CT series.[15]

Revision of type Ia endoleak post-EVAS can be cumbersome because no regular extension cuff can be placed. Revision of a type Ia endoleak can be done by graft explantation, proximal extension with Nellix-in-Nellix, or embolisation with coils and Onyx (Medtronic).[16,17] Experience with endovascular techniques to revise a type Ia endoleak post-EVAS is anecdotal so far, and little is known about long-term results of these solutions.

## Conclusion

EVAS with the Nellix endosystem allows treatment of concomitant iliac artery aneurysms >25mm. One year follow-up data show high patency of the devices with low incidence of type I or II endoleak. However, longer-term results are required to assess its durability.

## Summary

- EVAS with the Nellix endosystem allows treatment of concomitant iliac aneurysms >25mm within the instructions for use.

- Successful outcome depends on complete seal and exclusion of the entire common iliac artery aneurysm.

- Completion angiographies in multiple angles and without stiff guidewires is key to appreciate endoleaks or misalignment of the distal end of the Nellix stent frames.

- Longer term results are warranted to assess the sustainability of EVAS in treatment of common iliac artery aneurysms.

# References

1. Hobo R, Sybrandy JE, Harris PL, Buth J. Endovascular repair of abdominal aortic aneurysms with concomitant common iliac artery aneurysm: outcome analysis of the EUROSTAR Experience. *J Endovasc Ther* 2008; **15** (1): 12–22.

2. Thompson MM, Heyligers JM, Hayes PD, *et al.* Endovascular aneurysm sealing: early and midterm results from the EVAS FORWARD Global Registry. *J Endovasc Ther* 2016; **23** (5): 685–92.

3. Donayre CE, Zarins CK, Krievins DK, *et al.* Initial clinical experience with a sac-anchoring endoprosthesis for aortic aneurysm repair. *J Vasc Surg* 2011; **53** (3): 574–82.

4. van den Ham LH, Zeebregts CJ, de Vries JP, Reijnen MM. Abdominal aortic aneurysm repair using Nellix endovascular aneurysm sealing. *Surg Technol Int* 2015; **26**: 226–31.

5. Karthikesalingam A, Cobb RJ, Khoury A, *et al.* The morphological applicability of a novel endovascular aneurysm sealing (EVAS) system (Nellix) in patients with abdominal aortic aneurysms. *Eur J Vasc Endovasc Surg* 2013; **46** (4): 440–45.

6. Ter Mors TG, van Sterkenburg SM, van den Ham LH, Reijnen MM. Common iliac artery aneurysm repair using a sac-anchoring endograft to preserve the internal iliac artery. *J Endovasc Ther* 2015; **22(6):** 886–88.

7. Krievins DK, Savlovskis J, Holden AH, *et al.* Preservation of hypogastric flow and control of iliac aneurysm size in the treatment of aortoiliac aneurysms using the Nellix endovascular aneurysm sealing endograft. *J Vasc Surg* 2016; **64** (5): 1262–69.

8. Rayt H, Bown M, Lambert K, *et al.* Buttock claudication and erectile dysfunction after internal iliac artery embolization in patients prior to endovascular aortic aneurysm repair. Cardiovasc Intervent Radiol 2008; **31** (4): 728–34.

9. Wong S, Greenberg RK, Brown CR, *et al.* Endovascular repair of aortoiliac aneurysmal disease with the helical iliac bifurcation device and the bifurcated-bifurcated iliac bifurcation device. *Journal of Vascular Surgery* 2013; **58** (4): 861–69.

10. Parlani G, Verzini F, De Rango P, *et al.* Long-term results of iliac aneurysm repair with iliac branched endograft: a 5-year experience on 100 consecutive cases. *Eur J Vasc Endovasc Surg* 2012; **43** (3): 287–92.

11. Karthikesalingam A, Hinchliffe RJ, Malkawi AH, *et al.* Morphological suitability of patients with aortoiliac aneurysms for endovascular preservation of the internal iliac artery using commercially available iliac branch graft devices. *J Endovasc Ther* 2010; **17** (2): 163–71.

12. Böckler D, Holden A, Thompson M, *et al.* Multicenter Nellix endovascular aneurysm sealing system experience in aneurysm sac sealing. *J Vasc Surg* 2015; **62** (2): 290–98.

13. van Zeggeren L, Gonçalves FB, van Herwaarden JA, *et al.* Incidence and treatment results of Endurant endograft occlusion. *J Vasc Surg* 2013; **57** (5): 1246–54.

14. Boersen JT, Schuurmann RCL, Slump CH, *et al.* Changes in aortoiliac anatomy after elective treatment of infrarenal abdominal aortic aneurysms with a sac anchoring endoprosthesis. *European Journal of Vascular and Endovascular Surgery* 2016; **51** (1): 56–62.

15. Holden A, Savlovskis J, Winterbottom A, *et al.* Imaging after Nellix endovascular aneurysm sealing: A consensus document. *J Endovasc Ther* 2016; **23** (1): 7–20.

16. Donselaar EJ, Holden A, Zoethout AC, *et al.* Feasibility and technical aspects of proximal Nellix-in-Nellix extension for late caudal endograft migration. *J Endovasc Ther* 2016. Epub.

17. Ameli-Renani S, Das R, Weller A, *et al.* Embolisation of a proximal type I endoleak post-nellix aortic aneurysm repair complicated by reflux of onyx into the nellix endograft limb. Cardiovasc Intervent Radiol 2015; **38** (3): 747–51.

# Peripheral arterial consensus update—Pathways of care

# Intermittent claudication & lifestyle

# Tobacco cessation and arterial reconstruction

## S McKeever and MR Smeds

## Introduction

Smoking is the single most important modifiable risk factor in almost all vascular diseases and remains an important cause of preventable death and disability.[1,2] Also while nearly 70% of smokers have expressed an desire to stop smoking and 44% actually attempt to quit each year, only 4–7% will be successful if unaided.[1,3,4] That so few people manage to cease smoking without help may be attributed to a lack of support and guidance from healthcare professionals. Indeed, a large percentage of patients who present to vascular surgeons have poorly controlled modifiable risk factors, including smoking.[5]

Furthermore, compared with those who continue to smoke, vascular surgery patients who cease smoking have a reduced risk of major complications during surgery, increased graft patency, fewer amputations, and a lower risk of arterial disease progression.[6–10] Therefore, surgeons are in a unique position to be able to advise patients on stopping smoking—one in 12 successful attempts to quit smoking relate to an operation and patients scheduled to undergo an invasive procedure are more likely to quit.[11,12]

Although vascular surgeons do routinely advise patients to quit smoking, many may not know how extensive the advice needs to be or which prescriptions for smoking cessation medication need to be provided to prompt behavioural change.[13,14] Those who provide smoking cessation counselling typically do not spend a significant amount of time with the patients despite evidence suggesting there is a dose response to behavioural therapy.[15] Also, a recent study (performed by vascular surgeons) indicates that patients are more likely to consider stopping smoking if smoking cessation medication is prescribed alongside advice.[16]

The goal of this chapter is to describe the effects of cigarettes on the vascular system and provide vascular surgeons with information on smoking cessation approaches so that they can help their patients stop smoking.

## The neurobiology behind tobacco addiction

Nicotine is absorbed in the central nervous system rapidly and in high concentrations. It then binds to nicotinic acetylcholine receptors, causing release of dopamine, norepinephrine, glutamate, vasopressin, and serotonin among other neurotransmitters. These substances stimulate the mesolimbic system resulting in a generalised behavioural arousal, pleasure, reduced stress/anxiety, and improved concentration.[4] Upregulation of these receptors occurs, resulting in greater concentrations of nicotine needed to have the same effects over time.

Understanding the reasons why people become physically addicted to nicotine is important for understanding the available methods for smoking cessation. Given the rapid delivery of nicotine by cigarettes, the aim of nicotine-replacement products is to provide nicotine at lesser doses to gradually break down the physical dependence on the drug while lessening the "urge" for it. Furthermore, smoking cessation medications such as varenicline (Champix, Pfizer) and bupropion (Zyban, GlaxoSmithKline) work on the receptors that have been upregulated.

It should also be recognised that few smokers will be successful (in the long term) with their first attempt to quit. Therefore adjustments in medication may be needed and behavioural support should be continued in the clinical setting until the desired outcome is met.

## Effect of cigarette smoking on the vascular system

Smoking causes a nicotine-mediated increase in sympathetic tone, leading to increased heart rate, blood pressure and myocardial oxygen demand and is known to alter the function of endothelial cells and cause increased platelet aggregation.[17] A procoagulant state is created by altering the coagulation cascade, causing abnormalities in the fibrinolytic system, and impairment of the release of tissue plasminogen activator.[6,18] Vasomotor dysfunction, inflammation, and modification of lipids are the components of initiation and progression of atherosclerosis associated with smoking. There is increased endothelial production of endothelin-1, which is a potent vasoconstrictor. Cigarette smoke decreases nitric oxide availability, which is primarily responsible for the vasodilatory function of endothelium as well as regulation of inflammation, leukocyte adhesion, and thrombosis.[18]

Atherosclerosis is, in part, accelerated by an inflammatory response. Recruitment of leukocytes to the surface of endothelial cells is an early event in the development of atherosclerosis, and smoking increases proinflammatory cytokines responsible for this activation and cell interaction. Effects on patients' lipid profiles are thought to promote plaque formation in smokers, with higher levels of cholesterol and low-density lipoproteins seen.[19] This accelerated atherosclerosis, in turn, has effects on many arteries in the body.

### Peripheral arterial disease

Cigarette smoking is a major risk factor for peripheral arterial disease, with smokers being twice as likely to develop the disease as they are to develop coronary artery disease.[20] Also, smoking is an independent predictor of atherosclerosis progression and has been shown in multiple studies to increase the risk of intermittent claudication and rest pain. Patients who successfully quit smoking have improvement in claudication symptoms and increased walking distance as well as decreased major adverse cardiovascular events and limb loss.[8–10]

Smokers develop peripheral arterial disease, on average, 10 years earlier than do non-smokers, and there is a direct relationship between smoking and the development of this disease—as well as to the progression to more severe symptoms, including critical limb ischaemia.[21,22]

Of patients who undergo bypass procedures for the management of peripheral arterial disease, those who smoke have an increased risk of graft failure. One meta-analysis found that smokers had a threefold increased risk of graft failure. It also found that of those who smoked and who had graft failure, smoking could be directly attributed as the cause in 57%.[10] Patients who successfully quit smoking had a similar graft patency rate to that of patients who never smoked.

Smoking has also been demonstrated to increase the risk of major amputation after revascularisation, with rates being directly associated with smoking intensity. Examining outcomes at three years amongst smokers and non-smokers who underwent revascularisation demonstrated an amputation rate of 21% in heavy smokers compared with 2% in moderate and light smokers.[23]

In another study with five-year follow-up, people who continued to smoke more than 15 cigarettes per day were five times more likely to undergo amputation at two years after revascularisation than those who smoked 15 cigarettes or fewer.[17] Finally, smoking cessation has been associated with improved overall survival in patients with peripheral arterial disease; patients who quit smoking have twice the survival rate at five years than those who continued to smoke.[9]

## Aneurysmal disease

Smoking is the most significant modifiable risk factor in aneurysmal disease, with ongoing smoking associated with an increased risk of abdominal aortic aneurysm expansion.[20] Compared with patients who report having never smoked (on a regular basis), patients who were current smokers had a 13 times' increased risk of having an aneurysm detected during follow up.[16] Both the duration of smoking and the number of cigarettes smoked per day increased the risk of aneurysm rupture. Nearly 90% of patients with aneurysms have a history of tobacco use, with almost 50% being active smokers.[24]

## Carotid artery disease

Current smoking is associated with development of carotid artery stenosis as well as development of carotid stroke.[25] It is associated with increased intimal media thickening progression rate and decreasing luminal diameters of the internal carotid artery, both of which slow with cessation of tobacco use.[26] Patients who continue to smoke following carotid endarterectomy are more likely to have an ipsilateral stroke or a transient ischaemic attack, and those who undergo stenting are more likely to suffer stroke, myocardial infarction or death within 30 days of the procedure.[27,28]

# Smoking cessation approaches

The US agency for Healthcare and Quality recommends that clinicians identify and document tobacco use and treat every patient identified with a combination of counselling and cessation medications. A central first step is to start a dialogue with patients about their tobacco use. Clinicians frequently ask their patients about smoking status but rarely spend the time to discuss quitting options or barriers.[2]

However, during such conservations, clinicians should incorporate the following "5 As". These are:

1. Ask the patient about tobacco use
2. Advise the patient to quit
3. Assess willingness to consider quitting

4. Assist the patient to quit by offering pharmacotherapy/behavioural counselling

5. Arrange follow-up.[2]

For those patients who are reluctant to quit, the "5 Rs" should be used to help patients identify reasons to quit. These include:
1. Relevance of quitting to them
2. Risks of tobacco use
3. Rewards of stopping tobacco
4. Roadblocks of quitting
5. Repeating the previous questions at every clinical encounter.

Patients are more likely to support initiatives that they have helped to create, so allowing them to identify these benefits will help create a partnership rather than a confrontational relationship. It is then important to understand patient's feelings about quitting, their confidence in their ability to do so, and their fears. With this information, along with a patient willingness to make an effort, a clinician can tailor treatments that are the most appropriate.

Combination medical therapy with motivational counselling is the recommended technique for smoking cessation; thus, once the patient has agreed to attempt to quit smoking, medications should be offered to assist in their efforts. There are seven medications approved by the United States Food and Drug Administration (FDA) as first-line pharmacotherapy for tobacco cessation, including five nicotine replacement therapies, varenicline and bupropion. Second-line therapy includes clonidine and nortriptyline.

### Nicotine replacement

Nicotine replacement therapy uses nicotine patches, gum, nasal spray, vapour inhalers, or lozenges to cover nicotine cravings and prevent withdrawal symptoms. In the USA, patches, gum and lozenges are available over the counter, while a prescription is required for the nasal spray or inhaler. Combination therapy of these products can be used to allow a baseline level of nicotine in the blood with extra doses use to cover cravings or withdrawal symptoms. Patches are an example of long-acting products and have been shown in studies to increase the chances of cessation while products such as gum, nasal spray, inhalers and lozenges are short-acting products that enter the blood stream more rapidly and help with cravings. A nicotine patch should be approached in a graded fashion, with the initial dose determined based on the estimated amount of nicotine consumed per day. A cigarette averages approximately 1mg of nicotine, so matching the number of cigarettes smoked per day to the patch size available is a good place to start. For example, a smoker who smokes one pack (20 cigarettes) per day should be given a 21mg patch. Patches are available in 7mg, 14mg and 21mg strengths, and multiple patches may be used for heavy smokers. Once prescribed, the patient needs to have frequent follow-up either in clinic or by phone. Ideally, follow-up should be frequent during the first two weeks following the patient's quit date, as studies have shown that abstinence from smoking during the first two weeks of patch therapy is highly predictive of long-term abstinence.[29] Doses of the nicotine patch can be safely increased for patients experiencing irritability, anxiety, or loss of concentration, and after four weeks of therapy, the dose can be gradually tapered down over several weeks. Duration of therapy is variable, but most patients use the patch for four to eight weeks.

## Pharmacological adjuncts

In addition to nicotine replacement, neurobehavioral medications can be used to treat addiction and assist with cessation of smoking. Bupropion is a monocyclic antidepressant that inhibits the reuptake of both norepinephrine and dopamine, which is similar to the positive reinforcement that comes with cigarette smoking. Treatment with bupropion in combination with nicotine replacement has been shown to increase long-term rate of abstinence. Initial treatment begins with 300mg per day with tolerable side-effects. Bupropion has been shown to attenuate weight gain associated with smoking cessation, which can be relayed to the patients as well. Varenicline is another drug that may be used; it is a partial nicotine agonist and antagonist that blocks nicotine from binding to the receptor and also partially stimulates receptor mediated activity, which ultimately leads to the release of dopamine. This reduces cravings and nicotine withdrawal symptoms. It is given at a dose of 0.5mg once daily for three days, followed by 0.5mg twice daily for four days and then 1mg daily. The patient should be educated that the quit date is day eight (the day that 1mg dosing is begun), and length of treatment can persist for 12 weeks. There are some side-effects with the drug that the clinician should be aware of—nausea and vivid dreams being the most common.

The above medications are FDA-approved first-line pharmacotherapies for smoking cessation but there are other options if they are ineffective. Tricyclic antidepressants such as nortriptyline have been shown to increase abstinence from smoking compared to control groups, along with behavioural support.[9]

## Counselling

Just as important as the above interventions is behavioural counselling. Often in busy vascular surgical practices, it is impractical to spend lengthy amounts of time discussing smoking cessation. Therefore it is helpful to have knowledge of outside resources that can be provided for your patient. The simplest way is for clinicians to encourage patients to use a tobacco quit line, (i.e., 1-800-QUITNOW in the USA). Additionally, many hospitals have smoking cessation specialists and they may be able to provide additional support for your patient.

## Conclusion

Patients frequently present to vascular surgeons' offices with poorly controlled risk factors. Knowledge in and provision of both behavioural counselling and the appropriate medications to support cessation efforts in vascular patients can result in desirable outcomes in both decreased progression of vascular disease and increased patency of repairs.

## Summary

- The majority of smokers want to quit smoking but if unaided, only a small percentage will be successful.

- A significant number of vascular surgery patients present to vascular surgeons' offices with poorly controlled risk factors including tobacco use.

- Provision of behavioural counselling and cessation medications/nicotine replacement can improve cessation success rates.

- Patients who are able to quit smoking will demonstrate decreased morbidity and mortality associated with vascular surgery procedures, increased patency of surgical and endovascular repairs, and decreased progression of disease.

# References

1. Burke M V, Ebbert JO, Hays JT. Treatment of tobacco dependence. Mayo Clin Proc 2008; **83** (4): 474–79.
2. Fiore MC, Jaen CR BT *et al*. Treating Tobacco Use and Dependence: 2008 Update. Rockville, MD: US Department of Health and Human Services, Public Health Service; 2008.
3. Fiore MC, Baker TB. Clinical practice. Treating smokers in the health care setting. *N Engl J Med* 2011; **365** 1222–31.
4. Hurt RD, Ebbert JO, Hays JT, McFadden DD. Treating tobacco dependence in a medical setting. *CA Cancer J Clin* 2009; **59** (5): 314–26.
5. Bianchi C, Montalvo V, Ou HW, *et al*. Pharmacologic risk factor treatment of peripheral arterial disease is lacking and requires vascular surgeon participation. *Ann Vasc Surg* 2007; **21** (2): 163–66.
6. Pittilo RM. Cigarette smoking and endothelial injury: a review. *Adv Exp Med Biol* 1990; **273**: 61–78.
7. Sorensen LT, Karlsmark T, Gottrup F. Abstinence from smoking reduces incisional wound infection: a randomized controlled trial. *Ann Surg* 2003; **238** (1): 1–5.
8. Quick CR, Cotton LT. The measured effect of stopping smoking on intermittent claudication. *Br J Surg* 1982; **69** (Suppl): S24–26.
9. Armstrong EJ, Wu J, Singh GD, *et al*. Smoking cessation is associated with decreased mortality and improved amputation-free survival among patients with symptomatic peripheral artery disease. *J Vasc Surg* 2014; **60** (6): 1565–71.
10. Selvarajah S, Black JH 3rd, Malas MB, *et al*. Preoperative smoking is associated with early graft failure after infrainguinal bypass surgery. J Vasc Surg 2014; **59** (5): 1308–14.
11. Hoel AW, Nolan BW, Goodney PP, *et al*. Variation in smoking cessation after vascular operations. *J Vasc Surg* 2013; **57** (5): 1334–38.
12. Shi Y, Warner DO. Surgery as a teachable moment for smoking cessation. Anesthesiology 2010; **112** (1): 102–07.
13. Ozturk O, Yilmazer I, Akkaya A. The attitudes of surgeons concerning preoperative smoking cessation: a questionnaire study*. Hippokratia* 2012; **16** (2): 124–29.
14. Owen D, Bicknell C, Hilton C, *et al*. Preoperative smoking cessation: a questionnaire study. *Int J Clin Pract* 2007; **61** (12): 2002–04.
15. Quinn VP, Stevens VJ, Hollis JF, *et al*. Tobacco-cessation services and patient satisfaction in nine nonprofit HMOs. *Am J Prev Med* 2005; **29** (2): 77–84.
16. Newhall K, Suckow B, Spangler E, *et al*. Impact and duration of brief surgeon-delivered smoking cessation advice on attitudes regarding nicotine dependence and tobacco harms for patients with peripheral arterial disease. *Ann Vasc Surg* 2017; **38**: 113–21
17. Cryer PE, Haymond MW, Santiago J V, Shah SD. Norepinephrine and epinephrine release and adrenergic mediation of smoking-associated hemodynamic and metabolic events. *N Engl J Med* 1976; **295** (11): 573–77.
18. Willigendael EM, Teijink JAW, Bartelink M-L, *et al*. Smoking and the patency of lower extremity bypass grafts: a meta-analysis. *J Vasc Surg* 2005; **42** (1): 67–74.
19. Lindholt JS, Heegaard NH, Vammen S, *et al*. Smoking, but not lipids, lipoprotein(a) and antibodies against oxidised LDL, is correlated to the expansion of abdominal aortic aneurysms. *Eur J Vasc Endovasc Surg* 2001; **21** (1): 51–56.

20. Ockene IS, Miller NH. Cigarette smoking, cardiovascular disease, and stroke: a statement for healthcare professionals from the American Heart Association. American Heart Association Task Force on Risk Reduction. *Circulation* 1997; **96** (9): 3243–47.

21. Black JH 3rd. Evidence base and strategies for successful smoking cessation. *J Vasc Surg* 2010; **51** (6): 1529–37.

22. Willigendael EM, Teijink JAW, Bartelink M-L, *et al.* Influence of smoking on incidence and prevalence of peripheral arterial disease. *J Vasc Surg* 2004; **40** (6): 1158–65.

23. Lassila R, Lepantalo M. Cigarette smoking and the outcome after lower limb arterial surgery. *Acta Chir Scand* 1988; **154** (11-12): 635–40.

24. Powell JT, Worrell P, MacSweeney ST, *et al.* Smoking as a risk factor for abdominal aortic aneurysm. *Ann N Y Acad Sci* 1996; **800**: 246–48.

25. McNally JS, McLaughlin MS, Hinckley PJ, *et al.* Intraluminal thrombus, intraplaque hemorrhage, plaque thickness, and current smoking optimally predict carotid stroke. *Stroke* 2015; **46** (1): 84–90.

26. Hansen K, Ostling G, Persson M, *et al.* The effect of smoking on carotid intima-media thickness progression rate and rate of lumen diameter reduction. *Eur J Intern Med* 2016; **28**: 74–79.

27. Rong X, Yang W, Garzon-Muvdi T, *et al.* Risk Factors Associated with Ipsilateral Ischemic Events Following Carotid Endarterectomy for Carotid Artery Stenosis. *World Neurosurg* 2016; **89**: 611–19.

28. Doig D, Turner EL, Dobson J, *et al.* Predictors of Stroke, Myocardial Infarction or Death within 30 Days of Carotid Artery Stenting: Results from the International Carotid Stenting Study. *Eur J Vasc Endovasc Surg* 2016; **51**(3): 327–34.

29. Hays JT, Croghan IT, Schroeder DR, *et al.* Over-the-counter nicotine patch therapy for smoking cessation: results from randomized, double-blind, placebo-controlled, and open label trials. *Am J Public Health* 1999; **89** (11): 1701–07.

# Acute and critical ischaemia consensus update

# Guidelines for superficial femoral artery intervention

K Dwivedi and T Cleveland

## Introduction

The combination of the burden of atherosclerotic disease and the anatomy of the superficial femoral artery makes it an almost unique environment in terms of challenges for endovascular intervention. The atherosclerotic material in the superficial femoral artery is often highly calcified and considerably bulky, particularly against a background of diabetes or renal failure (Figure 1). Additionally, restenosis appears to be more aggressive compared to other parts of the vascular system (notably the coronary or even iliac arteries). Indeed, Ida et al[1] showed that when nitinol stents are used during endovascular therapy, restenosis peaks late at approximately 12 months.

The anatomy of the superficial femoral artery is also very different from other territories. This segment is prone to compression (from muscle groups and external forces) and both elongation and torsion during the flexion and extension of the hip and knee joints. Therefore balloon-mounted stents, which do not have the characteristics to accommodate such forces, have not been used in this region, except in the early days of endovascular stents when there was little else available.

For these reasons, bypass has remained the gold standard in terms of durability for superficial femoral artery disease, as demonstrated by the BASIL (Bypass vs. angioplasty in severe ischaemia of the leg) trial.[2] This is particularly so when the disease pattern has been complex, often with a combination of complete occlusions, or there is long segment disease. In recent times, there have been a number of technical advances to the endovascular options for treating superficial femoral artery disease. Building on traditional plain balloon angioplasty, these advances have included the development of nitinol bare metal stents, drug-eluting balloons and stents, covered stents, cryoplasty, atherectomy (including laser) and even more recently, temporary stents.

There is, therefore, a bewildering range of potential options, making it very difficult for interventionalists to be certain about which devices to use for any individual patient. As a result, published guidelines are extremely useful for ensuring some consistency in what constitutes the standard of care that should be offered to patients. Also, a number of these devices are costly to purchase and healthcare systems need reassurance that they are delivering a treatment that is as cost-effective as possible.

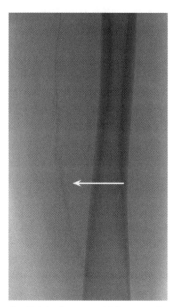

**Figure 1:** Heavy calcification (arrow), which is often seen with femoropopliteal disease.

## Guidelines

At the time of writing (January 2017), the UK National Institute for Health and Care Excellence (NICE) Guideline (CG147) Peripheral arterial disease: diagnosis and management,[3] published in August 2012, was due to be updated. The intended timeline for the evidence to be checked was three years after publication.

NICE guidance for treatment of patients with intermittent claudication is in relation to those who have:

- Received advice on the benefits of risk factor modification
- Not had satisfactory improvement in symptoms from a supervised exercise programme
- Imaging that has confirmed that angioplasty is suitable for the person.

Under such circumstances, primary stent placement is not recommended for treating patients with intermittent claudication caused by aortoiliac disease (except complete occlusion) or femoropopliteal disease. The guidance also states that bare metal stents are recommended when stenting is used for treating patients with intermittent claudication.

When a patient has critical limb ischaemia, the endovascular options recommended for patients are almost exactly the same, with consideration of primary stent placement when the critical limb ischaemia is caused by complete aortoiliac occlusion (rather than stenosis). It is recommended not to offer primary stent placement for treating people with critical limb ischaemia caused by femoropopliteal disease. The guidance indicates that bare metal stents should be used if needed as an adjunct to balloon angioplasty.

The standards of practice guidelines[4] from the Cardiovascular and Interventional Radiology Society for Europe (CIRSE) are directed specifically at superficial femoral and popliteal artery angioplasty and stenting. These state that typical indications for stent use include:

- Post angioplasty recoil or a residual stenosis of >30%
- Flow-limiting dissection
- Anatomically complex lesions including eccentric calcified plaques, long segment stenoses, and occlusions.

These standards also indicate that balloon angioplasty with provisional stent placement remains the standard of endovascular care, and that primary nitinol stent placement may reduce vessel restenosis, thereby reducing the need for repeat procedures in the mid-term. The authors recognise that literature reviews from 2009 and 2010 indicate that primary stent placement remained controversial at that time.

The CIRSE standards also indicate that if stents are used in a situation of "bailout", then they should be used in the areas of primary angioplasty failure, rather than used throughout the entire diseased segment (this practice is commonly described as "spot stenting"). However, if stents are used primarily, they should be selected to allow for full lesion coverage. Moderate vessel wall calcification and TASC (Trans-Atlantic Inter-Society Consensus) type D lesions[5] were noted to be positive predictors of the increased need for femoropopliteal stenting.

The CIRSE standards, which were published more recently (2014) than the NICE guidance, made note of the high incidence of the formation of neointimal hyperplasia following femoropopliteal interventions. This problem is seen more often in long segments of disease (occlusions or stenosis) and after the placement of multiple stents. The high incidence of restenosis and neointimal hyperplasia in this segment has led to the development and use of drug-eluting stents, drug-coated balloons and covered stents, and these have all been used in the femoropopliteal segment.

Whilst the CIRSE standards do not give guidance as to the specific role of placement for these treatment options, they do acknowledge the proof-of-concept animal studies and several multicentre, randomised controlled trials that have shown a difference in vessel restenosis associated with such interventions. On the other hand, they note that laser and directional atherectomy have no proven benefit compared with standard balloon angioplasty and stenting.

NICE has also issued guidance with regard to laser atherectomy,[6] considering the evidence adequate to recommend normal arrangements for the use of percutaneous laser atherectomy as an adjunct to balloon angioplasty (with or without stenting). However, the committee remained uncertain about whether laser atherectomy confers any advantages over balloon angioplasty alone and, if so, in which patients. Careful multidisciplinary team patient selection was recommended, with the evidence on efficacy and safety considered adequate to support the use of laser atherectomy with normal arrangements in place for clinical governance, consent and audit.

Conversely, NICE IPG3808 also reviewed the evidence for the use of percutaneous atherectomy of femoropopliteal arterial lesions with plaque excision devices in 2011, and concluded that the evidence on the efficacy of atherectomy with plaque excision devices was inadequate in quality.[7] Additionally, the evidence on safety was also considered to be inadequate, particularly with regard to the risk of distal embolisation. The recommendation was that the procedure should only be used with special arrangements for clinical governance, consent and audit or research. Further research was recommended and there was a stated intention to review the procedure on publication of further evidence. The guidance has not yet been updated.

More recently, as a part of the Medtech innovation briefings, NICE has issued information relating to the Lutonix (Bard) drug-coated balloon for peripheral arterial disease.[8] This drug-coated balloon is a paclitaxel-coated angioplasty balloon indicated for treating peripheral arterial disease. The briefing documented that the balloon has a lower paclitaxel concentration than alternative devices, and a drug delivery that is claimed to be novel. The majority of the data presented in the submission was from the LEVANT I and LEVANT II studies[9,10] that compare the Lutonix balloon with standard balloon angioplasty in symptomatic femoropopliteal disease. NICE indicated uncertainty around the use of late lumen loss as a primary outcome, as this was considered to be a technical outcome, particularly as to how it impacts on clinical success. Additionally, NICE indicated awareness of other CE-marked devices which, it considered, fulfil a similar function to the Lutonix drug-coated balloon, and these included:

- InPact Admiral (Medtronic)
- Stellarex (Spectranetics)
- Ranger (Boston Scientific)
- Passeo-18 Lux (Biotronik)
- Legflow (Cardionovum)
- Freeway (Eurocor Endovascular)
- Advance 18 PTX (Cook Medical).

Within the briefing document, it was noted that the additional cost of a drug-coated balloon, in relation to balloon angioplasty, was the cost of the drug-coated balloon itself (£580), a guidewire, a needle introducer and some contrast. It was also recognised that in the 2015/16 NHS England enhanced tariff option, as a high cost device, drug-coated balloons can be paid for through a separate price negotiation. Thus, an individual organisation can recoup the costs from purchasers. At a Medtech briefing, specialist commentators gave their views and comments, but no guidance on clinical scenario usage was offered as a part the briefing.

## Conclusion

Where does that leave interventionalists when it comes to making decisions on how to treat an individual patient? Clearly, appropriate clinical assessment must be made, preferably in a multidisciplinary team environment, to consider if and when endovascular treatment is appropriate to suggest to a patient. Following this, a full discussion with the patient is essential. However, once NICE guidance is published, UK health professionals are expected to take it fully into account when exercising their judgment. If, having considered the guidance, it is judged that a treatment not recommended in the guidance is reasonable to offer, this can be recommended by a healthcare professional. However, if departing from the guidance, a documented full discussion with the patient would be prudent. The Medical Defence Union concludes: "Ignorance of NICE Guidance is a poor defence, but a reasoned and reasonable decision to reject the guidance in an individual case, together with a good record made at the time, may be acceptable."[11] On the other hand, Samanta et al[12] argue that in the UK, guidance from NICE is likely to emerge as "a reasonable body of opinion" for the purpose of litigation, and medical practitioners who deviate from them should be ready to explain why they have done so.

The conundrum that then exists for an interventionalist is what to do when there are authoritative guidelines such as those issued by NICE, which, for an individual patient, are not considered to be appropriate by the doctor. Such a circumstance may arise when the doctor considers that evidence has come to light that was not taken into account in the guidance process, and which alters the best available treatment for the individual patient. This may result in a clinical judgment that potentially justifies deviation from the guidelines. As the guidance becomes less up to date, or even overdue for updating, this might become an increasing possible scenario. In such circumstances, consideration by a body of experts (such as a multidisciplinary meeting) that takes into account the available evidence, may result in a recommendation to the patient that is outside the published guidance. In such circumstances, an open discussion and contemporary documentation would appear to be prudent.

## Summary

- Superficial femoral artery disease intervention is uniquely challenging because of both anatomical and pathophysiological factors.

- There are a number of endovascular options for treating femoropopliteal disease.

- Both positive and negative evidence about the the use of newer technologies is accumulating at a rapid rate.

- There are a variety of levels of guidance from government bodies, Learned Societies and local purchasers.

- Interventionalists are obliged to be aware of guidance and take it into account.

- Guidance takes into account the best evidence available at the time of their formulation, is intended to be useful for patients and doctors, but may become rapidly out of date.

- Deviation from guidance may be reasonable, but should be carefully considered, discussed with patients and the reasons documented.

# References

1. Lida O, Uematsu M, Soga Y, *et al.* Timing of the restenosis following nitinol stenting in the superficial femoral artery and the factors associated with early and late restenoses. *Catheter Cardiovasc Interv.* 2011; **78**: 611–17

2. Bypass vs. angioplasty in severe ischaemia of the leg (BASIL): multicentre, randomised controlled trial. Adam DJ, Beard JD, Cleveland T, *et al. Lancet* 2005; **366** (9501): 1925–34.

3. Peripheral arterial disease: diagnosis and management. www.nice.org.uk/guidance/cg147 August 2012

4. Katsanos K, Tepe G, Tsetis D, Fanelli F. Standards of Practice for Superficial Femoral and Popliteal Artery Angioplasty and Stenting. Cardiovasc. Intervent. Radiol 2014; **37**: 592–603.

5. Norgren L, Hiatt, WR, Dormandy JA, *et al*, on behalf of the TASC II Working Group. Inter-Society Consensus for the Management of Peripheral Arterial Disease (TASC II). *Eur J Vasc Endovasc Surg* 2007; **33**: S1eS70.

6. Percutaneous laser atherectomy as an adjunct to balloon angioplasty (with or without stenting) for peripheral arterial disease. Interventional Procedure Guidance, November 2012. www.nice.org.uk/guidance/ipg433

7. Percutaneous atherectomy of femoropopliteal arterial lesions with plaque excision devices. Interventional procedure guidance 2011. www.nice.org.uk/guidance/ipg380

8. Lutonix drug-coated balloon for peripheral arterial disease. Medtech innovation briefing. July 2016. www.nice.org.uk/guidance/mib72

9. Scheinert D, Duda S, Zeller T et al. The LEVANT I (Lutonix Paclitaxel-Coated Balloon for the Prevention of Femoropopliteal Restenosis) Trial for Femoropopliteal Revascularization. JACC: Cardiovascular Interventions Volume 7, Issue 1, January 2014

10. Rosenfield K, Jaff M, White C et al . Trial of a Paclitaxel-Coated Balloon for Femoropopliteal Artery Disease. N Engl J Med 2015; **373:**145–53

11. Colbrook P, Doctor Magazine special report, March 2002. www.forward-me.org.uk/Letters/Legal_context_nice_guidance.pdf

12. Samanta A,  Samanta J, and Gunn M. Legal considerations of clinical guidelines: will NICE make a difference? J R Soc Med. 2003 Mar; **96(3):** 133–38.

# Drug-coated balloon consensus update

# Vessel preparation before drug-coated balloon use in femoropopliteal artery disease

## T Zeller

## Introduction

Drug-coated balloon angioplasty of femoropopliteal TASC (Trans-Atlantic Inter-Society Consensus Document on Management of Peripheral Arterial Disease) II A and B lesions has shown promising mid-term results in randomised controlled trials.[1-4] However, depending on lesion complexity, bailout stent placement is indicated, in a significant percentage of interventions and patency failures that occur in particular, in calcified lesions.[5,6] Drug-coated balloon angioplasty has the same limitations as standard balloon angioplasty, specifically acute recoil including undilatable calcified lesions and severe dissections requiring provisional bare metal stenting.[5,7] Vessel preparation with debulking devices or plaque modulation devices might improve acute and longer term technical outcomes of drug-coated balloon angioplasty in native femoropopliteal arteries as suggested in small single-centre studies.[8-10] Even less in known with regard to vessel preparation for femoropopliteal in-stent restenosis, in particular in-stent reocclusions that have been shown to be at high risk for developing recurrent in-stent restenosis or reocclusion following plain balloon angioplasty, cutting balloon angioplasty and even drug-coated balloon angioplasty.[11-12]

## Vessel preparation for native femoropopliteal arteries

After drug-coated balloon angioplasty, approximately 15% of paclitaxel transfers from the balloon surface into the vessel wall.[13] Intimal intraluminal calcification can increase the loss of antiproliferative drug when advancing the coated balloon into the lesion—in particular if the lesion is not sufficiently predilated—which can impair uptake.[14] The role of Mönckeberg-type medial calcification—a common manifestation in patients with diabetes and end-stage renal insufficiency[15]—on the biological efficacy of drug-eluting balloons is still unknown. Fanelli *et al*[6] and Tepe *et al*[5] reported a significant drop in primary patency and increase in late lumen loss following drug-coated balloon angioplasty of femoropopliteal lesions with circumferential calcification independent of lesion length.

Atherectomy mechanically recanalises the vessel without overstretch, removes the perfusion barrier for a subsequent antirestenotic therapy with a drug-coated balloon, and reduces the likelihood of bailout stenting, even in calcified lesions and as a result preserves the native vessel. The DEFINITIVE Ca++ (Determination of safety and effectiveness of the SilverHawk peripheral plaque excision system for calcium and the SpiderFX embolic protection device for the treatment of calcified peripheral arterial disease in the superficial femoral and/or the popliteal arteries) single-arm trial demonstrated calcified disease can be treated effectively with directional atherectomy using an embolic protection device.[17] Directional atherectomy-related lumen gain was 2.2mm, the bailout stent rate was as low as 4.1%, and flow-limiting dissections were found in 1.5% only.

In a prospective, single-centre study including 30 patients with peripheral vascular disease, Rutherford categories 3–6 heavily calcified femoropopliteal lesions defined as fluoroscopic calcification on both sides of vessel wall longer than 1cm in length were treated with directional atherectomy.[9] All procedures included distal protection with the SpiderFX filter (Medtronic) and intravascular ultrasound (IVUS)-guided atherectomy with the TurboHawk peripheral plaque excision system (Medtronic). Once a <30% residual stenosis was achieved confirmed by IVUS and angiography, a drug coated balloon was used for postdilation. A <30% residual stenosis was achieved in all cases without procedure-related adverse events, the bailout stenting rate was 6.5%. After one year, duplex derived primary patency rate was 90% (27/30) and freedom from major adverse events 87% (26/30). The authors concluded that directional atherectomy and drug-coated balloon angioplasty may represent a potential alternative strategy for the treatment of femoropopliteal severely calcified lesions. These promising data and the considered hypothesis have to be confirmed in a multicentre randomised trial.

The investigator initiated DEFINITVE AR (Directional atherectomy followed by a Pacliaxel-coated balloon to inhibit restenosis and maintain vessel patency: A pilot study of antirestenosis treatment) trial did assess and estimate the effect of treating a vessel with directional atherectomy followed by a drug-coated balloon compared to treatment with a drug-coated balloon alone. The randomised study arm was supplemented by a registry arm treating severely calcified lesions with the combination therapy using the Turbohawk atherectomy catheter in conjunction with a distal protection filter. Overall, 121 patients were enrolled at 10 centres in Europe, 102 patients in the randomised study arm and 19 patients into the calcium registry. Mean lesion length in both study cohorts was about 10cm.

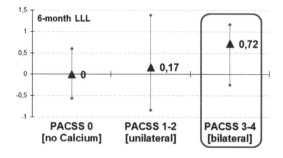

**Figure 1:** Retrospective corelab analysis of lesions included into the THUNDER trial[5] of the correlation of late lumen loss (LLL) and the degree of calcification (PACSS = peripheral arterial calcification scoring system).[16]

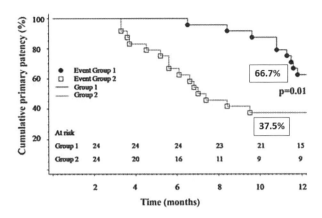

**Figure 2:** Plain drug-coated balloon angioplasty compared to vessel preparation using the excimer laser prior to drug coated balloon angioplasty:[20] 12-month primary patency rate 66.7% versus 37.5% (p=0.01).

The technical success, defined as ≤30% residual stenosis following the protocol-defined treatment at the target lesion as determined by the angiographic core laboratory, was achieved in 89.6% in the combination therapy cohort as compared to 64.2% in the drug-coated balloon angioplasty cohort (p=0.004). The stent rate was 0% in the combination therapy cohort and 3.7% in the drug-coated balloon cohort. Grade C and D dissections were significantly reduced in the combination cohort (2% *vs.* 19%; p= 0.009). At one year, there was no significant benefit for vessel preparation prior to drug-coated balloon angioplasty, the primary outcome of angiographic per cent diameter stenosis was 33.6±17.7% for directional atherectomy plus drug-coated balloon angioplasty *vs.* 36.4±17.6% for drug-coated balloon angioplasty only (p=0.48). Clinically-driven target lesion revascularisation was 7.3% for the combination therapy *vs.* 8% for drug-coated balloon angioplasty only. Duplex ultrasound patency was 84.6% for the combination therapy and 81.3% for drug-coated balloon angioplasty only. The study was not powered to show significant differences between the two methods of revascularisation in one-year follow-up. A larger adequately-powered randomised trial is warranted.

The REALITY trial (Directional atherectomy plus drug-coated balloon to treat long, calcified femoropopliteal artery stenoses) will evaluate the performance directional atherectomy plus drug-coated balloon angioplasty in a larger study cohort. However, the study is limited by its single-arm study design.

Stavroulakis *et al* published a retrospective single-centre experience comparing drug-coated balloon angioplasty *vs.* directional atherectomy with drug-coated balloon angioplasty for isolated lesions of the popliteal artery.[10] Seventy-two patients were treated with either drug-coated balloon angioplasty alone (n=31) or with the combination therapy (n=41). The technical success rate following drug-coated balloon angioplasty was 84% *vs.* 93% (p=0.24) after combination therapy. Bailout stenting was more common after drug-coated balloon angioplasty group (16% vs. 5%, P=0.13). The 12-month primary patency rate was significantly higher in the combination therapy group (82% vs. 65%, p=0.021), while freedom from target lesion revascularisation did not differ between the two treatment strategies (94% *vs.* 82%; p=0.072).

Data about combining vessel preparation with focal force balloons such as Angiosculpt (Spectranetics) or the Peripheral Cutting Balloon (Boston Scientific) are not yet published.

## Vessel preparation for femoropopliteal in-stent restenosis

Very little is known about the value of vessel preparation of in-stent restenosis prior to drug-coated balloon angioplasty. The EXCITE ISR study (Excimer laser randomized controlled study for treatment of femoropopliteal in-stent restenosis) compared plain balloon angioplasty with laser assisted balloon angioplasty in in-stent restenotic lesions with a mean lesion length of 19cm.[18] The combination therapy demonstrated superior procedural success (93.5% *vs.* 82.7%; p=0.01) with significantly fewer procedural complications. The combination therapy resulted in a significant higher six-month freedom from target lesion revascularisation of 73.5% *vs.* 51.8% (p<0.005) and was associated with a 52% reduction in target lesion revascularisation (hazard ratio [HR]: 0.48; 95% confidence interval [CI]: 0.31 to 0.74). It is well known that the main limitation of the treatment of in-stent restenosis is in-stent reocclussion according to the Tosaka classification, which defines in-stent restenosis lesion morphology by angiographic presentation into class I focal lesions (stenosis ≤50mm in length), class II diffuse lesions (stenosis >50mm in length) and class III total occlusions.[19] Accordingly, laser debulking resulted in the highest benefit in longer lesions.

To date, the only published study comparing plain drug-coated balloon angioplasty with vessel preparation using the excimer laser has been a small single-centre randomised study including 24 patients into each study arm.[20] Patients in the laser plus drug-coated balloon group demonstrated patency rates at six and 12 months of 91.7% and 66.7%, which are significantly higher than in the drug-coated balloon-only patients (58.3% and 37.5%, respectively.) The secondary outcome measure, target lesion revascularisation, was 16.7% at 12 months in the laser plus drug-coated balloon angioplasty group and 50% in the drug-coated balloon angioplasty alone group.

Theoretically, devices offering combined thrombectomy and atherectomy capabilities such as Jetstream (Boston Scientific) and Rotarex (Straub Medical) should be most effective in preparing in-stent reocclusions prior to drug-coated balloon angioplasty due to the unique composition of the occlusive material containing thrombus and neointima.

## Summary

- Drug-coated balloon angioplasty is limited by the shortcomings such as plain balloon angioplasty: elastic recoil and dissection.

- Vessel preparation prior to drug-coated balloon angioplasty using directional atherectomy for the treatment of femoropopliteal artery disease is safe according to the DEFINITIVE AR study.

- Vessel preparation prior to drug-coated balloon angioplasty using directional atherectomy significantly improves acute treatment outcomes such as residual stenosis, interventional success, and dissection rates.

- Despite significantly better acute outcome an underpowered prospective randomised trial (DEFINITIVE AR) did not proof superiority at one-year regarding technical and clinical outcomes for vessel preparation prior to drug-coated balloon angioplasty as compared to plain drug-coated balloon angioplasty.

- Lesion calcification and lesion length greater than 10cm were identified as potential predictors for superior outcomes for the combination therapy. A larger scale randomised controlled study focusing on such complex lesion types is warranted.

- A small, single-centre, randomised study comparing plain drug-coated balloon angioplasty with laser debulking prior to drug-coated balloon angioplasty in instent reocclusions resulted in significant better acute outcomes and one-year primary patency rate but no significant benefit for freedom from target lesion revascularisation.

- A larger scale randomised controlled study focusing on such complex lesion types is warranted.

# References

1. Tepe G, Zeller T, Albrecht T, *et al.* Local delivery of paclitaxel to inhibit restenosis during angioplasty of the leg. *N Eng J Med* 2008; **358** (7): 689-699.
2. Werk M, Langner S, Reinkensmeier B, *et al.* Inhibition of restenosis in femoropopliteal arteries: paclitaxel-coated *versus* uncoated balloon: femoral paclitaxel randomized pilot trial. *Circulation* 2008; **118** (13): 1358–65.
3. Tepe G, Laird J, Schneider P, *et al.* Drug-coated balloon *versus* standard percutaneous transluminal angioplasty for the treatment of superficial femoral and popliteal peripheral artery disease: 12-month results from the IN.PACT SFA randomized trial. *Circulation* 2015; **131** (5): 495–502.
4. Rosenfield K, Jaff MR, White CJ, *et al.* Trial of Paclitaxel-coated balloon for femoropopliteal artery disease. *N Eng J Med* 2015; **373**: 145–53.
5. Tepe G, Beschorner U, Ruether C, *et al.* Predictors of outcomes of drug-eluting balloon therapy for femoropopliteal arterial disease with a special emphasis on calcium. *J Endovasc Ther* 2015; **22** (5): 727–33.
6. Fanelli F, Cannavale A, Gazzetti M, *et al.* Calcium burden assessment and impact on drug-eluting balloons in peripheral arterial disease. *Cardiovasc Intervent Radiol* 2014; **37** (4): 898–907.
7. Scheinert D, Micari A, Brodmann M, *et al.* Drug-coated balloon treatment for femoropopliteal artery disease: The IN.PACT Global Study long lesion imaging cohort. *JACC Cardiovasc Interv* 2016 (submitted).
8. Sixt S, Carpio Cancino OG, Treszl A, *et al.* Drug-coated balloon angioplasty after directional atherectomy improves outcome in restenotic femoropopliteal arteries. *J Vasc Surg* 2013; **58** (3): 682–86.

9. Cioppa A, Stabile E, Popusoi G, *et al.* Combined treatment of heavy calcified femoro-popliteal lesions using directional atherectomy and a paclitaxel coated balloon: One-year single centre clinical results. *Cardiovascular Revascularization Medicine* 2012; **13** (4): 219–23.

10. Stavroulakis K, Schwindt A, Torsello G, *et al.* Directional Atherectomy With Antirestenotic Therapy vs Drug-Coated Balloon Angioplasty Alone for Isolated Popliteal Artery Lesions. *J Endovasc Ther* 2016. DOI: 1526602816683933.

11. Dick P, Sabeti S, Mlekusch W, *et al.* Conventional balloon angioplasty *versus* peripheral cutting balloon angioplasty for treatment of femoropopliteal artery in-stent restenosis: initial experience. *Radiology* 2008; **248** (1): 297–302.

12. Grotti S, Liistro F, Angioli P, *et al.* Paclitaxel-eluting balloon vs standard angioplasty to reduce restenosis in diabetic patients with in-stent restenosis of the superficial femoral and proximal popliteal arteries: three-year results of the DEBATE-ISR study. *J Endovasc Ther* 2016; **23**(1): 52–57.

13. Schnorr B, Kelsch B, Cremers B, *et al.* Paclitaxel-coated balloons—survey of preclinical data. *Minerva Cardioangiol* 2010; **58** (5): 567–82.

14. Schnorr B, Albrecht T. Drug-coated balloons and their place in treating peripheral arterial disease. *Expert Rev Med Devices* 2013; **10**(1): 105–14.

15. Jude EB, Eleftheriadou I, Tentolouris N. Peripheral arterial disease in diabetes--a review. *Diabet Med* 2010; **27**(1): 4–14.

16. Rocha-Singh KJ, Zeller T, Jaff MR. Peripheral arterial calcification: Prevalence, mechanism, detection and clinical implications. *Catheter Cardiovasc Interv* 2014; **83**: E212–20.

17. Clair DG, Roberts DK. Treatment of severely calcified femoropopliteal lesions with plaque excision and embolic protection- DEFINITIVE Ca++. *J Vasc Interv Radiol* 2011; **22**: 1785

18. Dippel EJ, Makam P, Kovach R, *et al,* EXCITE ISR Investigators. Randomized controlled study of excimer laser atherectomy for treatment of femoropopliteal in-stent restenosis initial results From the EXCITE ISR trial (Excimer laser randomized controlled study for treatment of femoropopliteal in-stent Restenosis). *JACC: Cardiovascular Interventions* 2015; **8**: 92–101.

19. Tosaka A, Soga Y, Iida O, *et al.* Classification and clinical impact of restenosis after femoropopliteal stenting. *J Am Coll Cardiol* 2012; **59**: 16–23.

20. Gandini R, Del Giudice C, Merolla S, *et al.* Treatment of chronic SFA in-stent occlusion with combined laser atherectomy and drug-eluting balloon angioplasty in patients with critical limb ischemia: a single-center, prospective, randomized study. *J Endovasc Ther* 2008; **20**: 805–14.

# Guidelines on drug-coated balloons

## I van Wijck, S Holewijn and MMPJ Reijnen

## Introduction

The prevalence of peripheral arterial occlusive disease increases alongside the growth in the ageing population. First-line treatment of the disease includes management of cardiovascular risk factors and, in case of intermittent claudication, supervised walking exercise. It is only for critical limb ischaemia or failed exercise training in patients with disabling intermittent claudication that an invasive treatment is justified. For decades, bypass surgery was the first-line treatment for complex lesions in the femoropopliteal artery whereas endovascular treatment was reserved for short lesions. Tremendous progress has been made with regard to endovascular treatment options for flow-limiting disease of the femoropopliteal artery. This has led to a broader acceptance of an endovascular-first strategy.

Plain balloon angioplasty is associated with a significant incidence of restenosis and is thus reserved for focal non-complex lesions. Bare nitinol stenting has improved short-term outcomes after endovascular treatment, but concerns persist about in-stent restenosis, stent fractures, and long-term outcomes. More recently, endovascular alternatives have been developed (including covered stents, drug-eluting stents, debulking devices, and drug-coated balloons), which may improve the results of endovascular therapy.

## Drug-coated balloon

Drug-coated balloons were designed to locally deliver a drug into the arterial wall to improve the durability of patency after endovascular treatment. This strategy avoids the risks associated with stenting such as in-stent restenosis and stent fractures. Each drug-coated balloon is unique with respect to drug dose, excipient molecule, balloon material, and balloon and coating technology used. The antiproliferative drug paclitaxel has evolved into the drug of choice for infrainguinal disease because it has proved to reduce cell proliferation and migration, and so reduce the formation of intimal hyperplasia. An excipient drug acts as a spacer, facilitates manufacturing, holds the drug in place during storage, and facilitates the paclitaxel transfer from the balloon to the vessel wall. Various excipients are in use, including urea (Medtronic), polysorbate and sorbitol (Bard), polyethylene glycol (Spectranetics), butyryltrihexyl citrate (BTHC, Biotronik), citrate ester (Boston Scientific) and shellac (Biosensors and Cardionovum). The coating process should be reliable, scalable and uniform. All aspects of the drug-coated balloon could influence their performance and as such results of randomised trials cannot be generalised.

# Guidelines

Most guidelines currently in use for the management of peripheral arterial occlusive disease do not include recommendations for drug-coated balloon treatment, because clinical evidence concerning these devices was lacking when these guidelines were formulated (mostly from 2007 to 2011). However, evidence on the use of drug-coated balloons has since been accumulating and there is clearly a need for continuous updating of the guidelines. Early studies with drug-coated balloons in the femoropopliteal arteries have already shown improved short-term patency rates compared to plain balloon angioplasty, but the limited data did not justify a general recommendation.[1] In 2011, the European Society for Vascular Surgery (ESVS) guidelines stated that drug-coated balloons were a promising technology for patients with critical limb ischaemia and infrapopliteal lesions, with a low level of evidence, while the use of drug-coated balloons in the femoropopliteal artery was left unmentioned.[2] One year later, the Guideline Development Group of the National Institute for Health and Care Excellence (NICE) guidelines on lower limb peripheral arterial disease noted that drug-coated balloons were amongst a number of novel technologies that were not considered within their scope, but they acknowledged their future potential. In 2014, drug-coated balloons were more extensively present in the Cardiovascular and Interventional Radiological Society of Europe (CIRSE) Standards of Practice guidelines and the Society for Cardiovascular Angiography and Interventions (SCAI) expert consensus statement for femoropopliteal arterial intervention appropriate use as these devices had already shown a significant inhibition of neointimal hyperplasia at six months of follow-up, expressed by a reduced late lumen loss.[3,4] In 2015, the TASC steering committee published an update on their consensus and acknowledged that results of drug-coated balloons *vs.* plain balloon angioplasty that were beginning to emerge were favourable for drug-coated balloons with regard to patency and target lesion revascularisation. Recommendations still did not include drug-coated balloon treatment, because of a lack of clinical and long-term data.[5] In the Society for Vascular Surgery (SVS) practice guidelines for atherosclerotic occlusive disease of the lower extremities from 2015, it was also acknowledged drug-coated balloons demonstrated improved patency compared to plain balloon angioplasty but that data were limited by small sample sizes, heterogeneous patient populations, and incomplete follow-up.[6] Although the FDA approved two drug-coated balloons for the treatment of occlusive lesions in the femoropopliteal artery, it remained to be shown how these devices would perform in comparison with other novel endovascular approaches.

The guideline of the Deutsche Gesellschaft für angiologie and Gesellschaft für gefäßmedizin, from 2015, concluded that when a reduced risk of restenosis and reinterventions was considered to be of clinical importance, drug-coated balloons should be used in the femoropopliteal artery. They emphasised that both the antiproliferative drug and the excipient play a significant role and that the evidence may not present a uniform "class effect" for all drug-coated balloons (www.awmf. org). Last year, the American Heart Association presented their guidelines on the management of patients with lower extremity peripheral artery disease and although drug-coated balloons were recognised as an available endovascular technique, they considered the assessment of appropriateness of specific endovascular techniques beyond the scope of their document.[7]

Last year an international positioning document acknowledged the time gap between the publication of guidelines and the appearance of new evidence. They concluded that according to the international definitions, the use of drug-coated balloons in TASC IIa and b *de novo* and restenotic lesions in the femoropopliteal artery would be highly recommended. It was recognised that long-term follow-up data were still lacking and that drug-coated balloons would need to meet a similar benchmark as was presented recently for drug-eluting stents.[8]

## Evidence from 2016

A major drawback of guidelines is that they are based on published evidence only and that considerable time may elapse between the original search for published evidence and their publication. Consequently, the most recent evidence may not be taken into account when guidelines are formulated. Last year, five meta-analyses (two on femoropopliteal[9,10] and three on infrapopliteal treatment)[11–13] and seven reviews were published on drug-coated balloon treatment. Of these, all but one by Peterson *et al* (which reviewed data for femoropopliteal lesions only) were for femoropopliteal and infrapopliteal lesions.[14–20]

### Femoropopliteal lesions

An updated meta-analysis showed that the evidence is clear that drug-coated balloons reduce target lesion revascularisation compared to plain balloon angioplasty, although different drug-coated balloons may have differential effects, emphasising the fact that each drug-coated balloon should prove its own efficacy.[9] The authors of the meta-analysis argued for randomised controlled trials comparing drug-coated balloons with other novel therapies such as drug-eluting stents. Furthermore, they reported that differences between plain balloon angioplasty and drug-coated balloon in terms of symptom and functional improvement were not delineated sufficiently and specific subgroups that might have greatest benefit from the use of drug-coated balloons are not yet defined.[9] A network meta-analysis in which the one-year outcomes of various treatment modalities were compared included 33 studies with data on 4,659 patients. The use of drug-eluting stents showed encouraging results at one year but bypass surgery still remained the principal intervention for long complex femoropopliteal lesions. The authors stated that drug-coated balloons might be an effective alternative to drug-eluting stents, in preventing the implantation of a foreign body, but that long-term efficacy has yet to be proven.[10]

Consistent conclusions were reported by the seven reviews on the use of drug-coated balloons for treatment of femoropopliteal lesions. They all showed favourable outcomes of drug-coated balloon over plain balloon angioplasty on short-term technical outcomes (primary patency, binary stenosis rate and target lesion revascularisation). Data for clinical outcomes (i.e. amputation, death, and change in ankle-brachial index or Rutherford classification) are, however, scarce and long-term data are lacking. At two years, drug-coated balloons still showed better technical outcomes than plain balloon angioplasty, but there are several challenges that accompany drug-coated balloon treatment, namely dissection, recoil, and calcifications.[18] None of the randomised controlled trials was powered to answer questions with regard to clinical outcomes, so future studies should shift their focus from technical to patient-centred outcomes.

The evidence on drug-coated balloons was further strengthened last year by original studies.[21–26] Two randomised controlled trials comparing drug-coated balloon with plain balloon angioplasty confirmed the favourable technical outcomes of drug-coated balloon over percutaneous transluminal angioplasty in *de novo* lesions.[21,23,24] Kinstner *et al*, who only included in-stent restenosis lesions, showed higher primary patency at one year for drug-coated balloons compared to plain balloon angioplasty—this finding was more evident in patients with TASC A/B lesions—without concomitant differences in clinical parameters.[23] Three registry studies were published on drug-coated balloons in 2016. One of them compared drug-coated balloon with a standard nitinol stent and interwoven nitinol stent in complex femoropopliteal lesions. All three treatments resulted in significantly improved clinical outcome and encouraging results for drug-coated balloon in short-term follow-up with comparable excellent effectiveness of both interwoven nitinol stent and drug-coated balloon at one year.[26] A retrospective analysis of two-year follow-up after drug-coated balloon treatment of complex femoropopliteal lesions showed that drug-coated balloons were effective in preventing restenosis, and in case there was restenosis, the lesion was shorter than the original lesion.[22] Finally, an Italian registry on long femoropopliteal lesions showed that drug-coated balloons with provisional stenting persistently resulted in clinical benefit at one-year follow-up.[25]

Data for long-term outcome are limited to the THUNDER trial that reported five-year outcomes. Although drug-coated balloon treatment was related to sustained better technical outcomes in terms of target lesion revascularisation and binary restenosis, follow-up was available only in a small proportion of patients. Clinical outcomes were similar with 57% of patients having a Rutherford classification of ≤2 at five-year follow-up.[27] Rutherford classification seemed to be somewhat worse in the drug-coated balloon group and differences were found between men and women, which was also mentioned in the PACIFIER trial.[27,28]

Most studies so far have focused on primary lesions and data on in-stent restenosis are limited and consequently not mentioned in the guidelines. Nevertheless, recent studies have shown a clear benefit for drug-coated balloons over plain balloon angioplasty in femoropopliteal in-stent restenenosis, but the results seem to be less favourable compared to primary lesions.[23,29–31]

### Infrapopliteal lesions

The treatment of infrapopliteal lesions is mostly performed in critical limb ischaemia and the primary goal is limb salvage. As a consequence, patency is less important than clinical outcomes, which include limb salvage and wound healing. The evidence for drug-coated balloons in infrapopliteal lesions is limited and sometimes conflicting. To date, only short-term outcomes are available on *de novo* lesions, showing that there could be a role for drug-coated balloons in infrapopliteal lesion treatment, but safety concerns also have been raised.[32]

Three meta-analyses reported on drug-coated balloon treatment of infrapopliteal lesions in 2016. Cassese *et al* showed favourable angiographic efficacy, but similar clinical outcomes at one year for drug-coated balloon *vs.* plain balloon angioplasty and drug-eluting stents.[11] Two network meta-analyses showed superiority of drug-eluting stents over drug-coated balloon for treatment of infrapopliteal lesions, but long-term data were lacking, as were data on clinical outcomes.[12,13] Six reviews reported on drug-coated balloon treatment of infrapopliteal lesions in 2016. Overall, no convincing evidence exists so far for the use of drug-coated balloons to treat infrapopliteal lesions.[14–16,18–20] More studies on the use of drug-coated balloons for infrapopliteal lesions are indicated with the right endpoints, such as wound healing, limb salvage, and functional and quality of life measures. Data for long-term outcome and cost-effectiveness are also gaps that need to be filled.

## Conclusion

There is increasing evidence that drug-coated balloons are associated with more beneficial technical outcomes compared to standard angioplasty with regard to binary restenosis, patency and target lesion revascularisation in the femoropopliteal artery, but data are mostly limited to one- or two-year follow-up. The benefit on clinical outcomes is less evident. Studies comparing drug-coated balloons with other novel alternatives, such as drug-eluting stents and debulking techniques are clearly needed, as are studies focusing on infrapopliteal arteries with appropriate clinical endpoints. There are many ongoing trials using drug-coated balloons and these results might shed further light on the long-term outcomes and clinical outcomes after drug-coated balloons treatment of femoropopliteal and infrapopliteal arteries. It would also work very well if the different guidelines could be harmonised and updated together. Having so many different guidelines on the same topic all over the world is rather time and resource consuming.

## Summary

- Drug-coated balloons outperform plain balloon angioplasty in *de novo* lesions of the femoropopliteal artery with regard to patency and target lesion revascularisation, but there are still limited data for long-term outcome.

- There is also scarce information on patient subgroups who may particularly benefit from these devices.

- The effect of drug-coated balloons is less evident in clinical outcome measures; future studies should shift their focus from technical to patient-centred outcomes.

- The evidence for the use of drug-coated balloons in infrapopliteal arteries is lacking and further studies with clinical endpoints are required.

- There is a need for head-to-head comparisons with other endovascular strategies.

- Evidence of the effectiveness of drug-coated balloon treatment of in-stent restenosis is increasing.

# References

1. Tendera M, Aboyans V, Bartelink ML, *et al*. ESC Guidelines on the diagnosis and treatment of peripheral artery diseases: Document covering atherosclerotic disease of extracranial carotid and vertebral, mesenteric, renal, upper and lower extremity arteries: the Task Force on the Diagnosis and Treatment of Peripheral Artery Diseases of the European Society of Cardiology (ESC). *Eur Heart J* 2011; **32** (22): 2851–906.

2. Setacci C1, de Donato G, Teraa M, *et al*. Chapter IV: Treatment of critical limb ischaemia. *Eur J Vasc Endovasc Surg* 2011; **42** (Suppl 2): S43–59.

3. Katsanos K, Tepe G, Tsetis D, Fanelli F. Standards of practice for superficial femoral and popliteal artery angioplasty and stenting. *Cardiovasc Intervent Radiol* 2014; **37** (3): 592–603.

4. Klein AJ, Pinto DS, Gray BH, *et al*. SCAI expert consensus statement for femoral-popliteal arterial intervention appropriate use. *Catheter Cardiovasc Interv* 2014; **84** (4): 529–38.

5. Jaff MR, White CJ, Hiatt WR, *et al*. An update on methods for revascularization and expansion of the TASC lesion classification to include below-the-knee arteries: A supplement to the inter-society consensus for the management of peripheral arterial disease (TASC II): The TASC steering committee. *Catheter Cardiovasc Interv* 2015; **86** (4): 611–25.

6. Conte MS, Pomposelli FB. Society for Vascular Surgery Practice guidelines for atherosclerotic occlusive disease of the lower extremities management of asymptomatic disease and claudication. Introduction. *J Vasc Surg* 2015; **61**(3 Suppl): 1S.

7. Gerhard-Herman, Gornik HL, Barrett C, *et al*. 2016 AHA/ACC guideline on the management of patients with lower extremity peripheral artery disease: A report of the American College of Cardiology/ American Heart Association Task Force on clinical practice guidelines. *J Am Coll Cardiol* 2016; Epub.

8. Cortese B, Granada JF, Scheller B, *et al*. Drug-coated balloon treatment for lower extremity vascular disease intervention: an international positioning document. Eur Heart J 2016; **37** (14): 1096–103.

9. Giacoppo D, Cassese S, Harada Y, *et al*. Drug-coated balloon *versus* plain balloon angioplasty for the treatment of femoropopliteal artery disease: An updated systematic review and meta-analysis of randomized clinical trials. *JACC Cardiovasc Interv* 2016; **9** (16): 1731–42.

10. Antonopoulos CN, Mylonas SN, Moulakakis KG, *et al*. A network meta-analysis of randomized controlled trials comparing treatment modalities for de novo superficial femoral artery occlusive lesions. *J Vasc Surg* 2016; **65** (1): 234–45.

11. Cassese S, Ndrepepa G, Liistro F, *et al*. Drug-coated balloons for revascularization of infrapopliteal arteries: A meta-analysis of randomized trials. JACC Cardiovasc Interv 2016; **9** (10): 1072–80.

12. Katsanos K, Kitrou P, Spiliopoulos S, *et al*. Comparative effectiveness of plain balloon angioplasty, bare metal stents, drug-coated balloons, and drug-eluting stents for the treatment of infrapopliteal artery disease: Systematic review and Bayesian network meta-analysis of randomized controlled trials. *J Endovasc Ther* 2016; **23** (6): 851–63.

13. Xiao Y, Chen Z, Yang Y, Kou L. Network meta-analysis of balloon angioplasty, non-drug metal stent, drug-eluting balloon, and drug-eluting stent for treatment of infrapopliteal artery occlusive disease. *Diagn Interv Radiol* 2016; **22** (5): 436–43.

14. Kayssi A, Al-Atassi T, Oreopoulos G, *et al*. Drug-eluting balloon angioplasty vs. uncoated balloon angioplasty for peripheral arterial disease of the lower limbs. *Cochrane Database Syst Rev* 2016; **8**: CD011319.

15. Herten M1, Stahlhoff S, Imm B, *et al*. Drug-coated balloons in the treatment of peripheral artery disease (PAD). History and current level of evidence]. *Radiologe* 2016; **56** (3): 240–53.

16. Naghi J, Yalvac EA, Pourdjabbar A, *et al*. New developments in the clinical use of drug-coated balloon catheters in peripheral arterial disease. *Med Devices (Auckl)* 2016; **9**: 161–74.

17. Peterson S, Hasenbank M, Silvestro C, Raina S. IN.PACT Admiral drug-coated balloon: Durable, consistent and safe treatment for femoropopliteal peripheral artery disease. Adv Drug Deliv Rev 2016.

18. Herten M, Torsello GB, Schönefeld E, Stahlhoff S. Critical appraisal of paclitaxel balloon angioplasty for femoral-popliteal arterial disease. *Vasc Health Risk Manag* 2016; **12**: 341–56.

19. Barkat M, Torella F and Antoniou GA. Drug-eluting balloon catheters for lower limb peripheral arterial disease: The evidence to date. Vasc Health Risk Manag 2016; **12**: 199–208.

20. Colleran R, Harada Y, Cassese S, Byrne RA. Drug coated balloon angioplasty in the treatment of peripheral artery disease. *Expert Rev Med Devices* 2016; **13** (6): 569–82.

21. Jia X, Zhang J, Zhuang B, *et al*. Acotec drug-coated balloon catheter: Randomized, multicenter, controlled clinical study in femoropopliteal arteries: Evidence from the Acoart I trial. *JACC Cardiovasc Interv* 2016; **9** (18): 1941–49.

22. Schmidt A, Piorkowski M, Görner H, *et al*. Drug-coated balloons for complex femoropopliteal lesions: Two-year results of a real-world registry. *JACC Cardiovasc Interv* 2016; **9** (7): 715–24.

23. Kinstner CM, Lammer J, Willfort-Ehringer A, *et al.* Paclitaxel-eluting balloon vs. standard balloon angioplasty in in-stent restenosis of the superficial femoral and proximal popliteal artery: One-year results of the PACUBA trial. *JACC Cardiovasc Interv* 2016; **9** (13): 1386–92.

24. Scheinert D, Schmidt A, Zeller T, *et al.* German center subanalysis of the LEVANT 2 global randomized study of the Lutonix drug-coated balloon in the treatment of femoropopliteal occlusive disease. *J Endovasc Ther* 2016; **23** (3): 409–16.

25. Micari A, Vadalà G, Castriota F, *et al.* One-year results of paclitaxel-coated balloons for long femoropopliteal artery disease: evidence from the SFA-long study. *JACC Cardiovasc Interv* 2016; **9** (9): 950–56.

26. Steiner S, Schmidt A, Bausback Y, *et al.* Midterm patency after femoropopliteal interventions: a comparison of standard and interwoven nitinol stents and drug-coated balloons in a single-center, propensity score-matched analysis. *J Endovasc Ther* 2016; **23** (2): 347–55.

27. Tepe G, Schnorr B, Albrecht T, *et al.* Angioplasty of femoral-popliteal arteries with drug-coated balloons: five-year follow-up of the THUNDER trial. *JACC Cardiovasc Interv* 2015; **8** (1 Pt A): 102–08.

28. Werk M, Albrecht T, Meyer DR, *et al.* Paclitaxel-coated balloons reduce restenosis after femoro-popliteal angioplasty: Evidence from the randomized PACIFIER trial. *Circ Cardiovasc Interv* 2012; **5** (6): 831–40.

29. Krankenberg H, Tübler T, Ingwersen M, *et al.* Drug-coated balloon vs. standard balloon for superficial femoral artery in-stent restenosis: the randomized femoral artery in-stent restenosis (FAIR) trial. *Circulation* 2015; **132** (23): 2230–36.

30. Grotti S, Liistro F, Angioli P, *et al.* Paclitaxel-eluting balloon vs standard angioplasty to reduce restenosis in diabetic patients with in-stent restenosis of the superficial femoral and proximal popliteal arteries: three-year results of the DEBATE-ISR study. *J Endovasc Ther* 2016; **23** (1): 52–57.

31. Stabile E, Virga V, Salemme L, *et al.* Drug-eluting balloon for treatment of superficial femoral artery in-stent restenosis. *J Am Coll Cardiol* 2012; **60** (18): 1739–42.

32. Zeller T, Baumgartner I2, Scheinert D, *et al.* Drug-eluting balloon vs. standard balloon angioplasty for infrapopliteal arterial revascularization in critical limb ischemia: 12-month results from the IN.PACT DEEP randomized trial. *J Am Coll Cardiol* 2014; **64** (15): 1568–76.

# Five-year results of laser and drug-coated balloons for in-stent restenosis

P Nicotera and JC van den Berg

## Introduction

New techniques and technologies have been developed over the last decades for the endovascular treatment of arterial occlusive disease affecting the superficial femoral artery and infrapopliteal arteries. Dedicated stents have been successfully used to deal with the problem of elastic recoil, flow-limiting dissection and residual stenosis after balloon angioplasty. As a result stenting has become the treatment modality of choice. Restenosis rates in various randomised controlled trials (with an average lesion length <10cm) was in the range of 20% at one year.[1,2] In daily practice treated lesion length is typically longer, so higher restenosis rates can be expected. Although there is a tendency to abandon the primary use of stents (and use drug-coated balloon angioplasty instead), stenting of the superficial femoral artery will not become obsolete (bailout stenting after drug-coated balloon angioplasty can be as high as 40% in long lesions). Therefore, the problem of in-stent restenosis will remain a problem affecting mid- and long-term outcome of superficial femoral artery stenting significantly.[3]

This chapter will provide an overview of the literature with the treatment of in-stent restenosis using various available techniques and will discuss the five-year results of combination therapy of laser debulking and drug-coated balloons.

## Treatment of in-stent restenosis

The major histological findings in in-stent restenosis can be summarised as follows:[4]

- In-stent restenotic lesions are complex and differ significantly from *de novo* atherosclerotic lesions
- In-stent restenotic lesions are heterogeneous and consist primarily of collagen and smooth muscle cells, with a high water content. They have an innermost intimal layer of dense smooth muscle cell tissue and an outermost intimal layer that can be described as a cell-poor scaffold or "sponge" comprised of collagen. This outermost intimal layer is the largest volume constituent of an in-stent restenotic lesion
- Calcium is rarely present in in-stent restenotic lesions.

The above described characteristics have important implications for the treatment of in-stent restenosis in the femoral artery. The luminal gain obtained with balloon angioplasty for in-stent restenosis in balloon-expandable stents involves three different mechanisms: tissue compression (by squeezing out the water content of the neointimal hyperplasia), extrusion of tissue out of the stent, and additional stent expansion. The latter may account for up to 56% of the total luminal gain.[5] Both tissue compression and extrusion can take place during percutaneous transluminal angioplasty of self-expanding stents as well, but additional stent expansion cannot be obtained (the stent being already fully expanded). In a volumetric analysis (using intravascular ultrasound, IVUS) of patients treated with percutaneous transluminal angioplasty for in-stent restenosis, it was found that after around 30 minutes, the intra-stent tissue volume had already increased by 32% (an intra-stent tissue volume decrease of 50% was noted immediately after percutaneous transluminal angioplasty).[6] In addition to the lack of further stent expansion and the quick recoil of the compressed tissue, the process of positive remodelling is not possible anymore after self-expandable stent placement.[7] Because of these factors balloon angioplasty will not be efficacious and thus the treatment of in-stent restenosis requires a completely different approach.[8,9]

Multiple therapeutic modalities have been used to deal with the problem of superficial femoral artery in-stent restenosis, including the combination of excimer laser debulking and drug-coated balloon angioplasty, the technique of which will be described hereafter.

## Technique of excimer laser debulking and drug-coated balloons

Either an ipsilateral, antegrade approach or a retrograde, contralateral approach with crossover can be used. After obtaining arterial access, a 4Fr introducer sheath is placed, and a diagnostic angiography of the whole affected limb is obtained. After successful crossing of the lesion with a hydrophilic guidewire (Glidewire, Terumo) a diagnostic catheter is advanced and contrast injected distally from the lesion to confirm intraluminal position. In case of a total occlusion, the lesion should preferably be crossed with the guidewire "looped" to avoid exiting of the wire through the struts of the stent in a "subintimal" fashion. The 4Fr introducer sheath can then be subsequently exchanged for a 5Fr or 6Fr sheath (depending on the size of the laser catheter that is to be used). Then the hydrophilic guidewire should be exchanged for a 0.014inch or 0.018inch guidewire, again depending on which type of laser catheter is used. A Turbo Elite laser catheter (Spectranetics, diameter ranging from 1.4mm to 2mm) is subsequently introduced while applying continuous saline flush on both the introducer sheath and through the laser catheter. The laser catheter is then slowly advanced through the lesion under fluoroscopic control (speed <1mm/sec). It is recommended to perform two passages with the laser catheter. Fluence and pulse repetition rate settings for the first passage should be intermediate, and this will allow for more efficacious ablation of any soft (thrombotic) material present; thus, minimising the risk of distal embolisation. The second passage will be performed using the maximum fluence and frequency (as set by the manufacturer). In this way, the vapour bubble formed around the tip of the catheter will be larger, increasing debulking efficiency. After removal of the laser catheter, balloon angioplasty of the treated segment is performed using standard angioplasty balloons, with a size 1mm less than the reference vessel diameter. This is followed by angioplasty using drug-coated balloons. The inflation time should be at least 60 seconds.[3] It is of utmost importance to avoid a so-called geographic miss; that is, a segment of the lesion not being treated with the drug-coated balloon. Bony landmarks, a ruler, or a road-map based technique can be used to ensure proper overlapping of the drug-coated balloons.

Alternatively the Turbo-Tandem system can be used for debulking. The Turbo Tandem (Spectranetics) requires a 7Fr sheath and consists of a guiding catheter with a ramp and a pre-mounted laser catheter that can be advanced onto the ramp allowing for an off-centre position of the laser catheter during ablation, allowing to obtain a larger luminal gain.[10] The Turbo Tandem catheter can only be used after creating a so-called pilot channel in the occlusion (the minimum diameter required is 2mm). The pilot channel can be obtained by using a small-size Turbo Elite catheter or predilation of the occlusion with an angioplasty balloon. After the first pass of the Turbo Tandem through the occlusion, the laser catheter is retracted off the ramp, the whole system is withdrawn, and in this way a total of four quadrant passes are performed. In cases where crossing of the stent in an antegrade fashion is not possible, either a puncture distally from the stent or a direct puncture of the stent can be performed and retrograde crossing of the occlusion can be attempted. After successful retrograde passage, the guidewire can be snared from above and the procedure can be completed in an antegrade fashion as described above.

## Results

A cohort of 25 patients (26 lesions; mean age 71.8 years) with in-stent restenosis or occlusion (not extending beyond the stent) of the superficial femoral artery and popliteal artery were followed up prospectively. In four patients, the occluded stent extended into the below-the-knee segment. The majority of patients had critical limb ischaemia (Rutherford class four: n=6; class five: n=7 and class six: n=2). The remaining 10 patients suffered from intermittent claudication (Rutherford class three). The average lesion length was 105.6mm (range 10–380mm). The majority of lesions were Tosaka class III (n=20), the remaining six lesions were Tosaka class I. Technical success was obtained in all cases. Two cases of distal embolisation were seen during the procedure, and both were treated successfully by endovascular means. Mean duplex follow-up was 35.1 months (range 4–77 months) and mean clinical follow-up was 37.3 months (range 10–78 months). The primary patency calculated as a Kaplan-Meier estimate at one, two, three, four and five years was 88%, 78.2%, 71.7%, 71.7% and 62.7%, respectively. The Kaplan-Meier estimates for freedom from target lesion revascularisation was 89.7%, 85.9%, 76.4%, 76.4% and 70% at one, two, three, four, and five years respectively. No amputations were needed during follow-up in the patients that suffered from critical limb ischaemia.

## Discussion

The results with combination therapy need to be compared to other treatment modalities that include conventional and cutting balloon angioplasty, covered stents, debulking techniques and drug-coated balloon angioplasty. The following overview is a summary from a recent review on the treatment of in-stent restenosis, and for a more detailed description the reader should refer to that article.[4]

In a randomised study that compared conventional balloon-angioplasty with peripheral cutting-balloon angioplasty in patients with in-stent restenosis, it was found that restenosis rates at six months with conventional percutaneous transluminal angioplasty was 73%, and with cutting balloon angioplasty slightly lower (65%). Likewise, the study by Tosaka *et al* showed that the rate of recurrence of in-stent restenosis after balloon angioplasty was significant, being the highest in class III lesions (84.8%) and lower in class II and I (53.3% and 49.9% respectively).

The results obtained with the Zilver paclitaxel-eluting stent (Cook Medical) in the treatment of femoral in-stent restenosis are better than those obtained with balloon angioplasty, with a primary patency rate at one year of 78.8% and the rate of freedom from target lesion revascularisation was 81% of 60.8% at one- and two years respectively. The results of the use of covered stents in superficial femoral artery in-stent restenosis, as described in the literature, are not equivocal, with a primary patency rate ranging from 48% (SALVAGE study) to 74.8% (RELINE study).

Several studies have evaluated the use of drug-coated balloons for the treatment of superficial femoral artery in-stent restenosis. The first study (registry by Stabile *et al*) that was published demonstrated a 92.1% primary patency rate at one year follow-up. At one year, no influence of lesion length on outcome was seen. The results of two-year follow-up showed a decrease in primary patency to 70.3% with a higher rate of recurrent restenosis in class II and III lesions than in class I lesions (33.3 % and 36.3 % respectively *vs.* 12.5%). The DEBATE-ISR study compared diabetic patients that were treated for femoropopliteal in-stent restenosis with drug-coated balloons, with a historical control group treated with conventional balloon angioplasty. At one year, restenosis was seen in 19.5% patients in the drug-coated balloons group *vs.* 71.8% in the conventional balloon angioplasty group. At three year follow-up, a complete catch-up was seen, without any difference between drug-coated balloon and conventional balloon angioplasty. More recently, two randomised trials (FAIR and PACUBA)[11] have been published. Both demonstrated a significant reduction in freedom from target lesion revascularisation and the incidence of recurrent restenosis at one year.

Mechanical atherectomy and laser debulking have been described as potential techniques. Primary patency rates at one year of directional atherectomy as stand-alone treatment range from 25% to 50%. All current (mechanical) atherectomy devices are contraindicated in the treatment of in-stent restenosis and this technique is, therefore, not recommended. Three large studies have been published on ablation with excimer laser (currently the only US Food and Drug Administration-approved device for in-stent restenosis). In the PATENT study, the primary patency at six months (64.1%) compared favourably to plain or cutting balloon angioplasty, but at 12 months the overall primary patency showed a drop to 37.8% (where class I performed better than class II and III lesions). In a non-randomised dual-centre study, laser atherectomy was associated with significantly lower rates of recurrent restenosis in class III lesions as compared to class I and II lesions at one year (54% *vs.* 91%) and two years of follow-up (69% *vs.* 100%). Similar results were obtained in the multicentre, prospective, randomised, controlled EXCITE-ISR trial, that evaluated laser atherectomy combined with percutaneous transluminal angioplasty and percutaneous transluminal angioplasty as stand-alone treatment. Six-month freedom from target lesion revascularisation was 73.5% for laser atherectomy and percutaneous transluminal angioplasty and 51.8% for percutaneous transluminal angioplasty alone. A particular benefit with combined treatment was seen in patients with long length in-stent restenosis.

The long-term results of most stand-alone therapies (except for covered stents) remain, however, suboptimal, especially in mid- to long-term follow-up. Therefore combination therapy of debulking and drug-coated balloons has emerged as alternative therapy. The first publications involved a small cohort of patients with short- and mid-term follow-up.[12,13] At a mean follow-up of 19.4 months, the primary patency was found to be 91.7%. Similar good results were seen in a study that involved 48 patients that were randomly assigned to treatment using a combination therapy of laser debulking and drug-coated balloon angioplasty, or drug-coated balloon angioplasty alone, with a follow-up of 12 months.[14] All patients were suffering from chronic critical limb ischaemia and presented with a Tosaka class III lesion with a lesion length of over 20cm. Primary patency at six and 12 months in the combined therapy group (91.7% and 66.7%, respectively) were significantly higher than in the drug-coated balloon group (58.3% and 37.5% respectively). Target lesion revascularisation at 12 months was 16.7% in the combination therapy group and 50% in the drug-coated balloon angioplasty only group. Also the number of major amputations was significantly reduced (8% *vs.* 46%; p=0.003). Ulcer healing was better in the patients that underwent combination therapy.

The data described herein present the long-term follow-up of a larger consecutive cohort of patients treated for isolated in-stent restenosis in the superficial femoral artery and is a continuation of the work published in 2014. It appears that after two years there is no significant drop-off in patency rates, with a Kaplan-Meier curve very similar to that seen in the five-year follow-up data of the ZILVER-PTX study,[15] suggesting an adaptation of the vessel to the presence of a stent, resulting in less restenosis trigger.

## Conclusion

Conventional balloon angioplasty, and cutting balloon angioplasty do not provide a solution for in-stent restenosis in the femoropopliteal arteries. Drug-coated balloon angioplasty provides good short-term results but a late catch-up is seen for long lesions after two years and for all lesions after three years. Covered stents have been demonstrated to yield good results at one year; however, long-term follow-up is not available. The burden of intima hyperplasia-associated in-stent restenosis in the peripheral arteries is quite considerable. Given the fact that the innermost layer of the substance that forms the in-stent restenosis consists of non-cellular material the cytotoxic effect of the drug paclitaxel may not be able to reach the cellular (outermost) layer, and this explains the catch-up seen after three years when using drug-coated balloons as stand-alone therapy. Debulking offers the possibility to remove the smooth muscle cell inner intimal layer and the aqueous outer intimal layer that mainly consists of extra-cellular matrix, thus making the cellular component accessible for the action of drug-coated balloons.

There is a growing body of evidence that by adding drug-coated balloon angioplasty to debulking, results can be achieved that compare favourably to those described in the literature that were obtained with standard balloon angioplasty, cutting-balloon angioplasty or debulking alone. Especially in long and complex lesions (Tosaka class III), this synergy is more pronounced, currently with no signs of late catch-up.

## Summary

- Superficial femoral artery in-stent restenosis differs significantly from *de novo* atherosclerotic lesions.

- The treatment of in-stent restenosis with conventional balloon angioplasty poor short-term results that can be improved by using drug coated balloon technology; the latter technique shows however a catch-up phenomenon after three years.

- Treatment of long femoral in-stent restenosis with a combination of laser debulking and drug-coated balloons shows excellent short-term results and good long-term results.

# References

1. Laird JR, Katzen BT, Scheinert D, *et al*. Nitinol stent implantation *versus* balloon angioplasty for lesions in the superficial femoral artery and proximal popliteal artery: twelve-month results from the RESILIENT randomized trial. *Circ Cardiovasc Interv* 2010; **3** (3): 267–76.
2. Schillinger M, Sabeti S, Loewe C, *et al*. Balloon angioplasty *versus* implantation of nitinol stents in the superficial femoral artery . *N Engl J Med* 2006; **354** (18): 1879–88.
3. Diehm NA, Hoppe H, Do DD. Drug eluting balloons. *Tech Vasc Interv Radiol* 2010; **13** (1): 59–63.
4. Van Den Berg JC. Management of in-stent restenosis in the superficial femoral artery. *J Cardiovasc Surg* (Torino) 2016; **57** (2): 248–56.
5. Mehran R, Mintz GS, Popma JJ, Pichard AD, *et al*. Mechanisms and results of balloon angioplasty for the treatment of in-stent restenosis. Am J Cardiol 1996; **78** (6): 618-22.
6. Albertal M, Abizaid A, Munoz JS, *et al*. A novel mechanism explaining early lumen loss following balloon angioplasty for the treatment of in-stent restenosis. Am J Cardiol 2005; **95** (6): 751–54.
7. Gyongyosi M, Strehblow C, Haumer M, *et al*. Vascular remodeling in atherosclerotic femoral arteries: three-dimensional US analysis. *Radiology* 2004; **233** (2): 366-75.
8. Dick P, Sabeti S, Mlekusch W, *et al*. Conventional balloon angioplasty *versus* peripheral cutting balloon angioplasty for treatment of femoropopliteal artery in-stent restenosis: initial experience. *Radiology* 2008; **248** (1): 297–302.
9. Tosaka A, Soga Y, Iida O, *et al*. Classification and clinical impact of restenosis after femoropopliteal stenting. *J Am Coll Cardiol* 2012; **59** (1): 16–23.
10. Schmidt A, Zeller T, Sievert H, *et al*. Photoablation Using the Turbo-Booster and Excimer Laser for In-Stent Restenosis Treatment: Twelve-Month Results From the PATENT Study. *J Endovasc Ther* 2014; **21** (1): 52–60.
11. Kinstner CM, Lammer J, Willfort-Ehringer A, *et al*. Paclitaxel-Eluting Balloon Versus Standard Balloon Angioplasty in In-Stent Restenosis of the Superficial Femoral and Proximal Popliteal Artery: 1-Year Results of the PACUBA Trial. *JACC Cardiovasc Interv* 2016; **9** (13): 1386–92.
12. Van Den Berg JC, Pedrotti M, Canevascini R. Endovascular treatment of in-stent restenosis using excimer laser angioplasty and drug eluting balloons. *J Cardiovasc Surg* (Torino) 2012; **53** (2): 215–22.
13. Van Den Berg JC, Pedrotti M, Canevascini R. In-stent restenosis: mid-term results of debulking using excimer laser and drug-eluting balloons: sustained benefit? *J Invasive Cardiol* 2014; **26** (7): 333–37.
14. Gandini R, Del GC, Merolla S. Treatment of chronic superficial femoral artery in-stent occlusion with combined laser atherectomy and drug-eluting balloon angioplasty in patients with critical limb ischemia: a single-center, prospective, randomized study. *J Endovasc Ther* 2013; **20** (6): 805–14.
15. Dake MD, Ansel GM, Jaff MR, *et al*. Durable clinical effectiveness with paclitaxel-eluting stents in the femoropopliteal artery: 5-year results of the Zilver PTX Randomized Trial. *Circulation* 2016; **133:** 1472–83.

# Outcomes of drug-coated balloons for TASC C and D lesions with calcifications, >15cm, and complete total occlusion

F Fanelli, A Cannavale, M Santoni and M Gazzetti

## Introduction

Based on the available evidence at the time of the first TransAtlantic Inter-Society Consensus (TASC) committee releases, surgical revascularisation was originally recommended for (TASC) D lesions.[1,2]

However, nowadays, endovascular treatment is not only recommended as the first-line approach for simple TASC lesions (A, B and C) but is also recommended for more complex lesions (TASC D) in selected cases.[3]

Drug-coated balloons have shown enticing results in claudicants with short lesions (TASC A and B), but the risk of late clinical failure due to restenosis, neointimal hyperplasia, or stent fractures is still a concern in more complex lesions and in patients with critical limb ischaemia.[4]

The theoretical advantages of drug-coated balloons in complex femoropopliteal lesions are a reduction of recurrent stenosis and reinterventions while limiting the use of metallic stents. The evidence for the use of drug-coated balloons in complex femoropopliteal stenosis and chronic total occlusions is building, but their use in this context is still a matter of debate.[5]

## Rationale of drug-coated balloon use in long/calcified lesions and chronic total occlusion

Complex and long femoropopliteal lesions represent a difficult environment because of the burden of atherosclerotic disease, presence of calcifications and the mechanical strains on the femoropopliteal segments. These factors may halt the early- and long-term technical and clinical success.[6]

In particular, the presence of heavily calcified lesions may be important as they may constitute a barrier for the navigation of the paclitaxel (the agent used for drug-coated balloons) into the vessel wall.[7,8]

Another limiting factor may by the type of recanalisation: subintimal *vs.* endoluminal, but no significant data are available.[9]

In complex settings such as total occlusions and calcified lesions, predilatation with undersized balloon is strongly recommended, as for indications for use (IFU), because it may protect the drug-coated balloon surface and contribute to increase the technical success (ability to cross and dilate the lesion).

Prolonged inflation up to three minutes is also advised to ensure an effective mechanical dilatation and sealing of eventual flow-limiting dissections.[10]

The use of a drug-coated balloon may limit the need for bailout stenting for residual stenosis; therefore, avoiding the extensive stenting that would expose the patient to a higher risk of stent fracture and/or stent thrombosis. This concept, introduced by Werk *et al,*[11] outlined that a higher acute residual stenosis was acceptable for drug-coated balloons compared with standard percutaneous transluminal angioplasty, apparently without compromising primary patency outcomes. This seems due to a delayed paclitaxel-induced regression of residual plaque following initial incomplete lumen expansion and moderate recoil.

Also in a retrospective study, Tepe *et al* found that the degree of residual stenosis after angioplasty with drug-coated balloon did not have a statistically significant influence on late lumen loss (r=−0.238).[7]

This study[7] also found that high calcium burden was a significant negative predictor for late lumen loss after drug-coated balloon angioplasty—confirmed by a study by Fanelli et al.[8] In particular, both studies showed that a high calcification score was correlated with less favourable late lumen loss, specifically with a high degree of circumferential calcification.

Regarding subintimal angioplasty, the DEBATE-SFA (Drug-eluting balloon in peripheral intervention for the superficial femoral artery) trial[12] showed that in TASC C/D lesions, drug-coated balloons and bare metal stents treatment yielded an advantage by significantly reducing the primary endpoint of binary restenosis at one-year compared with percutaneous transluminal angioplasty and bare metal stents. In particular in the subintimal recanalisation group, restenosis rate was 0% for drug coated balloons *vs.* 47.1% for percutaneous transluminal angioplasty (p=0.01).

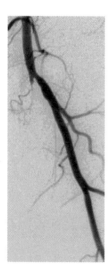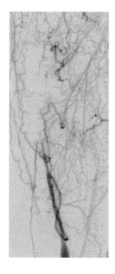

**Figure 1:** A 61-year-old male, with a smoking habit, presented with life-limiting claudication and ankle brachial index (ABI) of 0.5. (A) Angiogram showed a long (>15cm) complete occlusion of the superficial femoral artery. Endovascular recanalisation was successful; predilatation was performed with an Admiral balloon (Medtronic) 4x120mm. A drug-coated balloon (Inpact Admiral 5x120mm, Medtronic) was inflated for three minutes.

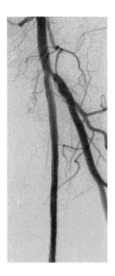
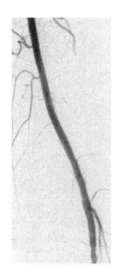

**Figure 2:** Follow-up angiogram at one year still shows patency of the femoropopliteal segment, with no recurrent stenosis. Post-procedure ABI remained stable at 0.9.

Although studies on this topic is sparse, the latest Cochrane review concluded that there is currently insufficient evidence to support subintimal angioplasty over other techniques.[13]

## Evidence and outcomes of drug-coated balloons

Analysis of drug-coated balloon efficacy has been also performed in complex TASC C and D lesions. Most of the current evidence for these lesions is from non-randomised multicentre studies, registries or subset analyses (level of evidence 2) rather than randomised controlled trials. The largest studies available on real-world complex lesions are the In Pact SFA and Lutonix Global registries.[14,15]

Lutonix Global[15] analysed long lesions (140–500mm) and of these, 42.1% were chronic total occlusions. The freedom from target lesion revascularisations was still similar for all lesions (93% in long lesions *vs.* 93.6% for all other lesions) as was the 30-day safety outcomes (99.3%). However, the rate of reinterventions for distal embolisation or thrombosis was slightly increased in long lesions compared to all lesions (2.3% for distal embolisation and 2.3% for target vessel thrombosis in long lesions *vs.* 0.6% and 1.3% in all lesions, respectively). Stents were provisionally implanted in 25.2% of cases.

A subset of long lesions was also analysed in the In.Pact Global Registry.[14] In this subset, 157 lesions were analysed with a mean length of 26.40±8.61cm (chronic total occlusions, 60.4%). The one-year primary patency rate was 91.1% (360 days) and 80.7% (390 days), and the one-year clinically-driven target lesion revascularisation was 6% with 40.4% provisional stenting.

The prospective, multicentre, single-arm SFA long study evaluated the In.Pact Admiral drug-coated balloon in 105 patients (60% diabetic; Rutherford class 2 27.6%; Rutherford class 3 61.9%; Rutherford class 4 8.6%; and Rutherford class 5 1.9%) with lesions longer than 150mm (chronic total occlusion 49.5%).[16]

Primary patency was 83.2% at 12 months, freedom from clinically-driven target lesion revascularisation was 96%, and provisional stenting occurred in 10.5% of cases (flow-limiting dissection occurred in 6.7% of patients). Allowing for one case of post-procedure thrombosis, no safety related adverse events were encountered.

Also another large registry analysed the In.Pact drug-coated balloon (Medtronic) and included 260 patients, with 288 lesions >10cm. The mean lesion length was 24cm, 65.3% were chronic total occlusions, 51.7% were *de novo* lesions, 11.1% were restenoses and 37.2% were in-stent restenoses. Kaplan-Meier estimated primary patency was 79.2±2.6% at one year and 53.7±3.4% at two years. Freedom from target lesion revascularisation was 85.4±2.1% for the entire cohort at one year and 68.6±3% at two years.[17] In the critical limb ischaemia group only, the amputation rate was 5.3% at one year and 7.9% at two years.

In a retrospective dual-centre study that compared the In.Pact balloon with the Zilver PTX stent (Cook Medical) in long lesions (chronic total occlusions, 52.7%), Zeller *et al* had similar results to the registry; they found that clinically-driven target lesion revascularisation was 15.6% for the drug-coated balloon *vs.* 19% for the Zilver stent at one year (p=0.54). The rate of provisional stenting was 18.3%; and in 9.9% of lesions, it was for flow-limiting dissection.[18]

## Evidence on combination therapy

To overcome the limits related to the disease burden in long/calcified lesions, drug-coated balloons have been combined with directional atherectomy.

The first study to look at this was by Cioppa *et al,* and this single-centre registry showed that directional atherectomy followed by an In.Pact drug-coated balloon was associated with a 90% primary patency at one year in 30 patients with long severely calcified femoropopliteal lesions (lesion length: 115±35mm). But, only four (13%) of these lesions were total occlusions.[18]

In the DEFINITIVE AR (Determination of effectiveness of a directional plaque excision system for the treatment of infrainguinal vessels) AR trial, 102 patients were randomised to receive treatment with either SilverHawk or TurboHawk directional atherectomy (Medtronic) followed by a drug-coated balloon (N=48; combination arm) or to treatment with a drug-coated balloon alone (N=54; control arm).[19] Lesion length was 11.2cm and 9.7cm respectively (p=0.05). Severe calcium was detected in 25% and 18.5% in the combination arm and control arm, respectively. Primary patency of 93.4% at one-year was shown in the combination arm compared with 89.6% for the control arm, but there was not a significant difference (P>0.05). The study may have been under powered, but a trend was noted favouring combination therapy *vs.* drug-coated balloon alone in long and severely calcified lesions.

## Conclusion

Drug-coated balloons represent a promising technique for the treatment of complex femoropopliteal stenoses and chronic total occlusions according to one-year results from large "real world" registries and large studies (Figures 1 and 2).

Although provisional stenting is always expected in complex femoropopliteal lesions, drug-coated balloons have the potential to reduce the stenting rate for residual stenosis. A potential limit for drug-coated balloons may be the delivery of drug due to presence of extensive calcifications or subintimal recanalisation, but these topics need further substantial research. Mechanical atherectomy may be considered a valid tool to overcome the limits of drug-coated balloons, but this technique also will need further studies show any advantage over drug-coated balloons alone.

Finally, due to the availability mainly of large registries and studies and lack of randomised controlled trials, drug-coated balloons in the treatment of TASC C-D femoropopliteal lesions have level of evidence 2.

## Summary

- The benefits of drug-coated balloons in long TASC C/D lesions and complete total occlusions would be to limit the high rate of recurrent stenosis and the provisional stenting.

- A higher threshold of acute residual stenosis may be acceptable for drug-coated balloon compared to standard percutaneous transluminal angioplasty.

- Different studies in long lesions have shown a one-year primary patency of 80% at least, lowest target lesion revascularisation of 6% and provisional stenting ranging between 10% and 40%.

- The combination of drug-coated balloon and atherectomy devices in long heavily calcified lesions is theoretically a promising option, but superiority to the drug-coated balloons alone has not been demonstrated yet.

# References

1. Dormandy JA, Rutherford RB. Management of peripheral arterial disease (PAD). TASC Working Group. TransAtlantic Inter-Society Consensus (TASC). *J Vasc Surg* 2000; **31**: S1–S296.
2. Norgren L, Hiatt WR, Dormandy JA, *et al.* Inter-Society Consensus for the Management of Peripheral Arterial Disease (TASC II). *J Vasc Surg* 2007; **45** Suppl S: S5–67.
3. Jaff MR, White CJ, Hiatt WR, *et al.* An update on methods for revascularization and expansion of the TASC lesion classification to include below-the-knee arteries: A supplement to the Inter-Society Consensus for the Management of Peripheral Arterial Disease (TASC II). *J Endovasc Ther* 2015; **22** (5): 663–77.
4. Elmahdy MF, Buonamici P, Trapani M, *et al.* Long-Term primary patency rate after nitinol self-expandable stents implantation in long, totally occluded femoropopliteal (TASC II C & D) Lesions: (Retrospective Study). *Heart Lung Circ* 2016. Epub.
5. Kayssi A, Al-Atassi T, Oreopoulos G, *et al.* Drug-eluting balloon angioplasty *versus* uncoated balloon angioplasty for peripheral arterial disease of the lower limbs. *Cochrane Database Syst Rev* 2016; (8): CD011319.
6. Nishibe T, Yamamoto K, Seike Y, *et al.* Endovascular Therapy for femoropopliteal artery disease and association of risk factors with primary patency: The implication of critical limb ischemia and TASC II C/D Disease. *Vasc Endovascular Surg* 2015; **49**: 236–41.
7. Tepe G, Beschorner U, Ruether C, *et al.* Drug-eluting balloon therapy for femoropopliteal occlusive disease: Predictors of outcome with a special emphasis on calcium. *J Endovasc Ther* 2015; **22**: 727–33.
8. Fanelli F, Cannavale A, Gazzetti M, *et al.* Calcium burden assessment and impact on drug-eluting balloons in peripheral arterial disease. *Cardiovasc Intervent Radiol* 2014; **37**: 898–907.
9. Klimach SG, Gollop ND, Ellis J, Cathcart P. How does subintimal angioplasty compare to transluminal angioplasty for the treatment of femoral occlusive disease? *Int J Surg* 2014; **12**: 361–64.
10. Zorger N, Manke C, Lenhart M, *et al.* Peripheral arterial balloon angioplasty: Effect of short *versus* long balloon inflation times on the morphologic tesults. *J Vasc Interv Radiol* 2002; **13**(4): 355–59.
11. Werk M, Albrecht T, Meyer DR, *et al.* Paclitaxel-coated balloons reduce restenosis after femoro-popliteal angioplasty: evidence from the randomized PACIFIER trial. *Circ Cardiovasc Interv* 2012; **5**: 831–40.
12. Liistro F, Grotti S, Porto I, *et al.* Drug-eluting balloon in peripheral intervention for the superficial femoral artery: the DEBATE-SFA randomized trial (drug eluting balloon in peripheral intervention for the superficial femoral artery). *JACC Cardiovasc Interv* 2013; **6**: 1295–302.

13. Chang Z, Zheng J, Liu Z. Subintimal angioplasty for lower limb arterial chronic total occlusions. *Cochrane Database Syst Rev* 2016;**11**: CD009418.

14. Scheinert D. In.PACT Global registry—oral presentation. EuroPCR 2015.

15. Fanellim F. Lutonix Global SFA Real-World Registry—oral presentation.  CIRSE 2016.

16. Ansel G. IN.PACT Global single-arm study—oral presentation. LINC 2016.

17. Schmidt A, Piorkowski M, Görner H, *et al.* Drug-Coated Balloons for Complex Femoropopliteal Lesions: 2-Year Results of a Real-World Registry. *JACC Cardiovasc Interv* 2016; **9**: 715–24.

18. Cioppa A, Stabile E, Popusoi G, *et al.* Combined treatment of heavy calcified femoro-popliteal lesions using directional atherectomy and a paclitaxel coated balloon: One-year single centre clinical results. *Cardiovasc Revasc Med* 2012; **13**: 219–23.

19. Zeller T. When DCB is not enough: Is there a need for a new DAART study?—oral presentation. LINC 2016.

# Stent use consensus update

# Swirling flow; producing better results in both primary stenting and in combination with DCB

PA Gaines, T Sullivan, M Lichtenberg and T Zeller

## Introduction

Atherosclerosis most frequently affects the superficial femoral artery, but attempted recanalisation has been hindered by a high rate of reocclusion. Difficulty inspires, and the last five years will be memorable for innovation in the battle against restenosis following peripheral intervention.

Failure of patency is important because it not only leads to recurrence of symptoms but any further intervention incurs both risk to the patient and financial cost to the healthcare provider. The clear majority of work leading to our current understanding of endovascular failure comes from the coronary literature. Lumen loss following angioplasty in coronary arteries typically occurs within the first 12 months and is due to immediate recoil, late negative remodelling (fibrosis of the adventitia) and restenosis. Restenosis is a complex process that is most probably driven by the inflammatory response that follows balloon barotrauma and stent implantation. That inflammatory response results in vascular smooth muscle cell proliferation and migration, extracellular matrix formation and the development of neointimal hyperplasia.[1]

That model of lumen loss, both early and late, lends itself to intervention at several levels. Early recoil and late negative remodelling should benefit from internal support. Stents within the coronary arteries reduced patency failure from up to 50% following angioplasty to 20–30% following bare metal stenting.[1] Similarly, within the superficial femoral artery, contemporary stents have been shown to improve short- to medium-term patency.[2,3]

The most dramatic change, however, has been on our ability to reduce restenosis by either changing the flow characteristics or directly delivering drugs to the vessel wall.

## Swirling flow

It is generally recognised that flow within an artery is laminar. Additionally, because of the non-planar curvature of arteries, flow is also swirling. This results in an increase in the velocity of blood against the vessel wall and a rise in the wall shear stress. It is now recognised that this increased shear stress results in a reduced risk of both atherosclerosis and restenosis.[4,5]

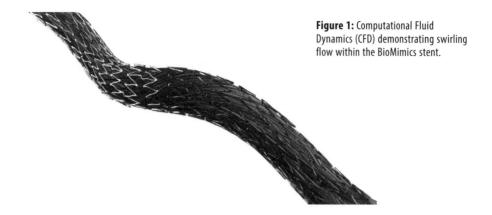

**Figure 1:** Computational Fluid Dynamics (CFD) demonstrating swirling flow within the BioMimics stent.

The BioMimics stent has true 3D helical curvature within the shape memory of the nickel-titanium alloy (nitinol) from which it is formed (Figure 1). The stent imparts non-planar curvature to the artery that produces swirling flow. Whether this could reduce the risk of restenosis was first tested in a porcine model where a straight stent was placed in one carotid artery and a helical stent in the other of the same animal. The study demonstrated that the swirling flow generated by the helical stent significantly reduced the development of restenosis, and that the degree of curvature matched the reduction in restenosis.[6]

The BioMimics 3D stent (Veryan) was subsequently tested in the first randomised controlled trial to directly compare two nitinol stents in the superficial femoral artery. The MIMICS trial was a multicentre, core-lab controlled, prospective, randomised trial in which the BioMimics 3D stent was compared to a conventional straight stent control (Lifestent, Bard) in 76 patients with symptomatic occlusive disease of the superficial femoral and proximal popliteal arteries.[7] Conventional radiographs and angiography confirmed that the BioMimics 3D stent imparts non-planar curvature to the diseased artery. Compared to a straight stent control, the BioMimics 3D stent had significantly better primary patency at two years. There was no change in clinically-driven target lesion revascularisation in the BioMimics 3D arm between 12 and 24 months whereas there was a three-fold increase in this outcome in the straight stent control arm over the same time period; a significant difference between the two stents (Figure 2).

## Drug-coated balloons

Current drug-coated balloons use paclitaxel, a powerful antiproliferative drug, to address the biological mechanisms leading to restenosis. The drug is combined with an excipient to provide uniform dosage and rapid transfer of the drug. Variations in the excipient, formulation and dosage of the paclitaxel result in different behaviours of the individual drug-coated balloons.

The pivotal trials showed improved performance over simple angioplasty but this was in a well-defined set of lesions and the importance of that in terms of generalisability of the value of drug-coated balloons deserves some attention.[8–12] Severe calcification and an inability to completely predilate the lesion were exclusions in these studies and effectively remove those lesions from any analysis. Furthermore, since only 12–26% of lesions were total occlusions, this non-calcified

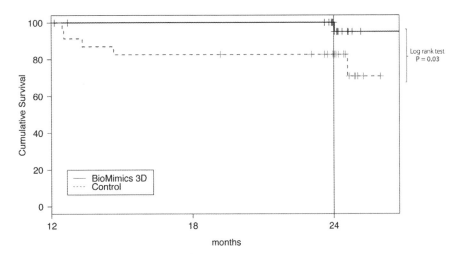

**Figure 2:** A landmark analysis of the data from the MIMICS trial, demonstrating ongoing clinically-driven target lesion revascularisation in the control (straight nitinol stent) arm but none in the BioMimics arm. This difference is significant (p=0.0263).

simple disease was unlikely to recoil after angioplasty resulting in a bailout stent rate of only 2.5–7%. When the same drug-coated balloons are used in more routine clinical practice, and documented within the global registries, the lesion patency and clinically-driven target lesion revascularisation rates remain good. This is because these more clinically generalisable cohorts are in fact measuring the outcome of drug-coated balloon plus stent. This everyday disease is more complex than those recruited to the pivotal trials, resulting in an average stent rate of 28–35.5%. The stent rate is clearly related to both lesion length and the chronic total occlusion rate. In IN.PACT Global, for instance, when the length of lesion exceeds 25cm, the stent rate is 53%, and in total occlusions the stent rate is 47%.

The Kaplan-Meier patency curves from the pivotal trials demonstrate that the improvement in patency and reduction in clinically-driven target lesion revascularisation over simply angioplasty occur between six and 12 months, but after this time the attrition rate is the same. This continued attrition is seen also in the global registries.

## The potential benefit of combining swirling flow with drug-coated balloons

There are clear limitations to the use of a drug-coated balloon in the superficial femoral artery: a "drug-coated balloon only" approach is not appropriate to clinical practice outside pivotal trials. Whilst the bailout stent rate was low in the pivotal trials, the global registries demonstrate that a much higher use of stents is required to maintain high patency and low clinically-driven target lesion revascularisation rates.

Loss of patency is a combination of recoil, late negative remodelling and restenosis. Drug-coated balloons alone clearly do not provide the scaffolding that a stent can to overcome the recoil and remodelling. Indeed, drug-coated balloons were intentionally tested in an environment that would avoid probable recoil; lesions were short, and both calcified lesions and lesions that demonstrated recoil after the initial predilatation were excluded in the pivotal trials.

The antiproliferative effects are necessarily time limited and yet contemporary data show that loss of patency due to restenosis in the superficial femoral artery occurs out to three to four years.[13] Something other than the drug is required to affect these late events.

It would appear, therefore, that in common clinical practice, a stent is required in a significant proportion of drug-coated balloon-treated lesions. If a stent is used to support a drug-coated balloon, it would appear sensible to use a device with good outcomes that would not only provide the scaffolding that drug-coated balloon-only therapy lacks, but could extend the period of low clinically driven target lesion revascularisation past the initial 12 months when drug-coated balloons are effective. The BioMimics 3D stent has been demonstrated, in a randomised controlled trial, to have a better patency and a reduced clinically-driven target lesion revascularisation rate when compared to a straight nitinol stent. Furthermore, as there was no clinically-driven target lesion revascularisation between 12 and 24 months in the BioMimics arm of the randomised controlled trial, this suggests that the use of a proven drug-coated balloon and BioMimics 3D might be the ideal combination.

## Conclusion

Both swirling flow and the use of antiproliferative drugs are effective at maintaining patency by inhibiting neointimal hyperplasia through complimentary mechanisms. In the management of routine disease with variably complex morphology, the use of a drug-coated balloon with the BioMimics 3D stent would appear to extend the prospect for durable clinical outcomes with benefit for both patient and health system costs.

## Summary

- In randomised controlled trials, both swirling flow and drug-coated balloons reduce restenosis.

- The BioMimics 3D stent has the added advantage of restricting recoil and late negative remodelling.

- In real-life lesions, stents are required to support drug-coated balloon in 28–35.5% of cases and are particularly needed in long lesions and total occlusions.

- A combination of drug-coated balloon and swirling flow should have additive benefit in the early (6–12 month) period.

- A combination of drug-coated balloon and swirling flow could give additional late benefit because of the improved 12–14 month clinically-driven target lesion revascularisation rate that is seen following the use of a BioMimics 3D stent.

# References

1. Jukema JW, Verschuren JJ, Ahmed TA, Quax PH. Restenosis after PCI. Part 1: pathophysiology and risk factors. *Nat Rev Cardiol* 2011; **9**: 53–62.

2. Laird JR, Katzen BT, Scheinert D, *et al.* Nitinol stent implantation vs. balloon angioplasty for lesions in the superficial femoral and proximal popliteal arteries of patients with claudication: three-year follow-up from the RESILIENT randomized trial. *J Endovasc Ther* 2012; **19**: 1–9.

3. Schillinger M, Sabeti S, Loewe C, *et al.* Balloon angioplasty *versus* implantation of nitinol stents in the superficial femoral artery. *N Engl J Med* 2006; **354**: 1879–88.

4. Caro CG. Discovery of the role of wall shear in atherosclerosis. *Arterioscler Thromb Vasc Biol* 2009; **29**: 158–61.

5. Carlier SG, van Damme LC, Blommerde CP, *et al.* Augmentation of wall shear stress inhibits neointimal hyperplasia after stent implantation: inhibition through reduction of inflammation? *Circulation* 2003; **107**: 2741–46.

6. Shinke T, Robinson K, Burke MG, *et al.* Novel helical stent design elicits swirling blood flow pattern and inhibits neointima formation in porcine carotid arteries. *Circulation* 2008; **118**: S1054.

7. Zeller T, Gaines PA, Ansel GM, Caro CG. Helical centerline stent improves patency: Two-year results from the randomized Mimics trial. *Circ Cardiovasc Interv* 2016; **9**: Epub.

8. Tepe G, Laird J, Schneider P, *et al.* Drug-coated balloon *versus* standard percutaneous transluminal angioplasty for the treatment of superficial femoral and/or popliteal peripheral artery disease: 12-month results from the IN.PACT SFA randomized trial. *Circulation* 2014; **131** (5): 495–502.

9. Laird JR, Schneider PA, Tepe G, *et al.* Durability of treatment effect using a drug-coated balloon for femoropopliteal lesions: 24-Month Results of IN.PACT SFA. *J Am Coll Cardiol* 2015; **66**: 2329–38.

10. Scheinert D, Schulte KL, Zeller T, *et al.* Paclitaxel-releasing balloon in femoropopliteal lesions using a BTHC excipient: twelve-month results from the BIOLUX P-I randomized trial. *J Endovasc Ther* 2015; **22**: 14–21.

11. Schroeder H, Meyer DR, Lux B, *et al.* Two-year results of a low-dose drug-coated balloon for revascularization of the femoropopliteal artery: outcomes from the ILLUMENATE first-in-human study. *Catheter Cardiovasc Interv* 2015; **86**: 278–86.

12. Rosenfield K, Jaff MR, White CJ, *et al.* Trial of a paclitaxel-coated balloon for femoropopliteal artery disease. *N Engl J Med* 2015; **373**: 145–53.

13. Iida O, Uematsu M, Soga Y, *et al.* Timing of the restenosis following nitinol stenting in the superficial femoral artery and the factors associated with early and late restenoses. *Catheter Cardiovasc Interv* 2011; **78**: 611–17.

# Beyond bare metal stent: The need for precision and durability

F Thaveau and E Girsowicz

## Introduction

Peripheral arterial disease is a public health issue, presenting an age-adjusted prevalence ranging from 12% to 20%.[1] The superficial femoral artery is the arterial axis affected by occlusive disease that most frequently causes intermittent claudication of the calf. Over the last 15 years, there has been a paradigm shift in its treatment, from conventional open surgical revascularisation to endovascular strategies, with continuous advances in imaging equipment and endovascular technologies. Since then, unprecedented improvements in outcomes have been obtained. Minimally invasive technologies have become the mainstay treatment strategy for all types of femoropopliteal occlusive disease. We are now equipped with devices designed specifically for the peripheral vasculature, from specialised crossing wires and catheters, to specific nitinol stents, drug-eluting stents and drug-coated balloons. Thanks to these improvements and the impressive growth in our understanding of the specificity and uniqueness of peripheral artery atherosclerosis, the annual treatment failure rates have been reduced from 20% to <3%.[2]

## Characterisation of the superficial femoral artery motion and stent behaviour

The superficial femoral artery presents unique anatomical characteristics because of its length and tortuosity with a reverse curvature shape ("S" shape) that induces disturbed haemodynamic patterns with low shear stress in the adductor hiatus region of the superficial femoral artery that lead to atherogenesis.[3] The artery's atherosclerotic lesions are also distinguished by unique features such as exuberant extracellular matrix proliferation and intimal and medial wall calcification that lead to a constrictive remodelling prone to restenosis.[4] Lastly, the superficial femoral artery sustains unique strains, from the haemodynamic radial distension of any artery to unique non-radial deformations. Additionally, it is located within a fibromuscular canal and is subjected to strong and multiple mechanical loads such as axial compression, flexion and torsion. In reality, little is known about the biomechanical environment of the artery.[5] Although there appears to be an abundance of data from studies conducted to characterise the superficial femoral and popliteal artery motion, there are a number of limitations and differences in those studies that stop the reader from having a precise understanding of those

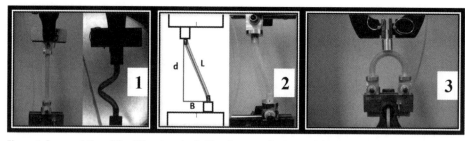

**Figure 1:** Representation of the different mechanical bench tests evaluating nitinol stents.

particular deformations. What is clear is that superficial femoral artery deformation with knee and hip flexion can result in stent-vessel interaction and stent fracture that could lead to clinical consequences, and that the amount of deformation varies depending on patient factors such as age or presence of atherosclerotic disease. Shortening of the artery seems to be greatest in the distal part and in the distal popliteal artery—the proximal part of the superficial femoral artery being more prone to axial twist. The arc of curvature is more important at the distal portion and least relevant in the middle portion, while local compression is greatest at the distal part of the artery. Those data are still incomplete, and a better understanding of artery deformation is needed to improve the development and evaluation of stents in the superficial femoral artery. Indeed, the knowledge and recognition of those unique characteristics have a major importance in order to develop patient-specific devices adapted to each individual biomechanical environment in order to ensure the best possible durability of the material used.

## Evaluation mechanical performance of stents

The growing interest in endovascular technologies has led to a steady increase on the number of stents available on the market. Apart from an evaluation of a stent's gross mechanical properties by the industry, there is no specific standard ISO test and no evaluation of their mechanical performance once deployed in an artery that reproduces the complex superficial femoral artery mechanical load. To ensure an adapted assessment of nitinol stents, we designed normal and pathological femoral artery models using 3D printing technology based on photo-polymerisation, providing precise resolution (up to 0.016mm), smooth surfaces and a transparent vessel wall.[6] The elasticity of the polymer enabled the model to sustain the different mechanical loads. Lastly, the wall thickness of the model was defined in order to match the radial deformation undergone in the superficial femoral artery as described in the literature. Two 5mm diameter models were created, one without stenosis and one simulating a stenosed artery. The stenosed model presented a 50% unique and focal stenosis representing an incomplete result following the first angioplasty. Three mechanical tests were created to reproduce the situations encountered in the superficial femoral artery. In order to reproduce those loads, experimentally, in the simplest possible way, the following combinations were carried out using a dynamometer: (1) bending-compression, (2) compression-torsion-bending and (3) multiple bending (Figure 1).

Judgment criteria were the determination of the level of kink of the stent-model couple, as well as the energy deployed to kink in Joules. An example of extension

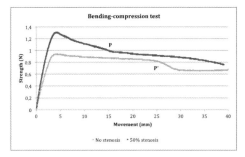

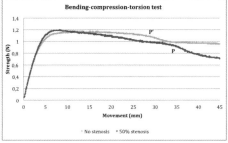

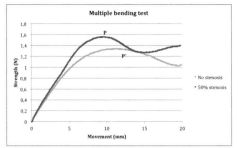

**Figure 2:** Evaluation of the Lifestent 6 x 80 mm. (P) plicature point for the normal model; (P') plicature for the 50% stenosed model; and (P") plicature for the stent alone. The secondary axis corresponds to the deployed strength during the test of the stents alone. (A) bending compression test; (B) bending compression and torsion test; and (C) multiple bending test.

curves obtained for the LifeStent 6x80mm (CR Bard) is shown on Figure 2. Each test permits to evaluate a characteristic of one stent, allowing an objective evaluation that could help the clinician to choose the correct material depending on the expected load in the deployment localisation. A comparison between the stent tested on its own or when deployed in a 3D-printed model highlights the importance of taking into account the coupling between the stent and the artery when evaluating an endovascular device. Indeed, when tested alone, no kink was observed; whereas when deployed in an artery model, a kink was observed with a deployed energy at plicature three to four times greater than when tested alone.

## Calcification in the superficial femoral artery

Another factor compromising the results of endovascular therapy in the superficial femoral artery is the calcium burden and its difficult assessment. Indeed, calcium is known for its ability to jeopardise the performance of endovascular procedures in the short and long term.[7] Vessel wall calcification represents a barrier to antiproliferative drugs, especially in lesions with circumferential calcifications. It also alters the morphology and compliance of the arterial wall, and potentially jeopardises the effect of stenting by increasing the risk of stent subexpansion, malposition and fractures. In our mechanical study, deployment of the Lifestent in the stenosed model led to malposition.[6] Indeed, the meshing cells positioned uncontrollably with an effective stent length different from the announced one (a difference up to 5% was observed), leading to an asymmetric positioning of the stent. This malposition alters the mechanical properties of the device and could jeopardise the patency and the long-term durability of the revascularisation.

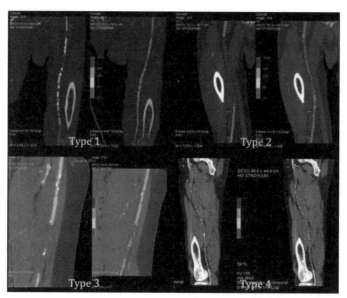

**Figure 3:** Examples of the four groups of patients in the proposed classification of superficial femoral artery occlusions based on quantitative CT angiography analysis.

Only a few studies proposed an evaluation of the arterial wall calcifications. We proposed a classification based on computed tomography (CT) angiography determining four types of complete total occlusion of the superficial femoral artery based on the diameter (> or <5mm) of the artery and the quantity of calcification (> or <4%) (Figure 3), but the relation between this classification and the clinical consequences are still to be determined.[8] Fanelli *et al* used CT angiography, digital subtraction angiography and intravascular ultrasound to measure calcium extension both longitudinally and circumferentially, confirming that the circumferential distribution of calcium is more important than its length in terms of endovascular revascularisation long-term efficacy.[9] On the basis of these facts, there has been a resurgence of atherectomy in order to prepare the artery and to facilitate its treatment, whether by drug-coated balloon, drug-eluting stents or standard nitinol stents. The use of atherectomy devices shows that we have a better understanding of the superficial femoral artery pathophysiology and biomechanics by trying to perform a treatment specific to the lesion. This approach will only lead to a reduction in the use of stents in the superficial femoral artery—the "leave noting behind" concept that will save the use of stents—in case of flow-limiting dissections or to scaffold long artery segments after complex long recanalisation.

## New treatment strategies for superficial femoral artery occlusive lesions

To date it has not yet been demonstrated which treatment strategy may improve the results for superficial femoral artery occlusive lesions. The tools currently available include drug-coated balloons, angioplasty with bailout stenting, primary stenting with a covered stent and drug-eluting stents. In a recent meta-analysis of randomised controlled trials comparing these treatment modalities, drug-eluting stents appears to be the most effective for primary patency at one year of follow-up.[10] The pharmacokinetic drug elution and delivery is a key point of this technology, and recent issues and development provide a promising strategy for treating superficial femoral artery lesions. The Zilver PTX randomised clinical study demonstrated superior outcomes compared with angioplasty and provisional bare metal stent placement at one year.[11] However, the study excluded lesions longer than 14cm, and the drug-eluting stent treatment strategy should be evaluated for severe and calcified lesions of the superficial femoral artery.

## Summary

- Bare metal stent treatment for superficial femoral artery lesions shows limitation.

- Precision and durability of new devices are mandatory to increase patency and effectiveness of severe occlusive lesions.

- Studies of the mechanical behaviour of stents with in-vitro tests should provide the industry with some answers.

- A real evaluation of calcification and a classification may help to choose between treatment strategies.

- A recent meta-analysis of randomised controlled trials shows a tendency towards superior primary patency for drug-eluting stents at one year for *de novo* superficial femoral artery occlusive lesions.

# References

1. Diehm C, Schuster A, Allenberg JR, *et al.* High prevalence of peripheral arterial disease and co-morbidity in 6880 primary care patients: cross-sectional study. Atherosclerosis 2004; **172:** 95–105.
2. Tepe G, Laird J, Schneider P, *et al.* Drug-coated balloon *versus* standard percutaneous transluminal angioplasty for the treatment of superficial femoral and popliteal peripheral artery disease: 12-month results from the IN.PACT SFA randomized trial. *Circulation* 2015; **131**: 495–502.
3. Wood NB, Zhao SZ, Zambanini A, *et al.* Curvature and tortuosity of the superficial femoral artery: a possible risk factor for peripheral arterial disease. J Appl Physiol 2006; **101:** 1412–8.
4. Banerjee S. Superficial femoral artery is not left anterior descending artery. *Circulation* 2016; **134**: 901–03.
5. Ansari F, Pack LK, Brooks SS, Morrison TM. Design considerations for studies of the biomechanical environment of the femoropopliteal arteries. *J Vasc Surg* 2013; **58**: 804–13.
6. Girsowicz E, Georg Y, Seiller H, *et al.* Evaluation of nitinol stents using a 3-dimensional printed superficial femoral artery model: a preliminary study. *Ann Vasc Surg* 2015; **30**: 1–10
7. Tepe G, Beschorner U, Ruether C, *et al.* Drug-eluting balloon therapy for femoropopliteal occlusive disease: predictors of outcome with a special emphasis on calcium. *J Endovasc Ther* 2015; **22:** 727–33.
8. Ohana M, El Ghannudi S, Girsowicz E, *et al.* Detailed cross-sectional study of 60 superficial femoral artery occlusions: morphological quantitative analysis can lead to a new classification. *Cardiovasc Diagn Ther* 2014; **4**: 71–79.
9. Fanelli F, Cannavale A, Gazzetti M, *et al.* Calcium burden assessment and impact on drug-eluting balloons in peripheral arterial disease. *Cardiovasc Intervent Radiol* 2014; **37**: 898–907.
10. Antonopoulos CN, Mylonas SN, Moulakakis KG, *et al.* A network meta-analysis of randomized controlled trials comparing treatment modalities for de novo superficial femoral artery occlusive lesions. *J Vasc Surg* 2017; **65** (1): 234–45.
11. Dake M, Ansel GM, Jaff MR, *et al.* Paclitaxel-eluting stents show superiority to balloon angioplasty and bare metal stents in femoropopliteal disease. Twelve-month Zilver PTX randomized study results. *Circ Cardiovasc Interv* 2011; **4**: 495–504.

# When a flexible stent is used with intravascular ultrasound

## JI Spark and RB Allan

## Introduction

Normal leg movements cause a range of dynamic forces to act on the superficial femoral artery and popliteal artery, including axial compression and extension, radial compression, bending and torsion. This is most pronounced at the transition between the adductor hiatus and popliteal fossa and becomes more marked with age.[1] These conditions result in the superficial femoral artery and popliteal artery being a hostile environment for stenting.

Conventional nitinol stents are not well suited in these arteries due to their relative rigidity and lack of compliance. This results in a transfer of arterial tortuosity distally with an increased risk of vessel kinking[2] and high stent fracture rates.[3] Although stenting is superior to plain angioplasty, the restenosis rate for stenting in the superficial femoral artery is still unacceptably high.[4,5] Better stent solutions are needed in the modern milieu of more aggressive endovascular treatment of complex lesions in these arteries.

## Flexible stents

Flexible stents are designed to mimic the flexibility found in the superficial femoral artery and popliteal arteries with the aim of coping with the wide range of extreme forces that are routine in these arteries. The two most commonly available flexible stents are the Supera (Abbott Vascular) and Tigris (Gore) stents. The Supera stent uses a closed end, braided design composed of six pairs of interwoven wires that offers flexibility with strong crush resistance and high resistance to fracture,[6] but requires precise deployment technique to avoid excessive elongation. Results have been promising with 78.9% primary patency at 12 months in shorter lesions[7] and 72.8% primary patency at 24 months in longer lesions (mean=126mm).[6] The Tigris stent is a hybrid design combining a nitinol wire frame and a heparin-bonded interconnecting expanded polytetrafluoroethylene (ePTFE) lattice. This design has great flexibility and allows the stent to move with the arterial wall with high resistance to longitudinal compression or elongation. Results with Tigris have been encouraging with 90% freedom from target lesion revascularisation at 12 months in shorter lesions[8] and 86% freedom from target lesion revascularisation at 12 month in a more high risk population (70% of patients with critical limb ischaemia, 74% with occlusions and a mean lesion length of 114mm).[9] A zero stent fracture rate has been achieved at two years.[10] The stent maintains its length on deployment with almost no elongation[10] making precise placement possible. We have treated 42

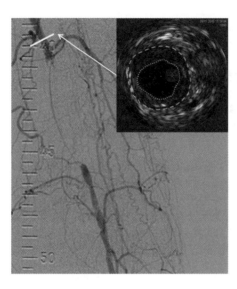

**Figure 1:** DSA image of occluded P1 segment (white bar shows "normal" proximal reference vessel). IVUS image at reference vessel level showing significant plaque burden, with 61% area reduction. Dashed line shows external elastic lamina and dotted line shows the lumen.

patients with Tigris stents. This was a higher risk group with critical limb ischaemia in 61% of cases, occlusion in 53% of cases, popliteal location in 82% of cases and a mean lesion length of 122mm. There was 100% immediate technical success and 12-month freedom from clinical directed target lesion revascularisation of 93% (unpublished data).

The improvement in stent design does not reduce the importance of optimal stent technique as poor technique may negate the benefits of the newer, more flexible stents. Imaging is an essential component of optimal stent technique by providing accurate and complete assessment of vessel anatomy and disease severity.

## Limitations of angiography guidance

Although digital angiography is the mainstay of imaging guidance for endovascular procedures, it has some fundamental limitations. Angiography produces a two-dimensional planar image or "lumenogram" of the contrast media within the lumen. This is intrinsically limiting when attempting to demonstrate the features of a complex three-dimensional structure such as the superficial femoral artery and provides little information about the vessel wall. The limitations of angiography have been demonstrated in comparative studies of angiography and anatomical specimens in the coronary and peripheral arteries [11, 12] that have revealed significant discordance in vessel size and disease severity.

## The need for IVUS

Intravascular ultrasound (IVUS) is an established technology that has been used extensively in the coronary arteries. Comparisons between angiography and IVUS in both the coronary and peripheral arteries have demonstrated the limitations of angiography, including unreliability of angiographic measurements caused by eccentric vessel shape,[13,14] underestimation of reference vessel diameters,[15–17] underestimation of the plaque burden,[17] underestimation of post treatment vessel size,[18] incomplete stent expansion[19, 20] and residual disease.[21] Randomised controlled trials carried out in the coronary arteries have shown that IVUS guidance of bare

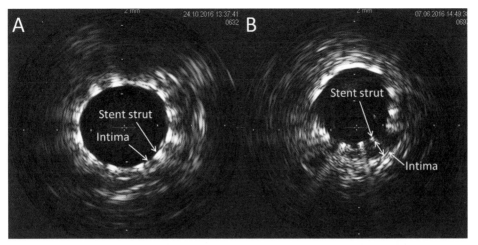

**Figure 2:** (A) Well apposed stent with struts in contact with intima around entire circumference. (B) Poorly apposed stent with 1/3 of stent struts not in contact with intima. Double-headed arrow shows the gap between outer surface of stent strut and intima.

metal stent implantation results in reduced rates of thrombosis, in-stent restenosis and target lesion revascularisation.[22] Although there is no prospective data for the peripheral arteries, retrospective registry evidence suggests that IVUS improves stenting outcomes in the femoropopliteal arteries.[23]

We are currently conducting a randomised controlled trial to investigate whether the routine use of IVUS improves endovascular interventional outcomes in the superficial femoral artery and popliteal arteries. From our experience in a pilot study[24] and the ongoing randomised controlled trial (unpublished data), we have found angiography and IVUS imaging findings disagreed in 66% of cases, predominately due to underestimation of vessel calibre and lesion length with angiography (mean difference in vessel calibre of 0.5mm and mean difference in lesion length of 43mm). This resulted in an increase in device size in 26% of cases and in length of treatment in 21% of cases. In 10% of cases residual disease seen with IVUS imaging resulted in additional treatment after apparently satisfactory angiography.

## How we use IVUS

From this experience we have integrated IVUS into our standard endovascular procedures. IVUS catheters are available in two varieties: a single transducer that rotates within the catheter at 1800rpm or a phased array transducer comprising 64 elements arranged around the catheter wall. Transducers operate in the 20–45MHz range and produce a 360-degree axial tomographic image with axial resolution in the range of 50–150 microns that can also be displayed as a longitudinal image by stacking the axial images. Catheters run on either a 0.014inch or 0.018inch guidewires and require 5Fr and 6Fr access sheaths, respectively. Image analysis software is available for measurement, tracking blood flow and radiofrequency analysis of plaque tissue types.

We prefer to use the phased array catheters as they are more robust. The rotational format is more prone to failure due to kinking when passage is

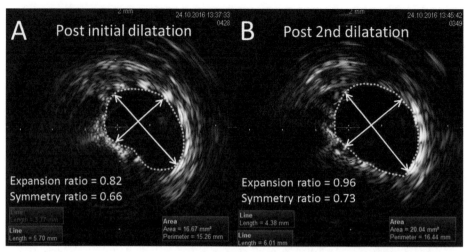

**Figure 3:** (A) IVUS image of Tigris stent after initial dilatation. Inadequate stent expansion and lumen symmetry according to the MUSIC stent criteria[26] (criteria for optimal expansion: expansion ratio [minimum in-stent lumen area/ average reference lumen area] ≥ 0.9 and symmetry ratio [minimum in-stent lumen diameter/maximum in-stent lumen diameter] ≥ 0.7). (B) IVUS image after second dilatation. Stent lumen larger and more symmetric: now within criteria. Dotted line shows lumen, double-headed arrows show minimum and maximum lumen diameters.

attempted through tight spaces that require increased forward force. Phased array catheters can easily be passed through an occlusion once crossing has been achieved without risk of transducer damage, allowing assessment of the lesion prior to commencing treatment.

Images can be obtained using manual or automated pullback. Automated pullback allows the acquisition of a more quantitative dataset but it is more time consuming. Excellent imaging can be rapidly accomplished with manual pullback and imaging of the entire superficial femoral artery can be performed in less than five minutes from placing the catheter onto the wire to removal. Imaging with fluoroscopy during the manual pullback and the use a radiopaque ruler allows for easy correlation between IVUS and angiographic appearances and assists in placement of devices. Additionally, the catheter can be move back and forward through areas of interest much like conventional ultrasound.

## IVUS-assisted stenting

We have found IVUS to be particularly useful in assisting stenting, with our approach to stenting being modified in just over half of cases. The high accuracy of vessel measurements results in very accurate stent sizing and fewer problems with under or oversized stents. IVUS has revealed that apparently normal vessel adjacent to the lesion on angiography often has considerable plaque burden (Figure 1). Relying solely on angiography can result in inadequate stent coverage with significant plaque being present beyond the end of a stent with the associated increased risk of edge restenosis. The combination of highly accurate IVUS imaging and the precise placement possible with the Tigris stent allows the interventionist to provide optimal coverage of lesions.

IVUS is better able to detect a non-apposed stent (Figure 2), which the coronary experience has shown to be associated with increased risk of thrombosis.[25] IVUS can also very accurately demonstrate incomplete stent expansion. It can determine residual stenosis from an under-expanded stent and then confirm that secondary angioplasty has achieved optimal stent expansion (Figure 3).

## Conclusion

Flexible stents are designed to cope better with conditions in the superficial femoral artery and popliteal artery. IVUS imaging provides additional imaging information and can assist in optimising stent deployment to treat lesions in these arteries. The combination of flexible stents and IVUS assisted angiography can improve outcomes for these difficult to treat lesions.

## Summary

- The superficial femoral and popliteal arteries represent a hostile environment for stenting.

- Newer, more flexible stents designed to cope with these conditions are now available and show promising results.

- Optimal stent techniques are still essential even with improved stent design.

- The superior imaging performance of IVUS can assist in optimising stent placement.

- More extensive use of IVUS is recommended to ensure that the advantages of new generation of flexible stents are maximised.

## References

1. Wensing PJ, Scholten FG, Buijs PC, et al. Arterial tortuosity in the femoropopliteal region during knee flexion: a magnetic resonance angiographic study. J Anat 1995; 187 (Pt 1): 133–39.
2. Arena FJ. Arterial kink and damage in normal segments of the superficial femoral and popliteal arteries abutting nitinol stents—a common cause of late occlusion and restenosis? A single-center experience. J Invasive Cardiol 2005; 17: 482–86.
3. Scheinert D, Scheinert S, Sax J, et al. Prevalence and clinical impact of stent fractures after femoropopliteal stenting. J Am Coll Cardiol 2005; 45: 312–15.
4. Laird JR, Katzen BT, Scheinert D, et al. Nitinol stent implantation versus balloon angioplasty for lesions in the superficial femoral artery and proximal popliteal artery: twelve-month results from the RESILIENT randomized trial. Circ Cardiovasc Interv 2010; 3: 267–76.
5. Schillinger M, Sabeti S, Loewe C, et al. Balloon angioplasty vs. implantation of nitinol stents in the superficial femoral artery. N Engl J Med 2006; 354: 1879–88.
6. Werner M, Paetzold A, Banning-Eichenseer U, et al. Treatment of complex atherosclerotic femoropopliteal artery disease with a self-expanding interwoven nitinol stent: midterm results from the Leipzig SUPERA 500 registry. EuroIntervention 2014; 10: 861–68.
7. Garcia L, Jaff MR, Metzger C, et al. Wire-interwoven nitinol stent outcome in the superficial femoral and proximal popliteal arteries: twelve-month results of the SUPERB trial. Circ Cardiovasc Interv 2015; 8: e000937.
8. Piorkowski M, Freitas B, Steiner S, et al. Twelve-month experience with the Gore Tigris vascular stent in the superficial femoral and popliteal arteries. J Cardiovasc Surg (Torino) 2015; 56: 89–95.
9. Parthipun A, Diamantopoulos A, Kitrou P, et al. Use of a new hybrid heparin-bonded nitinol ring stent in the popliteal artery: procedural and mid-term clinical and anatomical outcomes. Cardiovasc Intervent Radiol 2015; 38: 846–54.
10. Laird J. Novel nitinol stent for long lesions in the superficial femoral artery and proximal popliteal artery: 24 month results from the TIGRIS randomized trial. VIVA 2016: Vascular Interventional Advances Conference; Las Vegas 2016.

11. Kashyap VS, Pavkov ML, Bishop PD, *et al.* Angiography underestimates peripheral atherosclerosis: lumenography revisited. *J Endovasc Ther* 2008; **15**: 117–25.

12. Vlodaver Z, Frech R, Van Tassel RA, Edwards JE. Correlation of the antemortem coronary arteriogram and the postmortem specimen. *Circulation* 1973; **47**: 162–69.

13. Tabbara M, White R, Cavaye D, Kopchok G. In vivo human comparison of intravascular ultrasonography and angiography. *J Vasc Surg* 1991; **14**: 496–504.

14. Nissen SE, Gurley JC, Grines CL, *et al.* Intravascular ultrasound assessment of lumen size and wall morphology in normal subjects and patients with coronary artery disease. *Circulation* 1991; **84**: 1087–99.

15. Arthurs ZM, Bishop PD, Feiten LE, *et al.* Evaluation of peripheral atherosclerosis: A comparative analysis of angiography and intravascular ultrasound imaging. *J Vasc Surg* 2010; **51**: 933–39.

16. Cooper BZ, Kirwin JD, Panetta TF, *et al.* Accuracy of intravascular ultrasound for diameter measurement of phantom arteries. J Surg Res 2001; **100**: 99–105.

17. Briguori C, Tobis J, Nishida T, *et al.* Discrepancy between angiography and intravascular ultrasound when analysing small coronary arteries. Eur Heart J 2002; **23**: 247–54.

18. Nakamura S, Mahon DJ, Maheswaran B, *et al.* An explanation for discrepancy between angiographic and intravascular ultrasound measurements after percutaneous transluminal coronary angioplasty. *J Am Coll Cardiol* 1995; **25**: 633–39.

19. Schwarzenberg H, Muller-Hulsbeck S, Gluer CC, *et al.* Restenosis of peripheral stents and stent grafts as revealed by intravascular sonography: in vivo comparison with angiography. Am J Roentgenol 1998; **170**: 1181–85.

20. Van Sambeek MRHM, Qureshi A, van Lankeren W, *et al.* Discrepancy between stent deployment and balloon size used assessed by intravascular ultrasound. *Eur J Vasc Endovasc Surg* 1998; 15: 57–61.

21. Hitchner E, Zayed M, Varu V, *et al.* A Prospective evaluation of using ivus during percutaneous superficial femoral artery interventions. *Ann Vasc Surg* 2015; **29**: 28–33.

22. Parise H, Maehara A, Stone GW, *et al.* Meta-analysis of randomized studies comparing intravascular ultrasound *versus* angiographic guidance of percutaneous coronary intervention in pre–drug-eluting stent era. Am J Cardiol 2011; **107**: 374–82.

23. Lida O, Takahara M, Soga Y, *et al.* efficacy of intravascular ultrasound in femoropopliteal stenting for peripheral artery disease with TASC II class A to C lesions. *J Endovasc Ther* 2014; **21**: 485–92.

24. Allan RB, Wong YT, Puckridge PJ, Spark JI. Intravascular ultrasound modifies peripheral arterial endovascular interventions. Atherosclerosis 2014; **235**: e231–e2.

25. McDaniel MC, Eshtehardi P, Sawaya FJ, *et al.* contemporary clinical applications of coronary intravascular ultrasound. JACC: Cardiovascular Interventions 2011; **4**: 1155–67.

26. De Jaegere P, Mudra H, Figulla H, *et al.* Intravascular ultrasound-guided optimized stent deployment: immediate and 6 months clinical and angiographic results from the multicenter ultrasound stenting in coronaries study (MUSIC Study). Eur Heart J 1998; **19**: 1214–23.

# Popliteal aneurysm and angiosome concept

# Risk factors for poor outcome after endovascular repair of popliteal artery aneurysms

## A Cervin and M Björck

## Introduction

Popliteal aneurysm is a difficult disease to study due to its rarity. The prevalence has been reported to be approximately 1% in men in the age range 65–80 years.[1] The number of popliteal artery aneurysm repairs in 2009–2012 ranged between 3.4 and 17.6 per million inhabitants per year when eight countries participating in the Vascunet collaboration were assessed.[2] This background explains why most studies are based on small numbers, and why the approach to this disease has been surrounded by multiple controversies. Furthermore, very few publications report the patients in subgroups depending on their clinical presentation. Even so, the clinical consequences of these lesions include severe ischaemic manifestations secondary to embolisation and thrombosis, rupture, and compression of adjacent veins and nerves. This emphasises the importance of proactive and adequate treatment.

Fifty years ago there was a debate about whether a conservative or a more aggressive surgical approach was appropriate for asymptomatic popliteal aneurysms. Due to the higher risk of amputation in emergency cases (both in the acute setting and due to inferior patency at follow-up),[3,4] the more active approach was accepted; however, the exact criteria that would justify intervention remained controversial. The most accepted criterion for surgery is size, which should reflect the risk of rupture, but this is the indication for repair in only 2–4% of those treated.[5] The association of size with the probability of embolisation and thrombosis, which often occurs when the last crural artery is occluded, however, is not obvious. In some studies[6-8] size less than 2cm is associated with lower incidence of complications (0–9%); others also report acute complications in patients with small aneurysms.[5,9,10.] Galland and Magee, on the other hand, reported that size 3cm or larger, in combination with a distortion of more than 45 degrees, was correlated with acute ischaemia.[11] Thus, there are risk factors for acute complications of popliteal aneurysm that are not yet sufficiently investigated. This should be considered since most reports of outcome after surgery report from patients predominantly treated for asymptomatic popliteal aneurysms.

## Asymptomatic *versus* symptomatic popliteal aneurysms

The proportion of asymptomatic *vs.* symptomatic popliteal aneurysms varies substantially between different hospitals and countries. In the Vascunet report[2] published in 2014, evaluating on 1,471 popliteal aneurysm repairs from eight countries (Australia, Finland, Hungary, Iceland, New Zealand, Norway, Switzerland and Sweden), elective surgery dominated. It comprised 72% of all cases, but with great differences between the studied countries—only 26% in Hungary compared with 86% in Australia.

## Endovascular treatment

The traditional treatment of popliteal aneurysm is open surgery with medial or posterior approach and either a bypass or an interposition graft. In recent years, investigators have reported results after endovascular treatment with stent grafts. Again, there are great variations between hospitals and countries. In Finland and Switzerland, according to the aforementioned Vascunet report, no stent grafts were applied; whereas in Australia, the proportion was 35% and 30% in Sweden. The Society for Vascular Surgery Vascular Quality Initiative, a registry including 290 centres in the USA and Canada reported an increase of endovascular repair from 35% in 2010 to 48% in 2013.[12]

Questions remain about the durability of stent graft treatment for popliteal aneurysms. Again, most studies concern asymptomatic popliteal aneurysms, and the number of treated legs varies.[3,13] Few studies include more than 70 legs.[14,15] There is only one small randomised controlled trial that compared open and endovascular repair; it included only 30 legs all with asymptomatic popliteal aneurysms.[16] These studies report primary patency rates of 70–93% at one year and slightly higher secondary patency rates.[17,18]

Long-term data are scarce but two years secondary patency rates over 80% have been reported,[13,15] though a large proportion (10–51%) of the patients were lost to follow-up in those studies. Poor run-off (i.e. no or one vessel) is reported consistently to be a risk factor for worse outcome after endovascular repair.[4,19] In a study from the US Medicare administrative database, including 2,962 patients, endovascular treatment showed no benefit in terms of mortality or cost, but was associated with more reinterventions over time.[20]

There were attempts to identify when endovascular could be a better option than open repair. A Markov model study[21] suggested that even if open surgery with vein was the preferred strategy overall, patients at high risk for open repair should be considered for endovascular repair. It should be remembered, however, that this model was built on studies where the run-off vessels chosen for endovascular repair were not comparable to those chosen for open repair. The reports on open repair include patients with acute ischaemia as well as asymptomatic patients, while the papers reporting on endovascular repair are almost exclusively on asymptomatic patients. Obviously, this fundamental difference affects the anatomic configuration of the aneurysm, as well as the run-off, questioning the relevance of such a model, based on a comparison of "apples and oranges".

Two recent studies suggest that treatment of symptomatic popliteal aneurysm with endovascular repair has more complications, with primary patency at one year of only 54% and 43%, respectively.[4,18] Maragliano et al[22] reported a longer follow-up (mean 35 months) of 65 legs, of which 26 were symptomatic. There were 22 occlusions, with preoperative symptoms being the major risk factor for occlusion, although the numbers did not reach a statistical significance in a multivariable regression analysis.

## Open surgery

Results after open surgery are well studied.[23–26] Long-term data report secondary patency rates of 87–97%[25,27] in patients with mixed indications. Overall, the outcome is better with a venous graft. The indication of acute ischaemia is associated with inferior patency. However, the difference is rather small as in one-year data with secondary patency of 87% (acute) *vs.* 94% (asymptomatic) from Cervin *et al.*[18] Dorweiler *et al* found no differences when comparing symptomatic and asymptomatic patients treated with open repair,[25] while a systemic review and meta-analysis of acute thrombosed popliteal artery aneurysms reported one-year primary patency of 79%, but had no data on secondary patency rates, nor depending on bypass material.[28]

## Risk factors of potential importance

There are risk factors that, although not sufficiently well studied, may explain why endovascular repair has inferior patency, and even higher amputation risk, than open repair. When an aneurysm develops the artery often expands, not only in diameter but also in length. With open repair the artery can be shortened (with a posterior approach), restoring the natural anatomy, or by-passed (with a medial approach), but this is not possible when the patient is treated with a stent graft. The kinking that this results in is further emphasised when the knee is bent. Thus, it is very important to perform a completion angiogram with lateral projection and bending of the knee after endovascular repair.

Another issue that needs to be studied is the low flow situation associated with older and frail patients, who otherwise may seem ideal for endovascular repair. Low cardiac output, as well as immobilisation, may result in a low flow situation, increasing the risk of occlusion.

Another factor that needs to be better studied is the observation that occlusion of grafts and stent grafts after popliteal aneurysm repair is not so often associated with a risk of amputation, but quite often only with claudication. The main aim of popliteal aneurysm repair is actually to prevent embolisation, and in that respect both open and endovascular repair are effective, even if the risk of occlusion is much higher after endovascular repair.

## Conclusion

We still lack data on long-term outcome after endovascular repair of popliteal aneurysms, in particular in symptomatic patients. Poor run-off and acute ischaemia are associated with worse outcomes. The specific indications for endovascular repair still need to be defined.

## Summary

- Data for outcome after treatment with endovascular repair is mostly based on studies with asymptomatic popliteal aneurysm, with good run-off.

- Long-term data after endovascular repair is scarce.

- Reports on treatment with endovascular stent grafts in patients with popliteal aneurysm and acute ischaemia showed much lower patency, and significantly higher amputation rates than after open repair.

- Open surgery, on the other hand, has excellent long-term patency.

- We need more long-term data and better understanding of the mechanisms behind occlusion after endovascular repair, before the indication for this technique can be defined.

## References

1. Trickett JP, Scott RAP, Tilney HS. Screening and management of asymptomatic popliteal aneurysms. *Journal of Medical Screening* 2002; **9** (2): 92–93.
2. Bjorck M, Beiles B, Menyhei G, *et al.* Editor's Choice: Contemporary treatment of popliteal artery aneurysm in eight countries: A Report from the Vascunet collaboration of registries. *Eur J Vasc Endovasc Surg* 2014; **47** (2): 164–71.
3. Szilagyi DE, Schwartz RL, Reddy DJ. Popliteal arterial aneurysms. Their natural history and management. *Arch Surg* 1981; **116** (5): 724–28.
4. Huang Y, Gloviczki P, Oderich GS *et al.* Outcomes of endovascular and contemporary open surgical repairs of popliteal artery aneurysm. *J Vasc Surg* 2014; **60** (3): 631–38 e632.
5. Ravn H, Bergqvist D, Bjorck M. Nationwide study of the outcome of popliteal artery aneurysms treated surgically. *Br J Surg* 2007; **94** (8): 970–77.
6. Lowell RC, Gloviczki P, Hallett JW, Jr. *et al.* Popliteal artery aneurysms: the risk of nonoperative management. *Ann Vasc Surg* 1994; **8** (1): 14–23.
7. Whitehouse WM, Jr., Wakefield TW, Graham LM *et al.* Limb-threatening potential of arteriosclerotic popliteal artery aneurysms. *Surgery* 1983; **93** (5): 694–99.
8. Schellack J, Smith RB, 3rd, Perdue GD. Nonoperative management of selected popliteal aneurysms. *Arch Surg* 1987; **122** (3): 372–75.
9. Inahara T, Toledo AC. Complications and treatment of popliteal aneurysms. *Surgery* 1978; **84** (6): 775–83.
10. Ascher E, Markevich N, Schutzer RW *et al.* Small popliteal artery aneurysms: are they clinically significant? *J Vasc Surg* 2003; **37** (4): 755–60.
11. Galland RB, Magee TR. Popliteal aneurysms: distortion and size related to symptoms. *Eur J Vasc Endovasc Surg* 2005; **30** (5): 534–38.
12. Eslami MH, Rybin D, Doros G, Farber A. Open repair of asymptomatic popliteal artery aneurysm is associated with better outcomes than endovascular repair. *J Vasc Surg* 2015; **61** (3): 663–69.
13. Piazza M, Menegolo M, Ferrari A *et al.* Long-term outcomes and sac volume shrinkage after endovascular popliteal artery aneurysm repair. *Eur J Vasc Endovasc Surg* 2014; **48** (2): 161–8.
14. Tielliu IF, Verhoeven EL, Zeebregts CJ *et al.* Endovascular treatment of popliteal artery aneurysms: results of a prospective cohort study. *J Vasc Surg* 2005 ; **41** (4): 561–67.
15. Pulli R, Dorigo W, Castelli P, *et al.* A multicentric experience with open surgical repair and endovascular exclusion of popliteal artery aneurysms. *Eur J Vasc Endovasc Surg* 2013; **45** (4): 357–63.
16. Antonello M, Frigatti P, Battocchio P *et al.* Open repair *versus* endovascular treatment for asymptomatic popliteal artery aneurysm: results of a prospective randomized study. *J Vasc Surg* 2005; **42** (2): 185–93.
17. Mollenhoff C, Katsargyris A, Steinbauer M *et al.* Current status of Hemobahn/Viabahn endografts for treatment of popliteal aneurysms. *J Cardiovasc Surg* (Torino) 2013; **54** (6): 785–91.
18. Cervin A, Tjarnstrom J, Ravn H, *et al.* Treatment of Popliteal Aneurysm by Open and Endovascular Surgery: A Contemporary Study of 592 Procedures in Sweden. *Eur J Vasc Endovasc Surg* 2015; **50** (3): 342–50.

19. Garg K, Rockman CB, Kim BJ, *et al*. Outcome of endovascular repair of popliteal artery aneurysm using the Viabahn endoprosthesis. *J Vasc Surg* 2012; **55** (6): 1647–53.
20. Galinanes EL, Dombrovskiy VY, Graham AM and Vogel TR. Endovascular *versus* open repair of popliteal artery aneurysms: outcomes in the US Medicare population. Vasc Endovascular Surg 2013; **47** (4): 267–73.
21. Hogendoorn W, Schlosser FJ, Moll FL *et al*. Decision analysis model of open repair *versus* endovascular treatment in patients with asymptomatic popliteal artery aneurysms. *J Vasc Surg* 2014; **59** (3): 651–62.
22. Maraglino C, Canu G, Ambrosi R *et al*. " Endovascular Treatment of Poplital Artery Aneurysms: A Word of Caution after Long-Term Follow-Up". *Ann Vasc Surg* 2016. Epub.
23. Kropman RH, van Santvoort HC, Teijink J *et al*. The medial *versus* the posterior approach in the repair of popliteal artery aneurysms: a multicenter case-matched study. *J Vasc Surg* 2007; **46** (1): 24-30.
24. Johnson ON, 3rd, Slidell MB, Macsata RA *et al*. Outcomes of surgical management for popliteal artery aneurysms: an analysis of 583 cases. *J Vasc Surg* 2008; **48** (4): 845–51.
25. Dorweiler B, Gemechu A, Doemland M *et al*. Durability of open popliteal artery aneurysm  repair. *J Vasc Surg* 2014; **60** (4): 951–57.
26. Ravn H, Wanhainen A, Bjorck M. Surgical technique and long-term results after popliteal artery aneurysm repair: results from 717 legs. *J Vasc Surg* 2007; **46** (2): 236–43.
27. Huang Y, Gloviczki P, Noel AA, *et al*. Early complications and long-term outcome after open surgical treatment of popliteal artery aneurysms: is exclusion with saphenous vein bypass still the gold standard? *J Vasc Surg* 2007; **45**(4): 706–13.
28. Kropman RH, Schrijver AM, Kelder JC *et al*. Clinical outcome of acute leg ischaemia due to thrombosed popliteal artery aneurysm: systematic review of 895 cases. *Eur J Vasc Endovasc Surg* 2010; **39** (4): 452–57.

Below the knee

# Differences following open and endovascular management of critical ischaemia using fluorescence imaging

M Venermo and N Settembre

## Introduction

Non-invasive assessment of lower limb circulation is a cornerstone of the evaluation of the severity of peripheral arterial disease and the indications for revascularisation. As important is the perfusion assessment after the revascularisation to control the success of the revascularisation and its impact on perfusion. In daily clinical practice, ankle pressure, toe pressure as well as the indices derived from their comparisons with arm pressures, the ankle-brachial index and toe-brachial index, are the most used. Transcutaneous oxygen pressure and skin perfusion pressure are also used for measuring lower leg haemodynamics, and they measure the local perfusion as well. Indocyanine-green fluorescence imaging (ICG-FI) can also be used in the assessment of the perfusion of a foot. Although some publications exist on the use of this method in the assessment of the ischaemic foot, the technique is still relatively rare in vascular surgery. The assessment of perfusion with ICG-FI uses the time-intensity curve derived from the fluorescence imaging and parameters derived from the curve.

With revascularisation, we aim to increase arterial perfusion in a foot with severe chronic limb ischaemia and create adequate circumstances for the relief of rest pain or for wound healing. Today, the majority of the revascularisations are performed by endovascular means using percutaneous transluminal angioplasty combined with selective stenting. Severe chronic limb ischaemia patients usually require recanalisation of the occluded arteries. In the case of long occlusions, bypass surgery is still the first choice, especially when the patient has an autologous vein for the graft material and open surgery is not contraindicated. We measured the immediate increase in lower limb perfusion using ankle-brachial index, toe pressure as well as ICG-FI in patients who underwent surgical or endovascular revascularisation due to severe chronic limb ischaemia and present our experience and results in this chapter.

## ICG-FI imaging

Since haemoglobin absorbs visible light at a wavelength of 600nm or less and water absorbs light at a wavelength of 900nm or more in the body, the degree of

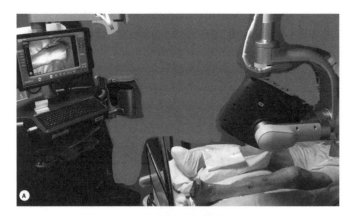

**Figure 1:** (A) The moving arm in the ICG-FI device allows the recording of the foot from different angles. After the ICG-injection, a time-intensity curve can be extracted from all regions of interest—for example, from (B) two different regions in the same leg or (C) from the same region before and after revascularisation.

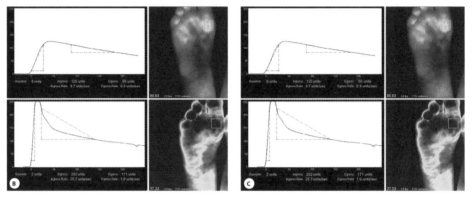

attenuation is small in the region of near-infrared light (600–900nm). This region is known as the optical window. This phenomenon is used in fluorescence imaging, since both the excitation light (760nm) and the fluorescence of ICG (845nm) are within the optical window and can thus penetrate the body.[1]

Indocyanine green dye was developed for near-infrared photography by the Kodak Research Laboratories in 1955 and was approved for clinical use as early as in 1956.[2] Indocyanine green has been used since the early 1970s in ophthalmology for imaging retinal blood vessels, which is called retinal angiography, and, more recently, in microsurgery and plastic surgery. The first publication on the use of ICG-FI in vascular surgery was presented by Unno in 2007, when he reported the intraoperative use of ICG-FI in nine patients.[3] Later on, techniques to extract numeric values from the ICG-FI were developed, and in 2012, Terasaki *et al* proposed the use of a time-intensity curve to extract numeric parameters for the quantitative evaluation of foot perfusion.[1] From the recorded images, signal intensity values were plotted against time as a time-intensity curve using a regions of interest analysis programme (Hamamatsu Photonics KK).[1,4]

The latest developments in the ICG-FI devices include built-in software for the time-intensity curve creation as well as the calculation of numeric parameters describing the foot perfusion.[5] With the patients in this study, we used Spy-Elite (Novadaq), which allows the recording of the foot from several angles using movable arm equipment and automatic reporting showing the time-intensity curve (Figure 1). The Spy device is equipped with an 806nm light-emitting diode as an excitation light source and a charge-coupled device camera covered with a lens that filters out light with a wavelength of 830nm. From the time-intensity curve, we extracted the maximum intensity and the intensity 10 seconds from the beginning of the curve. In our previous study, we analysed the repeatability of the time-intensity curve as well as the perfusion variables extracted from the curve and found the examination to be well repeatable when performed twice on the same patient.[4]

## ICG-FI in practice

The imaging takes place where there is no daylight. The patient lies in a supine position and the infrared camera is focused onto the foot. After a 15-minute rest, 5mg of indocyanine green is injected intravenously and, at the same time, the recording is started, continuing for three minutes. From the recorded image, perfusion can be measured from all possible areas of interest (Figure 2). In cases where another ICG-FI is needed from the same person, a 15-minute wait should be allowed between the examinations to avoid any indocyanine green residuals in the body. Because the indocyanine green is metabolised in liver, the examination is contraindicated in patients with severe liver dysfunction. Furthermore, although extremely rare, anaphylaxis due to indocyanine green is possible and has to be considered with every patient. The biggest limitation of ICG-FI is that it seems to be rather dependent on the individual, meaning that it is difficult to set "normal values" or a "threshold for severe chronic limb ischaemia". However, it is highly repeatable in one individual, which makes it useful in quality control and surveillance after revascularisation.

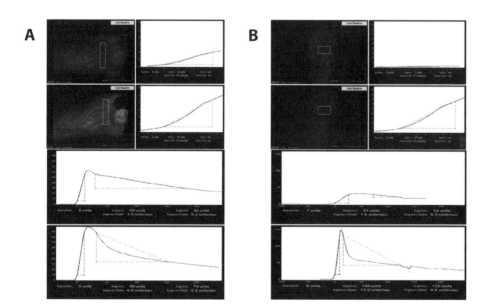

**Figure 2:** (A) Time-intensity curves before and after endovascular revascularisation (recanalisation of the anterior tibial artery) and (B) surgical revascularisation (bypass from the common femoral artery to the distal anterior tibial popliteal (ATP). (A) After endovascular revascularisation, the Spy10 increased from 22IU to 50IU, the maximum intensity from 63 to 98, and the intensity rate from 4 IU/s to 6.9 IU/s. (B) After crural bypass, the Spy10 increased from 1IU to 37IU, the maximum intensity from 31IU to 149IU, and the intensity rate from 1IU/s to 13.2IU/s.

## Change in perfusion after surgical bypass and endovascular revascularisation

Between September 2015 and March 2016, we measured foot perfusion with ankle-brachial index, toe pressure and ICG-FI in 101 patients and 104 limbs with severe chronic limb ischaemia before and after either endovascular (n=72) or surgical (n=32) revascularisation. The patients' demographics were typical of severe chronic limb ischaemia: the mean age was 76 years, and 54% had diabetes. In the majority of the cases, the most distal revascularised artery was the crural artery (60%), followed by the popliteal artery (30%) and the superficial femoral artery (10%). All bypass operations were technically successful; however, in nine (9.5%) of the endovascular recanalisations, an open line from the aorta to the foot was not achieved and, thus, these procedures were technically unsuccessful.

When analysing the foot perfusion, we set the regions of interest to both the dorsal and plantar side of the foot to get as comprehensive an evaluation as possible. To achieve this, we had to perform the imaging twice to get both sides, and a 15-minute break between the two imaging sessions was needed in order for the indocyanine green to disappear from the body. In the analysis, we used three parameters derived from the time-intensity curve: maximum intensity, which is the absolute value of the maximum intensity in the time-intensity curve; intensity rate, which is the value from the time intensity curve describing the increase in maximum intensity per second; and Spy10, which is the intensity achieved during the first 10 seconds after the foot starts to gain intensity. As we measured both the plantar and the dorsal side of the foot, we used the mean value of these two in the final analysis.

Ankle-brachial index measurement was unsuccessful in 58 (57%) legs, mostly due to uncompressible arteries at the ankle level, and toe pressure measurement was unsuccessful in 49 (48%) legs, mostly due to amputated toes or a large tissue lesion. ICG-FI was successful without complications in all patients. In cases with successful revascularisation (63 endovascular and 32 surgical), the haemodynamic parameters increased significantly: the mean ankle-brachial index increased from 0.41 to 0.85 and toe pressure from 29 to 49. The mean maximum intensity in ICG-FI, in turn, increased from 81IU to 120IU and the mean Spy10 from 26IU to 59IU. In the nine legs with technically unsuccessful revascularisation, no change was seen in haemodynamic parameters. When successful surgical and endovascular revascularisations were analysed separately, the increase in all ICG-FI parameters was greater after surgical bypass when compared to endovascular revascularisation. The maximum intensity in the open surgical group increased from 78IU (SD 50) to 134 (SD 52) (p=0.001) and in endovascular group from 83 (SD 46) to 113 (SD 56) (p=0.003). The corresponding increase for Spy10 was from 26.6 to 69.7 after surgery (p=0.003) and from 26.0IU to 54 after an endovascular procedure (p=0.000). Interestingly, there were six patients who underwent technically successful revascularisation, but whose postoperative ICG-FI parameters were worse. In the end, in five of the six legs, there was a revascularisation failure, which explained the worsened perfusion. In one patient, a substantial preoperative infection and inflammation explained the preoperatively high perfusion figures, which were milder postoperatively as the patient had been receiving antibiotic treatment.

# Conclusion

One of the most important but, at the same time, challenging tasks in the treatment of severe chronic limb ischaemia is to obtain an objective comparable measure of the foot perfusion. Ankle-brachial index and toe pressure are useful, but not without limitations as they are not available for a relatively high proportion of the patients. ICG-FI can be used despite these limitations, and, due to its high repeatability, it is useful in surveillance. We evaluated the increase in foot perfusion after endovascular revascularisation and surgical bypass. The mean increase in foot perfusion was significantly higher after bypass surgery when compared to endovascular revascularisation. This is well in line with clinical experience: after bypass, we see a "red-hot foot", which is not typical after endovascular revascularisation.

## Summary

- The goal of revascularisation is to increase arterial circulation in the foot; it is thus mandatory to measure this increase after revascularisation and to ascertain and control the success of the procedure.

- The traditionally used ankle-brachial index and toe pressure are useful, but not reliable nor available for a substantial proportion of the patients with severe chronic limb ischaemia.

- ICG-FI can be used in the assessment of perfusion in almost all patients, although it is not completely non-invasive.

- The increase in limb perfusion seems to be higher after surgical revascularisation than after endovascular revascularisation, which is in line with the clinical picture after revascularisation: the typical "red-hot foot" after bypass is seldom seen after endovascular revascularisation.

- Despite technical success in the completion angiogram, there may be immediate failure of the revascularisation, which emphasises the importance of early perfusion measurement after revascularisation, and patency control in cases with unchanged or impaired perfusion measures.

# References

1. Terasaki H, Inoue Y, Sugano N, et al. A quantitative method for evaluating local perfusion using indocyanine green fluorescence imaging. *Ann Vasc Surg* 2013; **27** (8): 1154–61.
2. Alander JT, Kaartinen I, Laakso, et al. A review of indocyanine green fluorescent imaging in surgery. *Int J Biomed Imaging* 2012; **27** (8): 1154–61.
3. N. Unno, M. Suzuki, N. Yamamoto, et al. Indocyanine green fluorescence angiography for intraoperative assessment of blood flow: a feasibility study. *Eur J Vasc Endovasc Surg* 2008; **35**: 205–07.
4. Venermo M, Settembre N, Albäck A, et al. Pilot assessment of the repeatability of indocyanine green fluorescence imaging and correlation with traditional foot perfusion assessments. *Eur J Vasc Endovasc Surg* 2016; **52** (4): 527–33.
5. Braun JD, Trinidad-Hernandez M, Perry D, et al. Early quantitative evaluation of indocyanine green angiography in patients with critical limb ischemia. *J Vasc Surg* 2013; **57** (5): 1213–18.

# Diabetic foot consensus update

# Point-of-care duplex ultrasound—a paradigm shift in the detection of peripheral arterial disease in diabetes

P Normahani, NJ Standfield and U Jaffer

## Introduction

Diabetic foot complications are frequent and challenging to manage, with potentially poor outcomes in terms of major lower limb amputation rates and overall mortality.[1,2] They also represent a common cause of diabetic admissions to hospital and cost the UK NHS more than £600 million per year.[3]

Peripheral arterial disease is prevalent in diabetes and is a major independent risk factor for the development of diabetic foot ulcers.[4,5] Its detection in the non-ulcerated foot is important for the correct identification of risk status and forward referral for higher-level surveillance and ulcer prevention. Moreover, the prompt and accurate detection of peripheral arterial disease is paramount for the ulcerated foot as time to revascularisation is an important determinant of ulcer healing.[6] Diagnosis of the condition in diabetes is not straightforward. Clinical history, examination and ankle-brachial pressure index (ABPI) measurements are often confounded by presence of neuropathy and arterial calcification. This poses a significant challenge to those at the front line of diabetic foot care who are in need of a reliable non-invasive bedside screening tool.

With the advent of high quality, affordable and compact ultrasound machines, growth of point-of-care ultrasonography in specialties with little previous experience in its performance has ensued.[7] This approach may be valuable in screening for peripheral arterial disease in diabetes by front-line healthcare workers.

## Detection of peripheral arterial disease in diabetes

Neuropathy masks symptoms of claudication and rest pain whilst arterial calcification hinders palpation of foot pulses. The European Working Group on Critical Leg Ischemia recommends that a non-invasive vascular test should be used in addition to pulse palpation for the assessment of patients with diabetes and foot ulceration.[8]

There is currently little evidence to support the use of any one non-invasive diagnostic modality over another.[9] ABPI measurement has been reported to have sensitivity as low as 54%.[10] Audible Doppler waveform assessment also has poor sensitivity in patients with diabetes (29.6%) as well as poor inter- and intra-rater observer reliability.[11,12] Limited evidence suggests that toe-brachial index (TBI), pulse oximetry and waveform analysis may be superior to ABPI measurements.[9] However, there are little data to support the use of any of these modalities routinely, highlighting a need for further development.

Continuous Doppler waveform assessment appears promising. Williams *et al* studied 130 limbs in 68 individuals and compared the diagnostic accuracy of foot pulses, ABPI, TBI and visual continuous Doppler waveform analysis of the distal tibial vessels using the Doppler assist device.[13] They concluded that loss of triphasic flow on continuous Doppler waveform analysis was the most effective screening tool of all the methods tested with a sensitivity of 100% in diabetics with no neuropathy and 92% in those with neuropathy. This methodology was, however, limited by its low specificity of 66% in patients with neuropathy. This is likely a limitation of the Doppler device; heavily calcified blood vessels in patients with neuropathy cannot be penetrated by ultrasound resulting in loss of signal.

This limitation is overcome by using colour duplex ultrasound, which allows for visualisation of the blood vessel and can, therefore, be used to find a calcium free window for pulsed wave Doppler spectral waveform analysis.

Current national and regional training recommendations for podiatrists endorse history, pulse palpation with or without audible Doppler waveform assessment and ABPI as part of the standard assessment for arterial insufficiency.[14–16] This is concerning in view of the unreliability of these methods as reported in the wider literature. Root cause analysis of 140 amputation in Sheffield highlighted that in 30 (21%) cases amputations were the result of delayed vascular referral, investigation or intervention highlighting a need to for development in peripheral arterial disease screening.[17]

## Point-of-care vascular ultrasound

Point-of-care ultrasound has been described as "ultrasonography brought to the patient and performed by the provider in real time".[7] This allows images to be obtained immediately and findings directly correlated with the patient's signs and symptoms allowing for rapid diagnosis at the bedside. Point-of-care ultrasound performed by non-radiologists has been shown to be feasible in clinical practice e.g. trauma (Focused assessment with sonography in trauma scan; FAST scan), aortic ultrasound and gallbladder ultrasound.[18–20]

Goal-directed or focused vascular ultrasound examinations may be beneficial in clinical situations where ascertainment of blood flow is necessary such as diabetic foot assessment.

Point-of-care vascular ultrasound may potentially improve time to diagnosis and allow for rapid triage of those requiring urgent vascular assessment. This may in turn reduce delays to revascularisation and improve diabetic foot outcomes. For the purpose of screening, a full arterial duplex ultrasound scan would be both time-consuming and technically challenging to learn and perform, and may not be required as a rule-out test for peripheral arterial disease. Instead, focused scanning of the distal tibial arteries (anterior and posterior) at the ankle provides

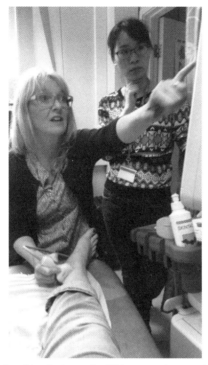

**Figure 1:** Podiatrist scanning of the distal posterior tibial artery under supervision of a vascular scientist.

information regarding the upstream state of the vasculature—the podiatry ankle duplex ultrasound scan (PAD-scan).

In a recent national survey of podiatrists, 92% (n=203/220) expressed a wish to receive point-of-care vascular ultrasound training for the assessment of diabetic foot. Seventy-six percent (n=165/220) believed that this non-invasive test could improve detection of arterial disease and 74% (162/220) reported that it could rationalise the number of patients needing further vascular assessment and imaging.

## Training

Ultrasound is a user-dependent technology and, therefore, requires the implementation of an appropriate training programme. Traditionally, training in duplex ultrasound has been associated with a lengthy apprenticeship model. We have previously demonstrated that novices can readily learn an abbreviated lower limb duplex ultrasound during a three-day intensive course incorporating simulation and hands-on training.[21]

More recently, we enrolled 13 newly qualified podiatrists to an intensive three-hour long simulation and hands-on training session (Figure 1). Participants were then assessed performing bilateral focused PAD-scans of three diabetic patients with peripheral arterial disease. A total of 156 vessel assessments were performed. The loss of triphasic flow was accurately detected in 145 vessels (92.9%) and the correct waveform was identified in 139 cases (89.1%). Additionally, participants achieved excellent scores in technical proficiency and image acquisition quality (manuscript in submission).

## Future work

Our group is launching a quality improvement initiative to pilot a training curriculum for the PAD-scan. We will follow by assessing accuracy of the PAD-scan performed by front line diabetic healthcare workers. If successful training can be achieved, we hope to see improvement in key performance indicators including time from presentation to revascularisation, time to wound healing, amputation rate and economic cost.

## Summary

- Rapid and accurate detection of peripheral arterial disease is paramount in the management of the diabetic foot.

- The detection of peripheral arterial disease is challenging in diabetes and currently there are little data to support the use of any one non-invasive modality over another.

- Qualitative waveform assessment, using a Doppler assist device, has shown promise in detecting peripheral arterial disease in diabetes, albeit with a low specificity. A focused point-of-care duplex ultrasound examination can potentially enhance this assessment by allowing direct vessel visualisation.

- Focused point-of-care duplex ultrasound is readily learned and accurately performed by podiatrists who would be supportive of the adoption of this technology at a national level.

- Further work is required to validate this focused point-of-care duplex ultrasound and assess its impact on patient-centred outcomes.

## References

1. Al-Rubeaan K, Al Derwish M, Ouizi S, et al. Diabetic foot complications and their risk factors from a large retrospective cohort study. PLoS One 2015; **10** (5): e0124446.
2. Moulik PK, Mtonga R, Gill G V. Amputation and mortality in new-onset diabetic foot ulcers stratified by etiology. Diabetes Care 2003; **26** (2): 491–94.
3. Marion K. Foot care for people with diabetes: The economic case for change (2013). http://bit.ly/2lmYLwA (date accessed 22 February 2017).
4. Golomb BA, Dang TT, Criqui MH. Peripheral arterial disease: morbidity and mortality implications. Circulation 2006; **114** (7): 688–99.
5. Brand FN, Kannel WB, Evans J, et al. Glucose intolerance, physical signs of peripheral artery disease, and risk of cardiovascular events: The Framingham Study. Am Heart J 1998; **136** (5): 919–27.
6. Elgzyri T, Larsson J, Nyberg P, et al. Early revascularization after admittance to a diabetic foot center affects the healing probability of ischemic foot ulcer in patients with diabetes. Eur J Vasc Endovasc Surg 2014; **48** (4): 440–46.
7. Moore CL, Copel JA. Point-of-care ultrasonography. N Engl J Med 2011; **364** (8): 749–57.
8. Second European Consensus Document on chronic critical leg ischemia. Eur J Vasc Surg 1992; 6 Suppl A: 1–32.
9. Brownrigg JRW, Hinchliffe RJ, Apelqvist J, et al. Effectiveness of bedside investigations to diagnose peripheral artery disease among people with diabetes mellitus: a systematic review. Diabetes Metab Res Rev 2016; **32** Suppl 1: 119–27.

10. Clairotte C, Retout S, Potier L, *et al.* Automated ankle-brachial pressure index measurement by clinical staff for peripheral arterial disease diagnosis in nondiabetic and diabetic patients. *Diabetes Care* 2009; **32** (7): 1231–36.

11. Alavi A, Sibbald RG, Nabavizadeh R, *et al.* Audible handheld Doppler ultrasound determines reliable and inexpensive exclusion of significant peripheral arterial disease. Vascular 2015; 23 (6): 622–9.

12. Tehan PE, Chuter VH. Use of hand-held Doppler ultrasound examination by podiatrists: a reliability study. *J Foot Ankle Res* 2015; **8**: 36.

13. Williams DT, Harding KG, Price P. An evaluation of the efficacy of methods used in screening for lower-limb arterial disease in diabetes. Diabetes Care 2005; **28** (9): 2206–10.

14. North West Podiatry Services Diabetes Clinical Effectiveness Group. Guidelines for the Prevention and Management of Foot Problems for People with Diabetes (2014). http://bit.ly/2lKNrLW (date accessed 22 February 2017).

15. Diabetes UK. Putting feet first: national minimum skills framework (2011). http://bit.ly/2kYKXVJ (date accessed 22 February 2017).

16. TRIEPodD-UK. Podiatry Competency Framework For Integrated Diabetic Foot Care – A user's guide. (2012). http://www.diabetesonthenet.com/media/fduk/TRIEPodD-UL_compframe.pdf (date accessed 22 February 2017).

17. Diabetes UK. Fixing footcare in Sheffield: Improving the pathway (2015). http://bit.ly/2ln3BKs (date accessed 22 February 2017).

18. Quinn AC, Sinert R. What is the utility of the Focused Assessment with Sonography in Trauma (FAST) exam in penetrating torso trauma? *Injury* 2011; **42** (5): 482–87.

19. Moore CL, Holliday RS, Hwang JQ, Osborne MR. Screening for abdominal aortic aneurysm in asymptomatic at-risk patients using emergency ultrasound. *Am J Emerg Med* 2008; **26** (8): 883–87.

20. Ross M, Brown M, McLaughlin K, *et al.* Emergency physician-performed ultrasound to diagnose cholelithiasis: a systematic review. *Acad Emerg Med* 2011; **18** (3): 227–35.

21. Jaffer U, Normahani P, Matyushev N, *et al.* Intensive simulation training in lower limb arterial duplex scanning leads to skills transfer in real-world scenario. *J Surg Educ* 2016; **73** (3): 453–60.

# A diabetic foot service in a department of vascular surgeons

DT Williams, A Powell-Chandler and O Griffiths

## Introduction

Non-traumatic lower limb amputation is a worldwide problem, usually related to underlying circulatory compromise and infection. Diabetes and its complications, including diabetic foot disease, is an escalating burden that represents a significant healthcare challenge. Foot problems associated with diabetes are a major cause of limb loss.

The positive impact of a multidisciplinary approach to managing diabetic foot disease in preventing major amputation is well established.[1–5] Initiatives aimed at improving amputation rates have demonstrated variable effectiveness and there is wide variation nationally and internationally in reported amputation rates both in the diabetic and non-diabetic population.[6–7] Further, there is a paucity of recent published data regarding the robustness of service implementations that span several years and in particular, initiatives that have impacted on limb salvage with a focus on patients with diabetes.[8–13]

In 2012, a study published by our vascular unit at Ysbyty Gwynedd, Bangor, UK, demonstrated significant falls in major lower limb amputation rates in diabetes between 2006 and 2009 associated with the introduction of a diabetic foot service provided by a Department of Vascular Surgery serving a local population of 220,000.[14]

Prior to the service commencing, vascular surgeons typically only received referrals for management of diabetic foot disease when surgical intervention was required or there was proven arterial disease as per guidelines at that time.[15] Patients referred to hospital were admitted under a variety of specialties, including diabetology, general medicine, orthopaedics, general surgery and vascular surgery, with no clear focal point for referrals and management.

The small specialist team based in a district general hospital was created to address diabetic foot provision and has evolved over the last 10 years. We present here our experience over 10 years in developing our unit structure, its activity and associated outcomes for patients with diabetes (Figure 1).

## Service developments

Key changes in the provision of hospital services for patients with diabetic foot disease began with the employment of a vascular surgeon with an interest in wound

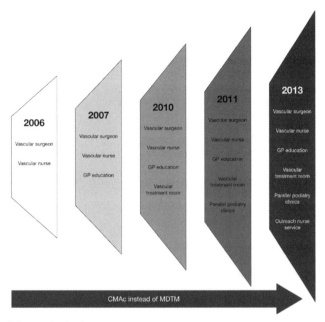

**Figure 1:** Key diabetic foot service developments.

healing in 2006. Figure 1 illustrates the major service changes that have occurred. Pivotal to the service development was that community healthcare professionals and other specialties, both in and outside the hospital setting, had an identifiable point of referral for any patient with a foot problem that was a concern. Thus, the service aimed to augment that already present in the community and change the pathways for escalation of care. The service was unusual in that, differing from the National Institute for Health and Care Excellence (NICE) clinical guidelines at that time, it was led by a vascular surgeon and promoted the vascular department, with its vascular ward and clinics, as the centre for managing and co-ordinating initial and ongoing care for patients with diabetic foot disease, regardless of underlying aetiology and presence of macrovascular disease. However, consistent with guidelines, working with senior podiatrists was key to effective service provision.[16]

In the current service, the two consultant vascular surgeons receive emergency referrals through face-to-face discussion, telephone or written referral throughout the week. Patients are generally seen and assessed by the consultant within 12 hours of referral. Those admitted to the ward, as a first phase of management, receive daily review by the same consultant together with wound assessments/ debridement to accurately determine initial and any ongoing tissue injury and response to interventions. The patient management is enhanced by a twice weekly combined consultant ward round. Once the extent of tissue injury has been fully determined and wound healing is demonstrated, the intensity of review reduces as a second phase of mobilisation and discharge planning commences. In partnership and as part of the continuous multidisciplinary approach, the ward and clinic nursing staff have developed enhanced skills in wound care and are integral to the service provision.

The service was initially developed by using staff already working at the hospital, rearranging clinical activity and clinics to facilitate improved communications and efficient cross-functional team working. Promotion of the service and developing a

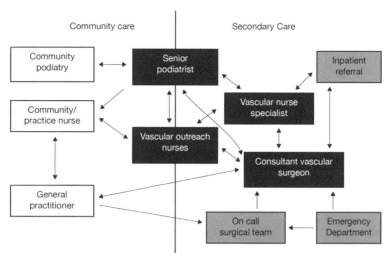

**Figure 2:** Pathways for communication and referrals for the patients with diabetic foot problems with core team members highlighted in black.

hospital at home provision were initial key progressive steps in service development. Following this, and precipitated by increasing workloads related to new referrals and continuity of care, the hospital at home service expanded further, using a vascular ward based treatment room for the review of patients attending the hospital most days of the week. The reconfiguration of vascular and diabetic podiatry clinics to run in parallel and in close proximity was the next major service enhancement.

The additional patient referrals and increasing numbers of patients with complex wounds created pressure on ward bed occupancy, community provision and the vascular nursing staff. This was the driver for a further service improvement, namely the creation of a vascular outreach nurse service. Two experienced nurses who previously worked on the vascular ward were recruited to provide specialised additional capacity to review patients both within hospital and in the community, liaising with district nurses and podiatrists. The outreach service facilitated earlier discharge from hospital for patients with complex wounds and increased capacity for patient reviews throughout the week. The outreach nurses are able to review patients both at hospital and in the community, continuing intensive wound monitoring and management. This additional capacity, working together with our senior podiatrists, has facilitated more streamlined and co-ordinated care for patients with diabetic foot disease (Figure 2). In late 2015, the emergency diabetic foot service expanded to receive patients from North East Wales, increasing the population served to 500,000.

## Outcomes

The age and gender profile for the population has remained relatively constant over the last 10 years, with a preponderance of males and mean age of males and females 67.3 and 73.4 years respectively in 2015. There were an estimated 9300 people with diabetes in our area in 2009. There has been an increase in the general population and an update on the increasing prevalence of diabetes since that time. A more recent estimate on the number of people with diabetes locally in 2010 is

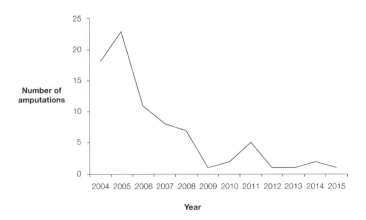

**Figure 3:** Total major amputations for patients with diabetes (estimated 11,500 local population with diabetes in 2010).

11,500. Figure 3 illustrates the major amputation rates per year over the last 12 years. The graph illustrates a reduction in major amputations (above and below knee proximal to the tarsometatarsal joints) following the introduction of the foot service in 2006, but also shows that significant reductions in amputations did not occur until 2009.

Retrospective data collection was required for 2004 and 2005 prior to the service commencing. Major amputations peaked at 24.6/10,000 in 2005 for patients with diabetes. We have managed to maintain the reduced rates of major amputation for patients with diabetes achieved in 2009, at 0.9/10,000 in 2012, 2013 and 2015.

Minor amputation and surgical debridement performed in theatre had been falling during 2004 to 2009 with a low point of 13 procedures in 2009. However, the department now routinely performs minor amputations and debridement in the ward treatment room and clinics. Although the number of theatre based minor procedures has remained static, these are generally for more radical procedures and include skin grafting. The total number of minor surgical procedures has risen to approximately 130 per year in 2015.

There has been no significant change in the number of endovascular or open arterial procedures performed over the last 10 years.

The number of new and review patients attending the service has risen markedly in recent years. Emergency admissions for patients with diabetic foot disease had been decreasing from 49 to 27 between 2004 and 2009, but in 2015 there were 83 admissions to the unit. The outreach service had over 1,000 patient attendances (patients with and without diabetes) in 2015 *vs.* 300 in 2014. Our two senior podiatry colleagues saw more than 1,300 patients with diabetes in their clinics in 2015. Hospital bed occupancy and length of stay for patients requiring emergency admissions continues to be an issue. However, the vascular ward cares for many patients who, prior to the service commencing, would have remained under several other specialties in acute and community hospitals across our region.

# Conclusion

The development of a diabetic foot service provided by the Department of Vascular Surgery and Wound Healing has been associated with improvements in major amputation rates for our population comparable to the best published figures. The number of vascular procedures has not increased, but rates of minor amputations and surgical debridement have risen. Patient new and follow–up appointments have increased markedly. Management of patients with diabetes by a service hosted within a Department of Vascular Surgery and Wound healing enables early, accurate assessment and targeted, timely and contiguous management of patients and their wounds by one core team. Within our district general hospital, there is continuous multidisciplinary activity with related specialties including radiology, anaesthetics, microbiology, nephrology, cardiology, diabetology, orthopaedics and pain teams. The constant dialogue between specialties negates the requirement of waiting for the outcome of fixed multidisciplinary team meetings. We are fortunate also to have ward and clinic staff that together with the administrative support staff are able to effectively co-ordinate bespoke care pathways.

Ultimately, the positive impact of the diabetic foot service by the Department of Vascular Surgery and Wound Healing is dependent upon colleagues from a range of disciplines who are able and willing to support our activities often at short notice, and the effective use of patient pathways. We are fortunate in having clinicians and managers who have embraced the service development. All the staff involved in the diabetic foot service are motivated by team achievements and positive feedback when managing patients with often complex, chronic and demanding conditions.

## Summary

- The incidence of diabetic foot problems continues to rise.

- A multidisciplinary approach in diabetic foot disease reduces major lower limb amputation rates.

- A vascular surgeon (with an interest in wound healing) has developed and led a provision for escalation of diabetic foot care.

- A Department of Vascular Surgery and Wound Healing has evolved over the last 10 years to provide and co-ordinate a lower limb service for patients with diabetes that has been associated with significant and sustained reductions in major amputation rates.

- Definitive initial assessment, treatment and continuity of care is provided seamlessly by a core group of clinical staff with continuous dialogue between specialties.

- A "hospital at home" service and senior hospital podiatrists link more effectively with community provision.

# References

1. Crane M, Werber B. Critical pathway approach to diabetic pedal infections in a multidisciplinary setting. *J Foot Ankle Surg* 1999; **38** (1): 30–33.

2. Dargis V, Pantelejeva O, Jonushaite A, *et al.* Benefits of a multidisciplinary approach in the management of recurrent diabetic foot ulceration in Lithuania: a prospective study. *Diabetes Care* 1999; **22** (9): 1428–31.

3. Larsson J, Apelqvist J, Agardh CD, Stenström A. Decreasing incidence of major amputation in diabetic patients: a consequence of a multidisciplinary foot care team approach? *Diabet Med* 1995; **12** (9): 770–76.

4. Canavan RJ, Unwin NC, Kelly WF, Connolly VM. Diabetes- and non-diabetes-related lower extremity amputation incidence before and after the introduction of better organized diabetes foot care: continuous longitudinal monitoring using a standard method. Diabetes Care 2008; 31 (3): 459–63.

5. Driver VR, Madsen J, Goodman RA. Reducing amputation rates in patients with diabetes at a military medical center: the limb preservation service model. *Diabetes Care* 2005; **28**: 248–53.

6. Vamos EP, Bottle A, Edmonds ME, *et al.* Changes in the incidence of lower extremity amputations in individuals with and without diabetes in England between 2004 and 2008. *Diabetes Care* 2010; **33** (12): 2592–97.

7. Lombardo FL, Maggini M, De Bellis A, *et al.* Lower extremity amputations in persons with and without diabetes in Italy: 2001–2010. *PLoS One* 2014; **9** (1): e86405.

8. Moxey PW, Gogalniceanu P, Hinchliffe RJ, *et al.* Lower extremity amputations—a review of global variability in incidence. *Diabet Med* 2011; **28** (10): 1144–53.

9. Krishnan S, Nash F, Baker N, *et al.* Reduction in diabetic amputations over 11 years in a defined U.K. population: benefits of multidisciplinary team work and continuous prospective audit. *Diabetes Care* 2008; **31** (1): 99–101.

10. Fortington LV, Rommers GM, Postema K, *et al.* Lower limb amputation in Northern Netherlands: unchanged incidence from 1991–1992 to 2003–2004. *Prosthet Orthot Int.*2013; **37** (4): 305–10.

11. Winell K, Niemi M, Lepantalo M. The national hospital discharge register data on lower limb amputations. *Eur J Vasc Endovasc Surg* 2006; **32** (1): 66–70.

12. Santosa F, Moysidis T, Kanya S, *et al.* Decrease in major amputations in Germany. *Int Wound J* 2015; **12** (3): 276–79.

13. Kolossváry E, Ferenci T, Kováts T, *et al.* Trends in major lower limb amputation related to peripheral arterial disease in Hungary: A nationwide study (2004–2012). *Eur J Vasc Endovasc Surg* 2015; **50** (1): 78–85.

14. Williams DT, Majeed MU, Shingler G, *et al.* A diabetic foot service established by a department of vascular surgery: an observational study. *Annals of Vascular Surgery* 2012; **26** (5): 700–06.

15. McIntosh A, Peters J, Young R, *et al.* Prevention and Management of Foot Problems in Type 2 diabetes: Clinical Guidelines and Evidence. Sheffield, University of Sheffield. 2003.

16. National Institute for Health and Clinical Excellence. Diabetic foot problems: Inpatient management of diabetic foot problems. NICE clinical guideline 119; 2011.

# Delay designates disaster for diabetic foot

K Noronen and M Venermo

## Introduction

Ulcer formation in an ischaemic limb is a sign of severe chronic limb ischaemia, the most severe form of peripheral arterial disease. The prevalence of severe chronic limb ischaemia and ischaemic ulcers is rising with the ageing population and the growing number of diabetics. According to estimates, peripheral arterial disease affects 9–24%[1–3] of diabetics during their lifetime and analogously 8–25%[1–4] of diabetics are estimated to develop a foot ulcer.

The primary care centres play a vital role in the early detection of inadequate arterial blood supply in a diabetic foot,[5,6] which is crucial for the patients' prognosis.[7,8] Once peripheral arterial disease is suspected, a vascular surgeon is usually consulted and further investigations are conducted, upon which the revascularisation plan is then based.

Diabetic foot ulcers and their treatment trajectories have been widely investigated, but studies concerning delay in revascularisation are scarce.[9,10] Specific target times for revascularisation are difficult to establish due to various referral patterns and very heterogeneous ulcers. The guideline for the timing of revascularisation according to previous studies could be summarised with the words "the sooner, the better".

According to the Finnish guidelines, a referral to vascular evaluation is made whenever tissue lesion of suspected ischaemic origin is detected; thus, the treatment process at the vascular outpatient clinic in Helsinki University Hospital (HUH) is started. Our aim has been to organise the first visit within one week from the referral for all these patients, including all diabetic patients with an ulcer. After ankle-brachial index and toe-pressure measurements in the vascular laboratory, vascular imaging—usually with magnetic resonance (MR) angiography—is scheduled, after which the decision on treatment is made and revascularisation is scheduled. If ischaemia is detected we consider the presence of an ulcer as a sign of severe chronic limb ischaemia and, therefore, revascularisation is scheduled within two weeks from the decision.

We performed a retrospective study on electively referred patients with suspected severe chronic limb ischaemia and tissue loss, including all patients with diabetic foot ulcers. The study provides a comprehensive analysis of the whole elective treatment process for patients with ischaemic ulcers.[11]

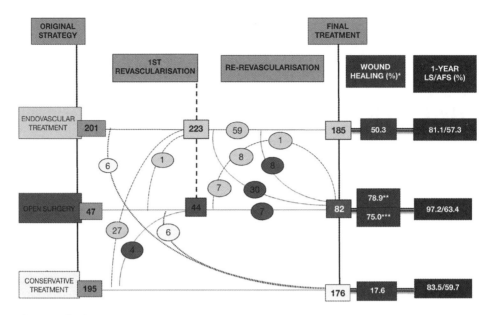

**Figure 1:** Delay designates.

## Patient population

During 2010–2011, 394 patients, with 449 affected limbs, visited a senior consultant at the vascular outpatient clinic for a suspected ischaemic ulcer. Diabetic patients (60%; n=235) formed the majority of the patient population. Diabetic patients tended to be younger than non-diabetic patients (75 years vs. 80 years) and lived more often at home independently (84% vs. 69%), but presented with no significant difference in mobility, only 29% vs. 26% of the patients had no walking aid in use.

## Treatment strategies

Revascularisation was scheduled for 233 (60%) patients with a total of 248 affected limbs (Figure 1). The majority of the patients (81%) were first assigned for endovascular treatment, but after reinterventions and changes in the treatment strategies, altogether 185 (69%) patients underwent endovascular treatment and 82 (31%) patients underwent open surgery. In diabetic patients, the final revascularisation rate was 68% for endovascular and 32% for open surgery.

For 195 (43%) of the affected limbs, including 114 diabetic feet, no revascularisation was planned, most commonly due to expected healing either spontaneously or after minor amputation or wound revision (62%; n=120).

## Delay in treatment

Each step of the treatment process was analysed from referral to revascularisation. The patient records revealed that on the first visit, many had had the wound already for a considerably long time; for less than half (48.4%) of the patients, the duration of the wound was reported to be less than two months. Reflecting this prehospital delay, there were 29 patients assigned from the first visit to urgent revascularisation and also 12 patients assigned for major amputation (Figure 2).

After vascular imaging and the decision on treatment, there were an additional 25 patients assigned for urgent revascularisation. These patients represent a delay in our own treatment process—they arrived in the emergency room because of a worsened wound or worsened overall condition while waiting for elective revascularisation. Even though infection was the reason for many (n=24) of the urgent revascularisations, only eight patients had clearly elevated C-reactive protein (>100mg/l) and only one of them a septic infection with fever. Other reasons for urgent procedures were gangrene (n=18) and increased pain (n=12).

For the entire treatment process, the overall delay from referral to revascularisation was 44 (interquartile range 27–62) days and for patients with diabetes analogously 45 [IQR 29–66] days.

## Limb salvage and amputation free survival

Overall, the one-year limb salvage was significantly better after open surgery with 92.7% compared with 81.1% after endovascular treatment (p=0.015) but no such difference was found in amputation-free survival between the treatment methods (p=0.348). To further assess limb salvage and amputation-free survival, we tested all the comorbidities, wound location and delay to treatment in a univariate analysis. Cox proportional hazards model was performed for all the factors reaching p value of <0.2.

Multivariate analysis was performed for the overall series as well as separately for diabetic and non-diabetic patients, and diabetes was found to be associated with inferior leg salvage (p=0.02) but no difference was seen in overall survival (p=0.1). When revascularisation was performed within two weeks, there was no difference in leg salvage between patients with diabetes and those without: 100% *vs.* 92.9% at 30 days; and 86.5% *vs.* 85.1% at 12 months, respectively. When the delay from

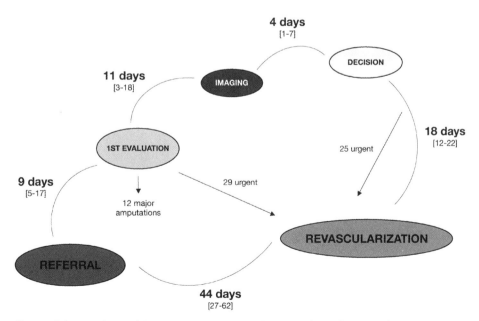

**Figure 2:** Delay on each step of the treatment process presented in median days with interquartile ranges.

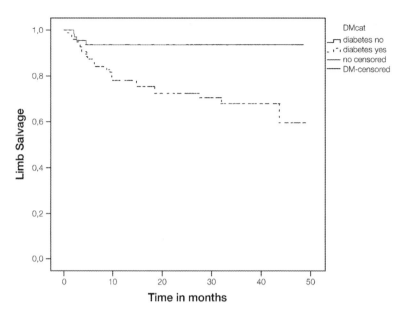

**Figure 3:** Limb salvage for diabetic patients and for patients with no diabetes after a delay >2 weeks from referral to revascularisation.

referral to revascularisation exceeded two weeks, leg salvage was significantly poorer in patients with diabetes (p<0.001) (Figure 3). A delay of over two weeks from the referral to revascularisation appeared to be an independent predictor for major amputation in diabetic patients (odd ratio [OR] 3.1, 95%; confidence interval [CI] 1.4–6.9), but not in non-diabetic patients.

## Wound healing

Of the patients undergoing revascularisation, 81.6% participated in surveillance afterwards, routinely, at least for one month. We determined the wound healing to be achieved when no further revascularisations were considered necessary and when the wound had healed entirely or almost and this was achieved in 60.7% (n=162) of the revascularised limbs. For the two treatment methods, wound healing was found to be significantly better after open surgery (p<0.001) (Figure 1). Failed endovascular treatment was found not to compromise the healing potential. There there was no significant difference in wound healing whether open surgery was chosen as the first-line treatment or as the secondary. Also no significant difference was found in wound healing for patients with or without diabetes (p=0.1)

Only a small proportion (26%) of the patients assigned for conservative treatment were assigned for surveillance, so their wound healing remains unclear and little emphasis can be placed on the low percentage (17.6%) of achieved healing.

## Conclusion

According to our retrospective analysis, wound healing was significantly better after open surgery than after endovascular treatment in the overall study population and in patients with diabetes. Diabetic patients also achieved wound healing rates and times equal to patients with no diabetes. However, diabetes was associated with inferior leg salvage if the delay before revascularisation exceeded two weeks. Therefore, timely revascularisation is crucial, especially in diabetic patients. Additionally, every vascular surgical unit should be aware of their delays and the possible consequences.

## Summary

- Pathway to treatment in patients with severe chronic limb ischaemia referred to a vascular surgeon is complex.

- Prehospital (patient or primary healthcare-related) delay is significant and leads to worsening of the tissue lesion in many patients, thus impairing the possibilities for leg salvage.

- Wound healing after open surgery is better than after endovascular treatment.

- Wound healing for diabetic patients after revascularisation is equal to patients without diabetes.

- Diabetes is associated with inferior limb salvage when delay from referral to revascularisation exceeds two weeks.

# References

1. Gregg E, Sorlie P, Paulose-Ram R, *et al.* Prevalence of lower-extremity disease in the US adult population >=40 years of age with and without diabetes: 1999-2000. National Health and Nutrition Examination Survey. *Diabetes Care* 2004; **27** (7): 1591–97.
2. Lavery L, Armstrong D, Wunderlich R, *et al.* Diabetic foot syndrome: evaluating the prevalence and incidence of foot pathology in Mexican Americans and non-Hispanic whites from a diabetes disease management cohort. *Diabetes Care* 2003; **26** (5): 1435–38.
3. Kallio M, Forsblom C, Groop P, *et al.* Development of new peripheral arterial occlusive disease in patients with type 2 diabetes during a mean follow-up of 11 years. *Diabetes Care* 2003; **26** (4): 1241–45.
4. Singh N, Armstrong D, Lipsky B. Preventing foot ulcers in patients with diabetes. **JAMA** 2005; **293** (2): 217–28.
5. Sanders A, Stoeldraaijers L, Pero M, *et al.* Patient and professional delay in the referral trajectory of patients with diabetic foot ulcers. *Diabetes Res Clin Pract* 2013; **102** (2): 105–11.
6. Yan J, Liu Y, Zhou B, Sun M. Pre-hospital delay in patients with diabetic foot problems: influencing factors and subsequent quality of care. *Diabet Med* 2014; **31** (5): 624–29.
7. Sanders L, Robbins J, Edmonds M. History of the team approach to amputation prevention: pioneers and milestones. *J Vasc Surg* 2010; **52** (3 Suppl): 3S–16S.
8. Rhim B, Harkless L. Prevention: can we stop problems before they arise? *Semin Vasc Surg* 2012; **25** (2): 122–28.
9. Faglia E, Clerici G, Caminiti M, *et al.* The role of early surgical debridement and revascularization in patients with diabetes and deep foot space abscess: retrospective review of 106 patients with diabetes. *J Foot Ankle Surg* 2006; **45** (4): 220–26.
10. Elgzyri T, Larsson J, Nyberg P, *et al.* Early revascularization after admittance to a diabetic foot center affects the healing probability of ischemic foot ulcer in patients with diabetes. *Eur J Vasc Endovasc Surg* 2014; **48** (4): 440–46.
11. Noronen K, Saarinen E, Albäck A, Venermo M. Analysis of the Elective Treatment Process for Critical Limb Ischaemia with Tissue Loss: Diabetic Patients Require Rapid Revascularisation. *Eur J Vasc Endovasc Surg* 2016; **53** (2): 206–13.

# Venous consensus update— Pathways of care

# Investigations of superficial and deep venous anatomy

# The place of ultrasound for deep venous assessment

F D'Abate

## Introduction

Venous ultrasonography is the primary recommended diagnostic tool for the detection of deep vein thrombosis in the extremities.[1] Despite yielding a diagnostic accuracy over 90% for proximal symptomatic deep vein thrombosis,[2] the accuracy for deep vein thrombosis affecting the distal and abdominal veins remains lower.[3-4] Furthermore venous ultrasonography is employed in monitoring the outcome of anticoagulative therapy by defining the amount of residual thrombus and patent lumen[5] and is helpful in determining the acuity of a thrombotic event.[6] Despite the fact that venous ultrasonography has proven to be an valid diagnostic tool in patients with deep vein thrombosis, limitations remain in the assessment of the abdominal and calf veins, in determining the acuity of the thrombus, and quantification of the residual thrombus. Early thrombus removal has proven to reduce the risk for future post-thrombotic syndrome, especially in iliofemoral deep vein thrombosis.[7] The optimal timing for treatment appears to be thrombus <2 weeks old; however, an accurate and standardised method for ageing deep vein thrombosis is not yet available. Even though several ultrasound criteria have been suggested[6] to determine the acuity of thrombus, in several cases, there is an overlap between the findings; also, ageing the acuity of thrombus is not possible. A standardised ultrasound method to age the thrombus is still not available. More than half of the patients with proximal deep vein thrombosis have residual vein thrombosis seen on venous ultrasound at six months to one year after diagnosis and completion of therapy. The presence of residual deep vein thrombosis has been shown to be a risk factor for recurrent venous thromboembolism and is, therefore, clinically useful.[5] Nevertheless, determining the presence of residual thrombosis can be difficult, particularly in the abdominal veins and in the distal veins where depth of the vessels and non-friendly ultrasound conditions (e.g. oedema, bowel gas, patient body habitus) may occur, reducing the lateral resolution of ultrasound. The quantification of residual thrombus and patent lumen remains operator dependent as a standardised ultrasound method is yet to be established. Several promising ultrasound related imaging techniques have emerged in an attempt to overcome the above mentioned limitations of venous ultrasonography, and these include techniques to define patency of lumen, residual thrombus size and acuity of thrombus in an objective, accurate and cost-effective manner that may be employed in a clinical setting.

## Patency of the venous system: New ultrasound techniques

Contrast-enhanced ultrasound involves the use of microbubble contrast agents and dedicated imaging techniques to accurately show the vascular architecture in real time. The main advantages include no risk of nephrotoxicity and no exposure to ionising radiation. Contrast-enhanced ultrasound has found main applications in echocardiography and has been used to enhance parenchymal tumour evaluation in clinical and research settings.[8] A few reports have recently suggested that there might be a role for contrast-enhanced ultrasound in the assessment of extremities and abdominal veins in patients with complicated deep vein thrombosis or in those patients where conventional ultrasound leads to diagnostic uncertainties.[9–10] Usually manual ultrasound venous compression, alongside with colour flow and spectral Doppler imaging techniques, increases the diagnostic accuracy of deep vein thrombosis; however, results still remain low, especially in obese patients, in the presence of local inflammation, oedema and/or with vessels at a greater depth. Also, compression ultrasound cannot be performed within the abdomen. Despite the potential that contrast-enhanced ultrasound may offer, there are only few studies in the literature regarding the venous application of contrast-enhanced ultrasound. Almost all these reports have been focused on portal vein thrombosis where contrast-enhanced ultrasound was recommended to differentiate between benign and malignant portal vein thrombosis in patients who had liver tumors.[11] A feasibility study[9] suggested that the use of contrast-enhanced ultrasound is "at least promising in the detection and characterisation of the deep venous system of the lower limb". This would be particularly beneficial towards the management of patients with high body mass index, local oedema or diffuse inflammation undergoing sonographic assessment for suspected deep vein thrombosis otherwise not definable by venous ultrasound.

Another application of venous contrast-enhanced ultrasound may be for venous stenting. Contrast-enhanced ultrasound may have the potential to increase the diagnostic accuracy of venous sonography in determining the presence of residual intra-stent thrombosis, thus playing a key role in the management of patients with recurrent intra-stent thrombosis; however, no data are yet available. Another non-Doppler imaging technique that may increase the accuracy of venous ultrasonography is B-mode blood flow (B-flow).[12] This technology has been mostly applied to the carotid arteries, arteriovenous fistulas and lower limb arteries with no reports to date on the venous assessment.[13] From our early experience, B-flow imaging appears to be more discriminatory in determining residual thrombus and patent lumen in patients with lower limb and abdominal deep vein thrombosis. Also in patients with iliac venous stents, B-flow appears to be more accurate in defining residual thrombus and patent lumen than compared to conventional venous ultrasonography. These techniques have the potential to improve visualisation of the lower limb venous system, reducing follow-up visits and diagnostic uncertainty. Further studies are needed to determine the role of these techniques in the clinical setting of patients with venous pathology.

## Ageing thrombosis

Despite several proposed ultrasound criteria to determine acuity of deep vein thrombosis, these are not always applicable and ageing of deep vein thrombosis remains based on patient symptoms. A recent review[14] highlighted the potential for non-invasive ultrasound related techniques for the classification of thrombus ageing, with elastography being the most promising of all techniques. Elastography is a non-invasive technique that differentiates between tissues of different elasticity based on an estimation of strain during tissue compression and expansion.[15] Both *in vivo* and clinical studies have assessed the potentials of elastography and have provided quantitative assessment of clot hardness. It was demonstrated that older clots were consistently harder and more regular than younger ones.[16] Ultrasound elastography could be implemented as a simple and cheap adjunct to venous ultrasonography to broadly distinguish between acute and chronic thrombi.[14] Another ultrasound related technique that was suggested to distinguish between acute and recent deep vein thrombosis is the assessment of the echogenicity of the thrombus. Gray-scale median analysis seemed to be the most reliable tool to objectively assess the echogenicity of thrombus and to differentiate between acute and recent deep vein thrombosis.[17]

Ultrasound-related techniques remain an operator dependent mode of analysis, which is dependent on both the image acquisition and quantification of the images. Reproducibility studies are needed to validate these techniques before being implemented in the clinical practice.

## Residual thrombus assessment

Residual vein thrombosis indicates a prothrombotic state and has been associated with an increased risk of thrombotic recurrence and risk of death.[5–18] In order to predict which patient will have a recurrence at the end of a trial of anticoagulative treatment, clinical decision guidelines and laboratory surrogate markers have been developed. Current markers, however, are poor in predicting individual recurrence risk and, therefore, better surrogate tests are needed.[19] One such test is the direct measurement of the presence of residual vein thrombosis. Although the definition of residual vein thrombosis has varied according to the technique used for its detection, there is current agreement on the persistence of a thrombotic burden of at least 4mm in diameter, as assessed with ultrasonography in the transverse section under maximum compressibility, in either the common femoral or the popliteal vein.[20] Current imaging techniques are limited in their ability to quantify thrombus burden, progression, resolution, and organisation over time in patients with acute deep vein thrombosis. These assessments are critical measures of therapeutic success when thrombolytic or thrombectomy treatment protocols are used for deep vein thrombosis. Amongst the emerging ultrasound related techniques to quantify residual vein thrombosis, 3D ultrasound imaging seems to be the most promising. A recent study from Zaho[21] and colleagues illustrated encouraging results on the use of 3D imaging for the quantification of residual vein thrombosis. Zaho concluded that 3D ultrasound reliably measures venous thrombus volume and "will be of increasing value as the appreciation for the deleterious effects of residual thrombus after deep vein thrombosis increases". Further large studies are needed to develop a standardised and accurate method to quantify residual vein thrombosis.

## Conclusion

Venous ultrasonography plays a key role in the diagnosis and management of patients with deep vein thrombosis. So far ultrasound has proved to be a reliable and accurate diagnostic tool in this cohort of patients. Limitations remain in the assessment of the abdominal veins and calf veins in determining the acuity of the thrombus and quantification of the residual thrombus; however, new promising emerging techniques show encouraging potential in overcoming the main restrictions of ultrasound.

## Summary

- Despite the fact that venous ultrasonography has proven to be a valid diagnostic tool in patients with deep vein thrombosis, limitations remain in the assessment of the abdominal and calf veins in determining the acuity of the thrombus and quantification of the residual thrombus.

- Several promising ultrasound-related imaging techniques have emerged in an attempt to define patency of lumen, residual thrombus size and acuity of thrombus in an objective, accurate and cost-effective manner that may be employed in a clinical setting.

- Contrast-enhanced ultrasound and B-flow imaging may have the potential to better define patency of vessels and residual thrombosis.

- Elastography appears to be the most promising ultrasound-related technique to determine age of thrombus.

- 3D ultrasound appears to be promising in quantifying the volume of residual thrombus in an objective and accurate manner.

- Further studies are needed to determine validation and reproducibility of these techniques.

## References

1. Foley WD, Middleton WD, Lawson TL, *et al.* Color Doppler ultrasound imaging of lower-extremity venous disease. *Am J Roentgenol* 1989; **152**: 371–76.
2. Behrouz K., Boissel JP, Cucherat M, *et al.* A systematic review of the accuracy of ultrasound in the diagnosis of deep venous thrombosis in asymptomatic patients. *Thromb Haemost* 2004; **91** (4): 655–66.
3. Kearon C, Julian JA, Newman TE, Ginsberg JS. Noninvasive diagnosis of deep venous thrombosis. McMaster Diagnostic Imaging Practice Guidelines Initiative. *Ann Intern Med* 1998; **128**: 663–77.
4. Tomkowski WZ, Davidson BL, Wisniewska J, *et al.* Accuracy of compression ultrasound in screening for deep venous thrombosis in acutely ill medical patients. *Thromb Haemost* 2007; **97** (2): 191–94.
5. Prandoni P, Prins MH, Lensing AW, *et al;* AESOPUS Investigators. Residual thrombosis on ultrasonography to guide the duration of anticoagulation in patients with deep venous thrombosis: a randomized trial. *Ann Intern Med* 2009; **150**: 577–85.
6. Murphy TP, Cronan JJ. Evolution of deep venous thrombosis: a prospective evaluation with US. *Radiology* 1990; **177**: 543–48.
7. Chong LY, Fenu E, Stansby G, *et al.* Management of venous thromboembolic diseases and the role of thrombophilia testing: summary of NICE guidance. *BMJ* 2012; **344**: 3979.
8. Yong Eun Chung, Ki Whang Kim Contrast-enhanced ultrasonography: advance and current status in abdominal imaging. *Ultrasonography* 2015; **34** (1): 3–18.
9. Spiss V, Loizides A, Plaikner M, *et al.* Contrast enhanced ultrasound of the lower limb deep venous system: a technical feasibility study. *Medical Ultrasonography* 2011; **13** (4): 267–71.
10. Smith A, Parker P, Byass O, Chiu K.Contrast sonovenography: Is this the answer to complex deep vein thrombosis imaging? *Ultrasound* 2016; **24** (1): 17–22.
11. Danila M, Sporea I, Popescu A, Şirli R. Portal vein thrombosis in liver cirrhosis: the added value of contrast enhanced ultrasonography. *Med Ultrason* 2016; **18** (2): 218–33.

12. Chiao RY, Mo LY, Hall AL. B-mode blood flow (B-flow) imaging. GE Med Syst Ultrasonics Symposium IIE; 2000: 1469–72.

13. D'Abate F, Ramachandran V, Young MA, *et al*. B-Flow imaging in lower limb peripheral arterial disease and bypass graft ultrasonography. *Ultrasound Med Biol* 2016; **42** (9): 2345–51.

14. Dharmarajah B, Sounderajah V, Rowland SP, *et al*. Aging techniques for deep vein thrombosis: a systematic review. *Phlebology* 2015; **30** (2): 77–84.

15. Gennisson JL, Deffieux T, Fink M, Tanter M. Ultrasound elastography: principles and techniques. *Diagn Interven Imag* 2013; **94**: 487–95.

16. Rubin JM, Xie H, Kim K, *et al*. Sonographic elasticity imaging of acute and chronic deep venous thrombosis in humans. *J Ultrasound Med* 2006; **25**: 1179–86.

17. Cassou Birckholz MF, Engelhorn CA, Salles-Cunha SX, *et al*. Assessment of venous thrombus time of progression by gray-scale median analysis. *Int Angiol* 2011; **30** (1): 79–87.

18. Young L1, Ockelford P, Milne D, *et al*. Post-treatment residual thrombus increases the risk of recurrent deep vein thrombosis and mortality. *Thromb Haemost* 2006; **4** (9): 1919–24.

19. Kyrle PA, Rosendaal FR, Eichinger S. Risk assessment for recurrent venous thrombosis. *Lancet* 2010; **376** (9757): 2032–9.

20. Palareti G, Cosmi B, Legnani C, *et al*. D-dimer to guide the duration of anticoagulation in patients with venous thromboembolism: a management study. *Blood* 2014; **124** (2): 196–203.

21. Zhao L, Prior SJ, Kampmann M, *et al*. Measurement of thrombus resolution using three-dimensional ultrasound assessment of deep vein thrombosis volume. *J Vasc Surg Venous Lymphat Disord* 2014; **2** (2): 140–47.

# Haemodynamic assessment of venous reflux and obstruction

## A Nicolaides

## Introduction

Reflux or obstruction, or a combination of both, are the main abnormalities responsible for chronic venous insufficiency and the post-thrombotic syndrome. Their presence and anatomic extent can be assessed by duplex ultrasound. Although an estimate of the severity of reflux in individual veins can be made by measurements of peak velocity in cm/sec or volume flow in ml/sec at peak reflux, measurements of reflux or functional outflow obstruction for the whole limb in absolute units can only be made using plethysmographic methods.

## Reflux

### Measurement of reflux using air-plethysmography

The effect of changes in posture and exercise on volume measurements have been studied in the past by foot volumetry[1] and strain gauge plethysmography.[2] More recently, air plethysmography has provided volume changes in the whole leg so that venous volume, ejected volume and residual venous volume can be measured in ml and reflux in ml/s, with ejection fraction and residual volume fraction as derived measurements.[3] The coefficient of variation for these measurements is less than 10%.

Figure 1 shows the volume changes in the leg as a result of several manoeuvres. Initially, the patient is in the horizontal position with the leg elevated (A) to empty the veins and obtain a baseline. On standing (B), the volume increases to a new plateau. The increase in volume represents the venous volume, which is 100–150ml in normal limbs. The venous filling index is defined as the ratio of 90% of the venous volume, divided by the time taken to achieve 90% of filling. Venous filling index is expressed in ml/s. In normal limbs, it is 1–2 ml/sec—being the inflow from the microvascular bed.[4]

It was shown by Christopoulos *et al* that the venous filling index rose with increasing severity from normal control participants, to patients with varicose veins, to those with post-thrombotic sequelae.[4] In a series of 134 limbs with chronic venous disease and a Comprehensive Classification System for Chronic Venous Disorders (CEAP) score of C1–C6, the prevalence of chronic swelling and skin change were both zero if venous filling index was <3ml/s. Prevalence was 12% and 19% when venous filling index was 3–5ml/s, 46% and 61% when venous filling index was 5–10ml/sec, and both 76% when venous filling index was greater than 10ml/sec.[5]

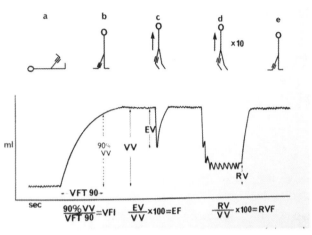

**Figure 1:** Diagrammatic representation of typical recording of venous volume changes during standard sequence of postural changes and exercise. (A) Patient in supine position with leg elevated 45 degrees; (B) patient standing with weight on non-examined leg; (C) single tiptoe movement; (D) 10 tiptoe movements; (E) return to resting standing position as B. VV = venous volume; VFT = venous filling time; VFI=venous filling index; EV=ejected volume; EF=ejection fraction; RV=residual venous volume; RVF=residual volume fraction

Venous filling index was also significantly higher in classes C2–C6 compared with C0–C1 in a study of 294 limbs by Nishibe *et al*, but they were unable to discriminate the clinical severity.[6] Similarly, the mean standard deviation of the venous filling index in a study by van Bemmelen *et al* was higher in limbs with ulcers (n=16; 5.4±3.8ml/s) and dermatitis (n=6; 7.7±4.6ml/s), compared with those with varicose veins (n=10; 2.6±1.7ml/s). The differences were significant between varicose veins *vs.* ulceration (p=0.003) and *vs.* dermatitis (p=0.034). However, there was a large amount of overlap between these groups.[7] In a study by Welkie *et al*, the venous filling index increased (p<0.0001) from control legs (n=94) to legs with varicose veins and mild swelling (n=109) to pigmentation with moderately severe swelling (n=67).[8] They noted that no additional haemodynamic deterioration occurred between the skin pigmentation stage and venous ulceration.

Neglen and Raju studied the morphologic distribution of venous incompetence (measured by erect duplex ultrasound and descending venography), results of ambulatory venous pressure measurement, venous refilling time, the Valsalva test and air-plethysmography for correlation with the clinical severity class as defined by the authors in 118 consecutive limbs (class 0, n=34; class 1, n=42; class 2, n=11; class 3, n=31).[9] There was pure deep incompetence in 29% of limbs with severe venous disease (class 2/3), only 6% had pure superficial disease, and the remainder had a combination. A history of previous thrombosis and the presence of posterior tibial vein incompetence were markedly common with ulcer disease (84% and 42%, respectively). The duplex Doppler ultrasound multisegment score correlated strongly with clinical severity classification (r=0.97). The venous refilling time and venous filling index had the highest sensitivity in identifying severe venous disease (class 2/3), and the ambulatory venous pressure had excellent specificity. The authors concluded that for non-invasive determination of reflux, a combination of venous filling index and duplex ultrasound scanning not only localised reflux but also separated severe from mild clinical vein disease, with high sensitivity and specificity.

## Abolition of reflux in limbs with isolated saphenous vein reflux

Park *et al* reported early haemodynamic results using air-plethysmography in patients treated for isolated superficial reflux in 1,756 limbs.[10] Ninety percent of the limbs were treated with high ligation and stripping and phlebectomy. All haemodynamic variables improved significantly at one month after surgery: venous volume, venous filling index, and residual volume fraction were reduced by 25.2%, 71.5%, and 29.9%, respectively, and ejection fraction increased by 20.3% (p<0.001). Improvement in the overall venous function was associated not only with abolition of venous reflux but also with improved calf muscle pump performance.

## Abolition of superficial reflux in limbs with deep venous reflux

Ting *et al* evaluated 102 limbs with combined superficial and deep vein incompetence by air-plethysmography after high ligation and stripping and found that the venous filling index decreased from 5.99±3.99ml/s to 1.82±1.21ml/s, the ejection fraction increased from 48% to 53%, and the residual volume fraction decreased from 50% to 36% after surgery.[11] Ejection fraction improved but did not normalise in this series. The proportion of limbs with deep vein incompetence on duplex ultrasound scanning at more than one site decreased from 70% to 44%, and the mean number of sites with deep vein incompetence significantly decreased from 2.14±0.96 to 1.52±1.21 after surgery (p<0.001).

Padberg *et al* studied 11 limbs by air-plethysmography and found that venous filling index decreased from 12±5ml/s to 2.7±1ml/s, ejection fraction increased from 43±11% to 59±3%, and the residual volume fraction decreased from 56% ± 15 to 33±16% one month after high ligation and stripping, suggesting a significant reduction in deep reflux and significant improvement of calf pump function, but that deep venous reflux was resolved in only three limbs (27%).[12]

In a study by Marston *et al,* significant improvement in venous filling index was documented after endovenous laser therapy for 75 limbs with both deep and superficial venous reflux.[13] Maximal reflux velocity was measured in the popliteal and femoral veins, and venous filling index was significantly more improved if maximal reflux velocity was less than 10cm/s compared with limbs with maximal reflux velocity greater than 10cm/s. In 35 limbs with deep venous reflux in the common femoral vein, the mean venous filling index decreased significantly from 6.54±3.9ml/s to 2.2±1.9ml/s, and in 40 limbs with deep venous reflux in the femoral and/or popliteal veins, venous filling index significantly improved from 6.2±3.8ml/s to 3.3±3ml (p<0.001). The authors concluded that patients with deep venous reflux in the femoral and/or popliteal veins were less likely to completely correct their venous haemodynamics as measured by venous filling index.

## Abolition of deep venous reflux

Valve reconstructive surgery can involve internal valvuloplasty, external valvuloplasty, external valve banding, transposition of the vein, axillary/brachial vein transplantation and creation of neovalve (Maleti technique)[14] or non-autologous artificial venous valves.

Raju *et al* reported a 100% normalised venous recovery time and significantly decreased venous drainage index after operation (3.1±2.4ml/s *vs.* 4.1±2.8ml/s), and the cumulative competency rates of 140 repaired sites were 84% at 12 months, 72% at 24 months, and 59% at 30 months.[15]

McDaniel *et al* suggested that venous reconstruction might be considered in patients with deep vein incompetence and venous filling index greater than 4ml/s as they have a 43% chance of recurrent ulceration at one year and of 60% at two years. But, if patients have a venous filling index of less than 4ml/s, deep venous reflux is probably less severe and these patients may not benefit from venous reconstruction.[16]

## Measurements of venous outflow obstruction

Simple leg elevation with the patient supine can provide an estimate of the resting venous pressure by observing the height of the heel above the heart level at which prominent veins in the foot collapse. A study that measured direct femoral vein pressures in patients with iliofemoral occlusion demonstrated by venography showed that the average resting pressure in the supine position in those with poor pelvic collaterals was 5.5±10.5mmHg higher than the unobstructed opposite limb, whereas, the gradient between the two limbs in those with good collateral veins was 0.6±1.4 mmHg.[17]

In the presence of a stenosis, a peak velocity ratio of >2.5 across the stenosis is the best criterion to use for the presence of a pressure gradient >3mmHg.[18]

Several methods have been used to quantify outflow obstruction or indirectly measure its severity-residual volume fraction during exercise, maximum venous outflow or outflow fraction, arm-foot pressure differential and venous outflow resistance.

### Venous volume during walking

In one study, they measured the residual volume fraction using air-plethysmography during walking on a treadmill in 12 normal limbs of healthy volunteers and seven limbs with axial vein reflux combined with severe outflow obstruction due to a previous deep vein thrombosis followed by poor recanalisation.[19] Walking speeds were 1, 1.5, 2 and 2.5km/h. In normal limbs, the residual volume fraction was 45% (95% CI 42% to 50%) at 1km/h decreasing to 42% (95% CI 37% to 48%) (p<0.05) at 2km/h. In limbs with severe outflow obstruction, residual

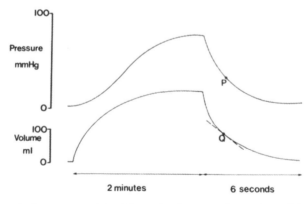

**Figure 2:** Pressure and volume venous occlusion inflow and outflow curves. Pressure is recorded with a needle in a vein in a foot vein and volume with the air-plethysmograph.

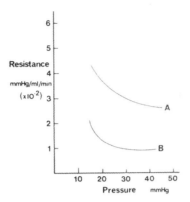

**Figure 3:** Resistance plotted against pressure for a limb with outflow obstruction (A) and a normal limb (B).

volume fraction was 68% (95% CI 62% to 74%) at 1km/h increasing to 79% (95% CI 73% to 86%) (p for trend=0.009). This residual volume fraction of 79% approximately corresponds to an air-plethysmography of 80mmHg.

## Gravitational venous drainage

The venous drainage index in ml/s is a recently introduced parameter of air-plethysmography.[20] It is the exact opposite of the venous filling index. The venous drainage index quantifies the rate of calf decompression from a position of dependency to elevation. It is intuitive that a slow rate of calf decompression, which occurs in obstruction, will have a poor response to gravitational drainage. This has been validated in healthy controls using graduated thigh-cuff pressures to simulate degrees of obstruction.[21] Using a tilt-table comparing healthy controls with patients of known obstruction, the cutoff point in determining presence of obstruction was a venous drainage index of <11ml/s.[22] In a subsequent study, venous drainage index was reduced significantly in response to iliac venous stenting.[23]

## Venous outflow resistance

Figure 2 shows inflow and outflow curves for calf volume and pressure obtained simultaneously.[5,24] Volume changes are obtained using air-plethysmography and pressure by direct puncture of a vein on the dorsum of the foot. Inflow curves are obtained by inflating a proximal thigh cuff to 80mmHg. After a plateau is reached, the thigh cuff is suddenly released and the outflow curve is recorded. Flow, "Q", can be calculated at any point on the volume outflow curve from the tangent at that point. The resistance, "R", is calculated by dividing the corresponding pressure, "P", from the pressure outflow curve by the flow Q (R=P/Q). The units are mmHg/ml/min. By calculating R at several points along the outflow curve and plotting them against pressure, it is possible to demonstrate how resistance changes with different pressures, which determine the cross-sectional area of the vein. Figure 3 shows two such plots, one from a patient with outflow obstruction (A) and the other from a normal limb (B). It can be seen that the resistance-pressure relationship is not linear. Resistance is low at high pressure when the veins and collateral channels are distended. As the pressure decreases, the vein wall becomes less stretched and eventually collapses reducing the cross-sectional area so that the resistance increases.[5]

## Combined quantitative measurements of reflux and outflow resistance

As indicated above, attempts to correlate individual venous haemodynamic measurements with symptoms and signs of chronic venous disease have produced poor or, at best, moderate results, probably because of lack of methods to quantitate obstruction. The authors of a recent study hypothesised that the combination of quantitative measurements of (A) overall reflux (superficial and deep) and (B) overall outflow resistance, i.e. including the collateral circulation would provide a haemodynamic index that should be related to the severity of the disease.[25] Twenty-five limbs with chronic venous disease and one limb from a healthy volunteer (Venous Clinical Severity Score, VCSS, 0-13) were studied. The clinical CEAP classification was C0 in one limb, C1 in two limbs, C2 in 10 limbs, C3 in three limbs, C4 in one limb, C5 in six limbs and C6 in three limbs. Air-plethysmography was used to measure reflux (venous filling index in mL/sec) when the patient changed from a horizontal to a standing position. Subsequently, outflow resistance was measured as described above. Outflow resistance increased markedly at pressures lower than 30mmHg due to decrease in vein diameter, so resistance at 30mmHg was used in this study. In a multivariable linear regression analysis with VCSS as the dependent variable, both venous filling index and outflow resistance at 30mmHg were independent predictors ($p<0.001$). Using the constant (0.333) and regression coefficients, the regression equation provided a haemodynamic index or estimated VCSS of 0.333+(venous filling index x 0.44)+(outflow resistance at 30mmHg x 158). Thus, haemodynamic index could be calculated for every patient by substituting venous filling index and outflow resistance at 30mmHg in the equation. Haemodynamic index or calculated VCSS was linearly related to the observed VCSS ($r=0.83$). The results indicate that the combination of quantitative measurements of reflux and outflow resistance provide a hemodynamic index which is linearly related to the VCSS. These findings need to be confirmed in a bigger series.

## Summary

- The measurements of reflux using air-plethysmography and outflow resistance using pressure and air-plethysmography volume changes were developed in the 1980s and 1990s when valve reconstruction was in its infancy and venous stenting for relief of obstruction was not available.

- At that time the need for clinical applications were limited.

- Now when valve reconstruction and stenting for iliac obstruction have not only been demonstrated to be feasible but have also become more widely used, it is advisable that reflux and resistance are measured before and after deep venous reconstruction so that objective criteria associated with clinical benefit can be developed.

- Such criteria will help us refine the indications for deep venous surgery.

# References

1. Thulesius O, Norgren L, Gjores JE. Foot-volumetry, a new method for objective assessment of edema and venous function. *Vasa* 1973; **2** (4): 325–29.
2. Barnes RW, Ross EA, Strandness DE, Jr. Differentiation of primary from secondary varicose veins by Doppler ultrasound and strain gauge plethysmography. *Surg Gynecol Obstet* 1975; **141** (2): 207–11.
3. Christopoulos DG, Nicolaides AN, Szendro G, *et al.* Air-plethysmography and the effect of elastic compression on venous hemodynamics of the leg. *J Vasc Surg* 1987; **5** (1): 148–59.
4. Christopoulos D, Nicolaides AN, Szendro G. Venous reflux: quantification and correlation with the clinical severity of chronic venous disease. *Br J Surg* 1988; **75** (4): 352–56.
5. Nicolaides AN. Investigation of chronic venous insufficiency: A consensus statement (France, March 5-9, 1997). *Circulation* 2000; **102** (20): E126–63.
6. Nishibe T, Kudo F, Miyazaki K, *et al.* Relationship between air-plethysmographic venous function and clinical severity in primary varicose veins. *Int Angiol* 2006; **25**(4): 352–55.
7. van Bemmelen PS, Mattos MA, Hodgson KJ, *et al.* Does air plethysmography correlate with duplex scanning in patients with chronic venous insufficiency? *J Vasc Surg* 1993; **18** (5): 796–807.
8. Welkie JF, Comerota AJ, Katz ML, *et al.* Hemodynamic deterioration in chronic venous disease. *J Vasc Surg* 1992; **16** (5): 733–40.
9. Neglen P, Raju S. A rational approach to detection of significant reflux with duplex Doppler scanning and air plethysmography. *J Vasc Surg* 1993; **17**(3): 590–95.
10. Park UJ, Yun WS, Lee KB, *et al.* Analysis of the postoperative hemodynamic changes in varicose vein surgery using air plethysmography. *J Vasc Surg* 2010; **51** (3): 634–38.
11. Ting AC, Cheng SW, Wu LL, Cheung GC. Changes in venous hemodynamics after superficial vein surgery for mixed superficial and deep venous insufficiency. *World J Surg* 2001; **25**(2): 122–25.
12. Padberg FT Jr, Pappas PJ, Araki CT, *et al.* Hemodynamic and clinical improvement after superficial vein ablation in primary combined venous insufficiency with ulceration. *J Vasc Surg* 1996; **24** (5): 711–18.
13. Marston WA, Brabham VW, Mendes R, *et al.* The importance of deep venous reflux velocity as a determinant of outcome in patients with combined superficial and deep venous reflux treated with endovenous saphenous ablation. *J Vasc Surg* 2008; **48** (2): 400–05.
14. Maleti O, Perrin M. Reconstructive surgery for deep vein reflux in the lower limbs: techniques, results and indications. *Eur J Vasc Endovasc Surg* 2011; **41** (6): 837–48.
15. Raju S, Berry MA, Neglen P. Transcommissural valvuloplasty: technique and results. *J Vasc Surg* 2000; **32** (5): 969–76.
16. McDaniel HB, Marston WA, Farber MA, *et al.* Recurrence of chronic venous ulcers on the basis of clinical, etiologic, anatomic, and pathophysiologic criteria and air plethysmography. *J Vasc Surg* 2002; **35** (4): 723–28.
17. Negus D, Cockett FB. Femoral vein pressures in post-phlebitic iliac vein obstruction. *Br J Surg* 1967; **54** (6): 522–25.
18. Labropoulos N, Borge M, Pierce K, Pappas PJ. Criteria for defining significant central vein stenosis with duplex ultrasound. *J Vasc Surg* 2007; **46** (1): 101-7.
19. Ibegbuna V. Haemodynamics in chronic venous disease. Vol. PhD Thesis. London: London University, 2002. pp. 221-235.
20. Lattimer CR, Kalodiki E, Mendoza E. Gravitational venous drainage is significantly faster in patients with varicose veins. *Phlebology* 2016; **31** (8): 546–53,
21. Lattimer CR, Doucet S, Kalodiki E, *et al.* Increasing thigh compression pressure correlates with a reduction in the venous drainage index of air-plethysmography (2nd prize) 16th annual EVF meeting St Petersburg, 2015.
22. Lattimer CR, Mendoza E. Simultaneous air-plethysmography and duplex scanning on a tilt-table in assessing gravitational venous drainage. *JVS: Venous and Lymph Dis* 2016; **4** (1): 151–52.
23. Lattimer CR, Kalodiki E, Azzam M, *et al.* Gravitational venous drainage improves significantly after iliac venous stenting but this may result in faster venous filling. *JVS: Venous and Lymph Dis* 2016; **4**(1): 137–38.
24. Labropoulos N, Volteas N, Leon M, *et al.* The role of venous outflow obstruction in patients with chronic venous dysfunction. *Arch Surg* 1997; **132** (1): 46–51.
25. Nicolaides A, Clark H, Labropoulos N, *et al.* Quantitation of reflux and outflow obstruction in patients with CVD and correlation with clinical severity. *Int Angiol* 2014; **33** (3): 275–81.

# Pelvic vein congestion and reflux

# Pelvic vein incompetence in women with chronic pelvic pain

DM Riding and CN McCollum

## Introduction

Chronic pelvic pain in women is a significant health problem, accounting for 20–30% of all UK gynaecology outpatient appointments.[1-3] The economic cost to the UK is £158 million per year.[4] Most women who present to their general practitioner are referred to a gynaecologist for further investigation. They then undergo a series of investigations including diagnostic imaging, hysteroscopy and laparoscopy. Common gynaecological disorders such as endometriosis, pelvic inflammatory disease (or secondary adhesions), uterine fibroids or polycystic ovarian syndrome are frequently diagnosed, but the majority of women (55%) never receive a diagnosis to explain their pain.[5]

For these patients, chronic pelvic pain ceases to be a symptom and becomes diagnosis in its own right. Treatment focuses on symptom management with opioids or non-opioid alternatives such as gabapentin or pregabalin. Hysterectomy is common, increasing both the risk to patients and healthcare costs without necessarily improving symptoms.[6] Persistent, debilitating symptoms of chronic pelvic pain have physical, psychosocial and psychosexual consequences with patients enduring a multitude of futile investigations and secondary-care assessments over many years.[3,5]

Incompetence of the ovarian and internal iliac veins, collectively known as pelvic vein incompetence, is increasingly recognised to be a possible cause of chronic pelvic pain. Other sequelae of pelvic vein incompetence—such as vulval varices, varicose veins in the thighs and legs and, in men, varicocoeles—are treated routinely, but the evidence base to support treatment of pelvic vein incompetence in women is non-existent. UK NHS commissioners have been understandably reluctant to approve investigation or treatment for pelvic vein incompetence.

The Manchester Pelvic Vein Study Group was set up three years ago to investigate the symptom profile of women with pelvic vein incompetence. Having reported that women with pelvic vein incompetence have a typical symptom profile with impaired quality of life, we secured a National Institute for Health Research award to set up a randomised controlled trial on whether coil/foam occlusion of incompetent pelvic veins reduces symptoms and improves quality of life in women with chronic pelvic pain thought to be due to pelvic vein incompetence. Subsequently, we obtained funding for a case-control study on the frequency of pelvic vein incompetence in chronic pelvic pain; this chapter presents interim data and reviews the relevant literature.

## Terminology

Just as the correlation between pelvic vein incompetence and chronic pelvic pain has yet to be fully accepted, there is no consensus on the nomenclature for either of these conditions. As we can define both pelvic vein incompetence and chronic pelvic pain, but not "pelvic congestion syndrome", we consider that this alleged syndrome should not, for now, be recognised.

## Characteristic symptoms of pelvic vein incompetence

The definition of chronic pelvic pain is clearly stated by the Royal College of Obstetricians and Gynaecologists in their "Green Top Guideline" and reads as follows: "Intermittent or constant pain in the lower abdomen or pelvis of a woman of at least six months in duration, not occurring exclusively with menstruation or intercourse and not associated with pregnancy."[7]

Pelvic congestion syndrome is less clear cut, with no accepted pathophysiological or diagnostic criteria. This makes analysis of the limited evidence challenging, with little consistency in the investigation and criteria for pelvic vein incompetence across the various studies. However, most clinicians using this nomenclature describe pelvic congestion as an alternative to chronic pelvic pain when it happens to coexist with incompetence of the ovarian or internal iliac veins. Occasionally, the clinical signs of pelvic vein incompetence can be clear, particularly when women develop large varices of the vulva or medial upper thigh.

Our experience is that most women present with chronic pelvic pain or recurrent varicose veins in the leg. Many patients have undergone numerous investigations to try to identify the cause for their symptoms, often including laparoscopy and even hysterectomy. Patient assessment should then seek to differentiate between pelvic vein incompetence-related pain and other potential causes. There is little published data to assist the clinician; dyspareunia is commonly reported,[8-10] which can be particularly severe in the perimenstrual period,[8-11] as are varicose veins of the legs and aching lower abdominal, pelvic or thigh pain that worsens throughout the day.[9,12]

## Symptom characterisation study

We performed a case-control study to explore symptoms experienced by women with pelvic vein incompetence, and to define the effect of the condition on quality of life and healthcare costs.[13] The cases were 40 premenopausal women aged 18–49 years with pelvic vein incompetence and lower limb varicose veins. There were two age-matched controls groups: (i) 40 healthy women with varicose veins but no pelvic vein incompetence; and (ii) 40 healthy women without varicose veins or with pelvic vein incompetence. Patients were asked to complete a structured questionnaire on disease specific outcomes, health status and use of healthcare resources.

Pelvic pain was reported by 38 of 40 (95%) pelvic vein incompetence cases, compared with 25 of 40 (62%) varicose vein controls, and 26 of 40 (65%) healthy controls (p=0.001). The median (range) EuroQol five dimensions questionnaire score for pelvic vein incompetence cases was 0.80 (0.29–1) compared with 0.80 (0.09–1) for varicose vein controls and one (0.62–1) for healthy controls (p=0.002). Of the 40 pelvic vein incompetence cases, 35 (88%) had visited a consultant in the previous 12 months compared with 12 of 40 (30%) varicose vein controls and 14 of 40 (35%) healthy controls (p<0.001). Typical symptoms experienced by women with pelvic vein incompetence were of vague aching sensation or dull pain in the lower abdomen, vagina or upper thighs which was worse on standing or prolonged sitting and which was relieved by lying down. Other symptoms associated with pelvic vein incompetence were premenstrual and menstrual pain and dyspareunia. Pelvic vein incompetence was not associated with abdominal bloating, lower back pain or dyschezia.

In conclusion, patients with pelvic vein incompetence were more likely to experience pelvic pain, have reduced health status, and incur greater healthcare costs than matched controls.

## The association between pelvic vein incompetence and chronic pelvic pain

Although the association between pelvic vein incompetence and chronic pelvic pain is assumed by many clinicians, there has been no robust case-control evidence to test the association. Most publications are from small, unpowered, non-matched cohorts or case series conducted by clinicians who have a financial interest in treating pelvic vein incompetence. These reports suggest that 11.2–28% of patients with chronic pelvic pain have pelvic vein incompetence.[14–16] The prevalence of pelvic vein incompetence in women with recurrent varicose veins of the leg has been reported to be in the range of 20–76%, with no reliable information on the frequency in healthy controls.[17,18] There have been no prospective cohort studies on the development of chronic pelvic pain in women with pelvic vein incompetence.

Beard *et al* is widely quoted and reports transfundal pelvic venography in 45 women with chronic pelvic pain and negative laparoscopy.[19] The frequency of pelvic vein incompetence is unclear, but the mean maximum pelvic venous diameter in women with chronic pelvic pain was 6.73mm compared with 3.25mm in healthy controls (p<0.01). However, 18 women were excluded from the study due to poor quality venography, and the cases and controls were not matched for age or parity.

The investigators then compared symptoms in women with pelvic vein incompetence and chronic pelvic pain with those experienced by women with chronic pelvic pain only. In this study, women with pelvic vein incompetence were more likely to report that walking, standing, lifting and bending exacerbated the pain. Additionally, they were more likely to experience back pain, vaginal discharge and headache.[20] The definition of pelvic vein incompetence in these studies was often unsatisfactory and based on venous diameter, the time taken for venous contrast to disperse or the radiological appearance of the venogram. Doppler technology was not available to assess the direction of flow in the relevant veins.

We initially used reflux of >0.5 seconds in the ovarian or internal iliac vein on colour duplex Doppler ultrasound to define pelvic vein incompetence, based on the diagnostic criteria for varicose veins. There remains a need for a well-powered epidemiological study with age and parity matched case-control pairs to define the criteria for clinically significant pelvic vein incompetence.

## The investigation of pelvic vein incompetence

There is an urgent need to standardise the investigation of and criteria for pelvic vein incompetence, to allow comparison between studies and to enable consistent clinical assessment. Champaneria *et al* correctly concluded that meta-analyses of studies on pelvic congestion syndrome could not be achieved with statistical credibility, due to the range of investigations and diagnostic criteria used.[21]

Diagnostic laparoscopy is mandatory in the investigation of chronic pelvic pain, and may reveal dilated, tortuous pelvic veins. However, as laparoscopy is normally performed with the patient head down, the pelvic veins are emptied during the procedure, which probably explains why the importance of pelvic varices has not been widely appreciated in gynaecology in the past. The positive pressure created by air insufflation during laparoscopy may further impede pelvic venous filling. If the pelvic veins could be reliably visualised using ultrasound, Duplex imaging would be ideal as it is inexpensive, minimally invasive, and it is entirely safe with no exposure to radiation or ionising contrast.

Barros *et al* performed transvaginal duplex in 249 patients with varicose veins of the legs and found pelvic vein incompetence in 150, with venography confirming pelvic vein incompetence in 156 patients. This data demonstrated that, in comparison to catheter venography, transvaginal duplex had a sensitivity of 96% (95% confidence interval=92–99%) and a specificity of 100% (lower 95% confidence interval=97%).[22] Unfortunately, the radiologists who assessed the venograms were not blinded to the results of the transvaginal duplex. There was also no clear definition of pelvic vein incompetence on duplex ultrasound or venography.

Park *et al* used combined transabdominal and transvaginal duplex ultrasound to assess women with pelvic congestion syndrome and healthy controls; mean left ovarian vein diameter was greater in pelvic vein incompetence than in controls (0.79cm +/- 0.23cm *vs.* 0.49cm +/- 0.15cm; p<0.001).[23] Retrograde flow was identified in all pelvic congestion patients compared with 25% of controls. All patients had pelvic varices. The authors did not explain why fewer than half the patients went on to have venography.

We use transvaginal high-definition colour duplex ultrasound as the first line investigation for pelvic vein incompetence. Following paired studies with retrograde venography, we have refined the definition of pelvic vein incompetence to reflux ≥0.7 seconds in any ovarian or internal iliac vein with reflux into a second order pelvic vein or into the thigh.

Not surprisingly, interventional radiologists consider catheter-directed fluoroscopic venography to be the "gold standard" as it allows the radiologist to empty and refill the venous system using a tilting table. Individual veins can be targeted for investigation and treatment can be offered at the same time.

## Our case-control study of pelvic vein incompetence in chronic pelvic pain

We designed a case-control study to explore the frequency of pelvic vein incompetence in women with non-gynaecological chronic pelvic pain compared with healthy age and parity matched controls. All premenopausal woman aged 18–54 who had undergone negative laparoscopy for chronic pelvic pain were invited to give fully informed consent to participate. Consenting chronic pelvic pain patients and their matched controls then completed a purpose-designed and validated symptom questionnaire before undergoing transvaginal duplex investigation for pelvic vein incompetence using a standardised protocol. The primary outcome measure was the frequency of pelvic vein incompetence defined as reflux >0.7 seconds into second order pelvic veins. Secondary outcomes included McGill short-form pain score, EuroQol five dimensions questionnaire three-level (EQ5D-3L) scores, and health economic assessments.

Interim analysis was conducted after recruitment of 44 matched case-control pairs. Pelvic vein incompetence was identified in 15 (34.1%) women, with chronic pelvic pain and in seven (15.9%) controls (p=0.046). Pelvic varices were found in 12 (27.3%) women with chronic pelvic pain and only one (2.3%) control (p<0.002). Of all women with pelvic vein incompetence (case or control), 12 (54.5%) experienced "dull" pain in the lower abdomen pelvis or thighs compared to 15 (22.7%) of those without pelvic vein incompetence. Mean EQ5D-3L health status scores were significantly lower in cases than controls for overall health evaluation (72.6% *vs.* 86.9%; p<0.001) and health state description (69% *vs.* 98%; p<0.001).

The frequency of pelvic vein incompetence in both healthy women and those with chronic pelvic pain was much higher than expected, with a strong statistical association between the two conditions. This study is continuing to recruit patients and we intend to publish interim data in an epidemiology journal when we have 50 matched case-control pairs. We will then ask epidemiologists to advise on the number of patients that need to be recruited as our initial power calculations were based on very much lower reported prevalences of pelvic vein incompetence.

Characteristic symptoms of dull lower abdominal, pelvic and thigh pain that persists throughout the day were more frequent in pelvic vein incompetence. Chronic pelvic pain is clearly associated with lower self-perception of health scores, and yet patients are often discharged back to their general physician before pelvic vein incompetence has been excluded.

Women with chronic pelvic pain and pelvic vein incompetence are now invited to participate in our concurrent, randomised controlled trial of transjugular occlusion of incompetent pelvic veins using coils and foam sclerosant. We aim to complete both studies in 2018.

## Conclusion

Large numbers of otherwise healthy women continue to experience debilitating symptoms due to chronic pelvic pain that may be caused by pelvic vein incompetence. These symptoms are a significant burden on the affected women, their families and health services.

Regrettably, the available evidence to guide clinicians and service commissioners is limited and of poor quality. We have now defined the symptoms experienced by women with pelvic vein incompetence and hope to be able to report on the frequency of this condition in chronic pelvic pain, and on the effectiveness of treating incompetent pelvic veins with coil/foam occlusion.

## Summary

- Chronic pelvic pain is a major health problem that confers a substantial burden on women, their families, and on health services; yet, 55% of women do not receive a diagnosis despite extensive investigation.

- Pelvic vein incompetence is likely be a cause of chronic pelvic pain, but the quality of existing studies is insufficient to guide investigation or treatment.

- Characteristic symptoms of pelvic vein incompetence and chronic pelvic pain include a dull pelvic pain or ache experienced throughout the month, radiating into the upper thigh, with exacerbation by prolonged standing or sitting. Dyspareunia is also common.

- Transvaginal duplex ultrasound involves no risk and is both sensitive and specific for pelvic vein incompetence. Retrograde catheter venography is obviously required for treatment.

- There is an urgent need for high quality case control studies defining the association between pelvic vein incompetence and chronic pelvic pain, and for randomised controlled trials on the efficacy of the available treatments.

## References

1. Zondervan KT, Yudkin PL, Vessey MP, *et al.* The community prevalence of chronic pelvic pain in women and associated illness behaviour. *Br J Gen Pract* 2001; **51** (468): 541–7.
2. Osman MW, Nikolopoulos I, Jayaprakasan K, Raine-Fenning N. Pelvic congestion syndrome. *The Obstetrician & Gynaecologist* 2013; **15** (3): 151–57.
3. Savidge C, Slade P, Stewart P, Li T. Women's perspectives on their experiences of chronic pelvic pain and medical care. *Journal of Health Psychology* 1998; **3** (1): 103–16.
4. Davies L, Gangar K, Drummond M, *et al.* The economic burden of intractable gynaecological pain. *Journal of Obstetrics and Gynaecology* 1992; **12** (suppl2): S54-S6.
5. McGowan L, Luker K, Creed F, Chew-Graham CA. 'How do you explain a pain that can't be seen?': The narratives of women with chronic pelvic pain and their disengagement with the diagnostic cycle. *British Journal of Health Psychology* 2007; **12** (2): 261–74.
6. Lamvu G. Role of hysterectomy in the treatment of chronic pelvic pain. *Obstetrics & Gynecology* 2011; **117** (5): 1175–78.
7. Gynaecologists RCoOa. The Initial Management of Chronic Pelvic Pain: Green Top Guideline No. 41. 2012.
8. Asciutto G, Mumme A, Marpe B, *et al.* MR venography in the detection of pelvic venous congestion. *European Journal of Vascular and Endovascular Surgery* 2008; **36** (4): 491.
9. Van Der Vleuten CJM, Van Kempen JAL, Schultze-Kool LJ. Embolization to treat pelvic congestion syndrome and vulval varicose veins. *International Journal of Gynecology and Obstetrics* 2012; **118** (3): 227–30.
10. Meneses L, Fava M, Diaz P, Andia M, *et al.* Embolization of incompetent pelvic veins for the treatment of recurrent varicose veins in lower limbs and pelvic congestion syndrome. *Cardiovascular and Interventional Radiology* 2013; **36** (1): 128–32.
11. Scultetus AH, Villavicencio JL, Gillespie DL. The nutcracker syndrome: its role in the pelvic venous disorders. *Journal of Vascular Surgery* 2001; **34** (5): 812.
12. Tropeano G, Di SC, Amoroso S, *et al* G. Ovarian vein incompetence: a potential cause of chronic pelvic pain in women. *European Journal of Obstetrics, Gynecology, and Reproductive Biology* 2008; **139** (2): 215.
13. Hansrani V, Morris J, Caress AL, *et al.* Is pelvic vein incompetence associated with symptoms of chronic pelvic pain in women? A pilot study. *European Journal of Obstetrics Gynecology and Reproductive Biology* 2016; **196**: 21–25.
14. Almeida ECS, Nogueira AA, Candido FJR, Rosa eJCS. Cesarean section as a cause of chronic pelvic pain. *International Journal of Gynaecology and Obstetrics* 2002; **79** (2): 101.

15. Hebbar S, Chawla C. Role of laparoscopy in evaluation of chronic pelvic pain. *Journal of Minimal Access Surgery* 2005; **1** (3): 116.

16. Lynn NEM, Thein HTS, Mya WW. Study of laparoscopic findings in patients with chronic pelvic pain in Central Women's Hospital, Yangon, Myanmar. *Journal of Obstetrics and Gynaecology Research.* 2015; **41**:104.

17. Marsh P, Holdstock J, Harrison C, *et al.* Pelvic vein reflux in female patients with varicose veins: comparison of incidence between a specialist private vein clinic and the vascular department of a National Health Service District General Hospital. *Phlebology* 2009; **24** (3): 108–13.

18. Geier B, Barbera L, Mumme A, Köster O, *et al.* Reflux patterns in the ovarian and hypogastric veins in patients with varicose veins and signs of pelvic venous incompetence. *Chirurgia* Italiana 2007; **59** (4): 481.

19. Beard RW, Highman JH, Pearce S, Reginald PW. Diagnosis of pelvic varicosities in women with chronic pelvic pain. *Lancet* 1984; **2** (8409): 946.

20. Beard RW, Reginald PW, Wadsworth J. Clinical features of women with chronic lower abdominal pain and pelvic congestion. *British Journal of Obstetrics and Gynaecology* 1988; **95** (2): 153–61.

21. Champaneria R, Shah L, Moss J, *et al.* The relationship between pelvic vein incompetence and chronic pelvic pain in women: Systematic reviews of diagnosis and treatment effectiveness. *Health Technology Assessment* 2016; **20** (5): 1–94.

22. Barros FS, Perez JMG, Zandonade E, *et al.* Evaluation of pelvic varicose veins using color Doppler ultrasound: comparison of results obtained with ultrasound of the lower limbs, transvaginal ultrasound, and phlebography. *Jornal Vascular Brasileiro* 2010; **9** (2): 15–23.

23. Park SJ, Lim JW, Ko YT, *et al.* Diagnosis of pelvic congestion syndrome using transabdominal and transvaginal sonography. *American Journal of Roentgenology* 2004; **182** (3): 683.

# Percutaneous valvuloplasty

## JC Ragg

## Introduction

The main feature of venous insufficiency is reflux, meaning that closure of one or several vein valves is not achieved during regular body movements. In late stages, the valve cusps are badly damaged or totally gone because of chronic inflammation; thus, surgical removal or endoluminal closure are the best options of treatment. However, in early stages, a valve may leak while the cusps are fully preserved and mobile. In this case, reduction of vein diameter could result in functional restoration. A first attempt to restore venous valves in case of insufficiency is extraluminal valvuloplasty; also called extraluminal stenting. A surgical tissue patch made from Dacron or polyurethane is wrapped around the surgically prepared vein and fixed with sutures like a coat. Thus, the diameter is reduced and the valves may work again. There are more than 15 years of positive functional experience with this method,[1-3] in spite of rather insufficient case selection due to former ultrasound limitations. However, the surgical approach usually requires general anaesthesia, it is even more extended than crossectomy and the result cannot be adjusted later on. The patch will be a lasting foreign body. Serious complications such as wound infection are rare, but may happen. Therefore, open surgery seems not to be the best option for the aimed treatment of early stages, in potentially younger people. Endoscopically guided procedures of valvuloplasty[4] have recognised that the procedure should be less invasive, but the technique was too complex to proceed to routine.

## Percutaneous valvuloplasty

The idea to shape veins or to reduce their diameter by injectable fluids is known and practised for more than 15 years when applying saline solutions in the perivenous space prior to thermal treatments of veins, called tumescent anaesthesia, based on a well-known supportive mode for liposuction.[5] In experienced vein centres, tumescent anaesthesia is performed strictly under ultrasound guidance. A cannula is advanced to the perivenous space in local anaesthesia and then fluid is injected in a way distributing it around the vein until sufficient reduction of vein diameter is accomplished. The effect of saline fluids is lost within days by resorption. The experience in precise ultrasound-guided vein shaping by perivenous fluids led our working group to the invention of percutaneous valvuloplasty in 2012; first choosing native hyaluronan gel of low viscosity to achieve proof of principle, and afterwards changing to more solid, cross-linked hyaluronan products to obtain more durable results.[6] Among many initial questions, one was aimed at the particle size to use—should it offer a maximum compression effect with large particles? Or should it be precise first of all and, thus, consist of small particles? In this chapter, we present a comparison of two evaluated substances with a two-year follow-up.

## Two initial studies comparing different hyaluronan products

Cases with proximal greater saphenous vein valve incompetence but preserved and mobile valve structures, according to 8–16MHz ultrasound analysis were included. In series A, 23 patients (15 female, eight male; 38–67 years, diameter range 7–11.5mm, mean 8.6mm) underwent percutaneous valvuloplasty using a hyaluronan gel consisting of large particles (>1mm; Macrolane, Galderma). In series B a smooth hyaluronan gel (particle diameter <0.2mm; Princess Volume, Croma/Stada) was chosen for 18 patients (12 female, six male; 34–69 years, greater saphenous vein diameter 7–11.8mm, mean 8.9mm). Injections were performed under sterile conditions with local anaesthesia from one single access using a patented safety cannula, consisting of a sharp tip to penetrate skin, fasciae and ligaments and, by turn of the handle, changed to a blunt tip to navigate in areas close to veins, to avoid incidental vessel puncture or intravascular injection. All procedures were performed strictly and continuously under ultrasound monitoring (Figures 1 and 2). Patient position was upright on a tilt table for marking, intermediate and final result control, and supine (0–20 degrees) during puncture and injections. Injections were carried out air-free to avoid disturbance of ultrasound signals. Treatment was terminated when the vein diameter was reduced to estimated normal or in case of proven elimination of reflux (Figure 3). Follow-up examinations with ultrasound were performed after three, six, 12, 18 and 24 months. Supplementary injections of hyaluronan were allowed.

## Results

Orthograde flow could be established in 22/23 cases of series A (95.6%) and 18/18 cases of series B (100%) in one session (A: 18, B: 17) or two sessions (A: 4, B: 1) (Figure 3). Gel volumina were 12–35ml (mean 19.4ml, series A) *vs.* 4–9ml (mean 6.9 ml, series B). After an initial learning curve, injections became more precise and effective. In two cases, a local overload of hyaluronan was successfully aspirated. There were no adverse reactions, in particular no sensation of local swelling or pressure, not even in cases with large volumina of hyaluronan. At

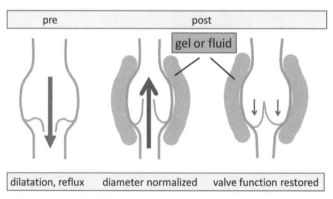

**Figure 1:** Principle of percutaneous valvuloplasty.

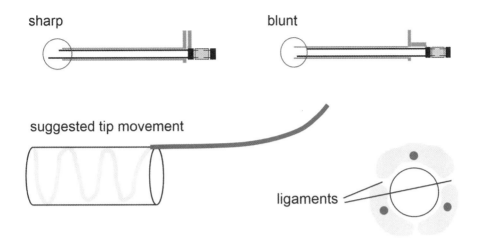

**Figure 2:** Flexible safety canula for percutaneous valvuloplasty and suggested way of injection.

one year follow-up, orthograde flow was present in 15/22 cases (68.2%, series A) *vs.* 14/18 cases (78.6%, series B). Cases with recurrent reflux (A: n=7, B: n=4) successfully received supplementary hyaluronan injections of the substance initially chosen, volumes were 2–6ml. After two years, orthograde flow was found in 14/22 cases (63.6%, series A) *vs.* 11/18 cases (61.1%, series B). Again, supplementary injections were performed with haemodynamic success in all cases but one (suspected valve damage, converted to thermal closure). A number of cases (A: n=7, B: n=4) had orthograde flow after two years without any supplementary injection. Both substances decreased with time, but the time curve was not clear as the depictability of hyaluronan got lost between months eight and 18 while a certain volume effect, according to the vein diameter, still existed.

## Discussion

Hyaluronan has been proven in large numbers of cases worldwide to reside within the human body with excellent biocompatibility, in particular after the introduction of non-animal based hyaluronic fillers.[7] The rate of adverse reactions is very low. Serious mistakes like intravascular injections[8] can be avoided by proper tools and technique. Macrolane is usually chosen for reasonable aesthetic large volume corrections, with drawbacks by interference of mamma augmentation with the early diagnosis of breast cancer. Other volume-increasing indications are still practised.[9] Princess is a smooth aesthetic product, among others, designed for the treatment of facial wrinkles.[10] It is obvious that small particles allow smaller tools and a more precise delivery,[11] in this study, as indicated by a much smaller gel consumption. Nevertheless, treatments in series B were more expensive as the costs per millilitre were approximately four-fold compared to Macrolane. Long-term results were not significantly different. So far, both types of hyaluronan are eligible for the (study-related) purpose of valvuloplasty, unless a manufacturer proceeds to provide a novel product with intermediate particle size and the product is subsequently is approved for commercial use.

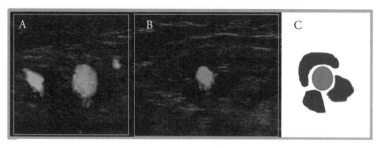

**Figure 3:** Cross-sectional ultrasound view of (A) dilated, refluxive vein, (B) after hyaluronan injection, (C) scheme. The horizontal gaps indicate the saphenous ligaments

The quality of valvuloplasty depends not so much on the technique, which is rather simple, but on inclusion criteria. Many valves considered "preserved and mobile" will show cellular aggregates, rough parts of the surface, increased thickness or even small structural defects when examined with the newest high-resolution ultrasound systems.

Besides the intention of functional restoration of vein valves (valvuloplasty), there might be a reason to consider venoplasty to achieve haemodynamic improvements in dilated zones when valves are missing or destroyed, potentially applicable to a much larger number of cases. However, a scientific basis is not yet provided.

The effects of valvuloplasty or veinoplasty or should last for years until the vein has gained stable healthy haemodynamics. This aim may be supported by further measures to fight stasis and congestion, like physical training, wearing of compression stockings, or medication. It is a fiction to eliminate venous insufficiency, since there are pathomechanisms (e.g. congenital valve defects, inflammation, degeneration) apart from simple dilatation, but there seems to be a relatively simple way to at least delay the onset of symptoms and varices.

## Conclusion

Percutaneous valvuloplasty is the first minimally invasive method to eliminate venous reflux while fully preserving the target vein. It is as feasible as with large-particle hyaluronan as with smoother gels. Small particle gels may be placed more precisely but are much more expensive when designed to be long lasting. Efforts are now focused on encouraging manufacturers to provide a definite substance for approval.

## Summary

- It may be assumed that many cases of venous insufficiency pass a stage characterised by reflux in one dilated valve zone, but still fully preserved and mobile vein cusps. This stage may exist for years, but is seldom recognised as it is usually long before symptoms or varicosities appear.

- In this stage, valvuloplasty is an effective principle to achieve functional restoration, proven by surgical wrapping.

- Percutaneous valvuloplasty by perivenous injection of biocompatible gels like hyaluronan is the first non-surgical modality for long-term vein diameter reduction. It can be exactly adjusted to the required diameter. Supplementary injections, if necessary, are easy to perform.

## References

1. Lane RJ, Cuzzilla ML, Coroneos JC et al. Recurrence rates following external valvular stenting of the saphenofemoral junction: a comparison with simultaneous contralateral stripping of the great saphenous vein. Eur J Vasc Endovasc Surg 2007; **34** (5): 595–603.

2. Belcaro G, Agus G, Errichi BM et al. Gore external valve support for superficial saphenous vein incompetence: a 10-year, follow-up registry. Panminerva Med 2011; **53** (3 Suppl 1): 35–41.

3. Sarac A, Jahollari A, Talay S et al. Long-term results of external valvuloplasty in adult patients with isolated great saphenous vein insufficiency. Clin Interv Aging 2014; **9**: 575–79.

4. Komai H, Juri M. Deep venous external valvuloplasty using a rigid angioscope. Surg Today 2010; **40**: 538–42.

5. Klein JA. The tumescent technique for liposuction surgery. AM J Cosmetic Surg 1987; **4**: 1124–32.

6. Ragg JC: A New Modality to Shape Enlarged Veins and Restore Valves by Perivenous Injection of Viscous Fluids. J Am Coll Cardiol Intv 2014; **7**: S33.

7. Ahn CS, Rao BK: The life cycles and biological end pathways of dermal fillers. J Cosmet Dermatol 2014; **13**(3): 212–23.

8. DeLorenzi C: Complications of injectable fillers, part 2: vascular complications. Aesthet Surg J 2014; **34** (4): 584–600.

9. Cerqua S, Angelucci F: Macrolane (large particle biphasic hyaluronic acid) filler injection for correction of defect contour after liposuction. J Cosmet Laser Ther 2013; **15** (4): 228–30.

10. Kopera D, Palatin M, Bartsch R et al. An open-label uncontrolled, multicenter study for the evaluation of the efficacy and safety of the dermal filler Princess VOLUME in the treatment of nasolabial folds. Biomed Res Int 2015:195328.

11. Kim YS, Choi JW, Park JK et al. Efficiency and durability of hyaluronic acid of different particle sizes as an injectable material for VF augmentation. Acta Otolaryngol 2015; **6**: 1–8.

# Varicose vein management

# Biomatrix sclerofoam as a rival for endothermal ablation

JC Ragg

## Introduction

Foam sclerotherapy, introduced in 1995 by Juan Cabrera,[1] has rapidly developed to become an alternative to surgery.[2] Today it is estimated to be the most frequently used modality to eliminate varicose veins. Cabrera-type sclerofoams are provided by mixing liquid sclerosant agents like Polidocanol (Aethoxysklerol, Asclera) or sodium tetra decyl sulfate (Fibrovein) with gases such as room air or $O_2/CO_2$, usually in a pair of syringes.[3] The application of sclerofoam by simple injection into a target vein is relatively easy, cheap and fast. Foam easily reaches remote and tortuous vascular structures. However, in comparison of primary and long-term results, foam sclerotherapy is inferior to thermo-occlusion or to surgery.[4,5] There are several reasons: common sclerofoams are very light (usually 80% gas), so they tend to float on blood. With increasing vein diameter they will not so much displace blood, but rather float on it, leaving zones of uncertain effects. Viscosity and stability are low, foams will collapse within 60–240 seconds and rapidly lose contact with the vein wall. Additionally, overdosage may lead to thrombosis and embolism.[6] Sclerosant and released transmitters like endothelin-1 appear quickly in the circulation, provoking systemic side-effects.[7]

When the first reports were published in 2008 on the deactivation of sclerosants by blood proteins,[8] we started to evaluate the interactions of heat-denatured whole blood or cell-reduced blood fractions with liquid sclerosants. We developed mixing mechanisms to prepare viscous and stable foams with an *in vitro* half-life of >60 minutes (Figure 1), yet rapidly disintegrating without particles >20 when arriving in the bloodstream. The novel foams, e.g. containing 20% denatured autologous blood, 40% liquid and 40% gas, were called "biomatrix sclerofoam". Negotiations with the local ethics committee led to establishment in 2015 of a safety setting for a first study in great saphenous veins. To exclude the risk of foam migration via the junction, the application was combined with short proximal thermo-occlusion, comparing to cases with total thermo-occlusion treatment (Figure 3).

## Patients and methods

In the study, 120 patients (78 females/42 males; mean age 32–81 years) with great saphenous vein insufficiency, diameters 6–24mm (mean: 10.3mm), and eligibility for thermo-occlusion and sclerotherapy were included. Cases were randomised into two diameter-equivalent groups, receiving different treatments: group A (n=60) first underwent junction segment closure by endovenous laser (810nm, ball tip; or

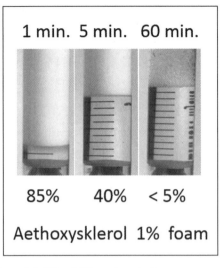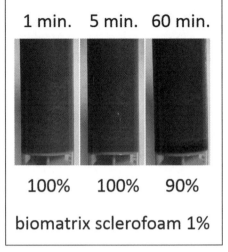

| 1 min. | 5 min. | 60 min. | 1 min. | 5 min. | 60 min. |
|--------|--------|---------|--------|--------|---------|
| 85% | 40% | < 5% | 100% | 100% | 90% |
| Aethoxysklerol 1% foam | | | biomatrix sclerofoam 1% | | |

**Figure 1:** Stability of different foams *in vitro.*

1470nm, slim/radial fibre, PhleboCath guide catheter 2.3mm Ø) in coaxial perivenous anaesthesia with varying segment lengths of 3–20cm. In this group, biomatrix sclerofoam (1% Aethoxysklerol, foam volumes 4–10ml) was then applied via the guide catheter after proven proximal closure (flushing with 5ml of "foamed saline") during catheter withdrawal under ultrasound monitoring, treating segments of 28–35cm in length. Group B (n=60) received endovenous laser for the whole insufficient vein length (38–55cm). Post-interventional examinations with standardised ultrasound were performed after two weeks and after two, six and 12 months by independent investigators.

## Results

Vein occlusion along the entire length intended to treat was obtained in all cases (120/120, visit week two) with both modalities in the first attempt. There were no adverse events; in particular, there were no thoracic or cerebral symptoms in the cases receiving sclerofoam. Group A cases required 38–77% less treatment time than those in group B, depending on the segment length. The investigators failed to discriminate modality-related intraluminal patterns of echogenicity or a borderline separating the modalities, except in a few cases (n=7) where high-energy 810nm laser left typical wall bruising. Vein diameter regression was similar (+/-12%) for laser and biomatrix sclerofoam. Both groups similarly showed mild post-interventional symptoms along the treated vein segments with no detectable difference related to the methods. In group B, veins with diameters >8 mm (n=11) showed no post-interventional symptoms.

During one-year follow-up, the laser-treated junction segments showed reperfusion in 2/60 cases in group A (3.33%) and in 1/60 in group B (1.6%). The thigh-to-knee segments showed partial reperfusion in 5/60 cases after biomatrix sclerofoam (8.33%, sources: junction n=2, side branches n=3) and in 6/60 cases after endovenous laser (10%, sources: junction n=1, perforator veins n=3, side branches n=2).

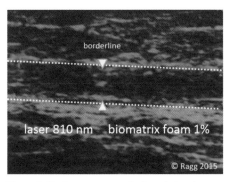

**Figure 2:** Similar appearance of vein occlusions by 810nm laser and biomatrix sclerofoam.

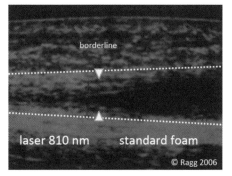

**Figure 3:** Inferiority of standard foam to 810nm laser: less diameter reduction, lower echogenicity indicating soft thrombus (study 2006).

## Discussion

The effect of stabilising foams by heated proteins is well known in the food and beverage industry, e.g. milk proteins for cappuccino. To use a blood protein matrix to provide a dense, viscous and stable sclerofoam may be a step further towards improving sclerotherapy. Foam placement, in particular when using catheters instead of cannulas, seems to be more precise with the novel composition, as blood replacement is more effective, and unintended foam washout is reduced. The biomatrix foam furthermore seems to be more effective than common foam, as contact time with the vein wall is increased. This is very different from recent attempts to provide an optimised sclerofoam in a constant quality from a pressurised dispenser (Varithena, BTG), as the concept still leans on the Cabrera principles with light and instable foams. It is no surprise that proof of progress is still missing.[9]

The first clinical application of a biomatrix sclerofoam presented in this report was surprisingly successful, as the effect on the target vein, according to closure rates, diameter reduction and echogenicity patterns was similar to laser-induced occlusion (Figure 2). This outcome was very different from earlier experience when our working group compared common Aethoxysklerol sclerofoam to endovenous laser in 2006 in a setting equivalent to this study, showing less lumen reduction and much higher rates of failure or relapse in foam-treated segments (32% after one year), so the strategy was abandoned (Figure 3). To replace thermo-occlusion by a foam-based modality is not just motivated by the redundancy of tumescent anaesthesia but also by the option to selectively include perforator veins and relevant side branches.

The junction is a difficult target for sclerofoam treatment as it is not possible to stop a foam column, expanding with the vein spasm, precisely at a certain spot without separate means. In most cases, the terminal valve is missing or destroyed, with the consequence of local turbulence and washout. Furthermore, epigastric vein inflow will flush the junction, limiting foam effects. Single or double balloon catheters have been proposed to stop foam propagation, and permanent or temporary occluding device (plugs) may become an alternative. Our group is currently developing a temporary occluding device integrated within a guidewire. Another project is vein lumen reduction by perivenous injection of hyaluronan[10] which could potentially provide a totally symptom-free regression phase even in very large saphenous diameters (>15mm diameter), competing with vein gluing. Focal hyaluronan injection, being more precise and durable than tumescent fluids, could also be used to achieve a low-cost blockage of the junction.

Future applications of the novel biomatrix foam could include saphenous veins of all diameters, but also short targets like vein stumps or perforator insufficiencies, large recurrent varicosities, abdominal varices, varicoceles and maybe even low-flow vascular malformations, and skipping expensive coils.

## Conclusion

According to these first results, biomatrix sclerofoam seems to be a safe and effective modality to provide vein closure. The primary and one year results are similar to endovenous laser, apart from the excluded junction segment. Future studies will include biomatrix sclerofoam application in the saphenous junction (stand-alone), with temporary or permanent blocking devices and hyaluronan vein compression, and comparison to common foam sclerosants.

## Summary

- To improve foam sclerotherapy for larger veins, the development of more viscous and stable sclerofoams is required

- Biomatrix sclerofoam, integrating autologous heat-denatured blood proteins, is a new way to provide foams with the desired properties

- Apart from the junction segments, the tested biomatrix sclerofoam performs at a quality level similar to thermo-occlusion, but without need for anaesthesia

- The novel foams could become an alternative as a stand-alone modality in veins up to 8mm diameter, and combined with thermo-occlusion, blocking device or hyaluronan compression for veins of any diameter

- Approval studies will be carried out as soon as manufacturers have succeeded to provide a reasonably priced single use foaming device

## References

1. Cabrera J, Cabrera J jr. Nuevo método de esclerosis en las varices troncolares. Patol Vasc. 1995; 4:55–73
2. Bergan JJ, Pascarella L. Severe chronic venous insufficiency: primary treatment with sclerofoam. *Semin Vasc Surg* 2005; **18** (1): 49–56.
3. Wollmann JC. The history of sclerosing foams. *Dermatol Surg* 2004; **30**: 694–703
4. Rasmussen LH, Lawaetz M, Bjoern L *et al.* Randomized clinical trial comparing endovenous laser ablation, radiofrequency ablation, foam sclerotherapy and surgical stripping for great saphenous varicose veins. *Br J Surg* 2011; **98** (8): 1079–87.
5. Van den Bos R, Arends L, Kockaert M. *et al.* Endovenous therapies of lower extremity varicosities: a meta-analysis. *J Vasc Surg.* 2009; **49**: 230–39.
6. Guex JJ, Allaert FA, Gillet JL. Immediate and midterm complications of sclerotherapy: Report of a prospective multicenter registry of 12,173 sclerotherapy sessions. *Dermatol Surg* 2005; **31**: 123–28.
7. Frullini A, Felice F, Burchielli S, Di Stefano R. High production of endothelin after foam sclerotherapy: a new pathogenetic hypothesis for neurological and visual disturbances after sclerotherapy. *Phlebology* 2011; **26** (5): 203–08.
8. Parsi KET, Connor DE, Herbert A, *et al.* The lytic effects of detergent sclerosants on erythrocytes, platelets, endothelial cells and microparticles are attenuated by albumin and other plasma components in vitro. *Eur J Vasc Endovasc Surg* 2008; **36**:216–2

9. Gibson K, Kabnick L on behalf of the Varithena Investigator Group. A multicenter, randomized, placebo-controlled study to evaluate the efficacy and safety of Varithena (polidocanol endovenous microfoam 1%) for symptomatic, visible varicose veins with saphenofemoral junction incompetence. *Phlebology* 2016. pii: 0268355516635386.

10. Ragg JC. Endovenous techniques: US-guided perivenous hyaluronan injection or saline tumescence? *Vein Therapy News* 2015; **9**:12–14

# Anti-venous thrombosis protocol—a proposed scoring system

SJ Goodyear, A Wagstaff and IK Nyamekye

## Introduction

Deep vein thrombosis is a recognised complication of endovenous procedures, even when performed under local anaesthesia.[1-4] Wide ranging incidence is reported (range 0–16%), with the upper figures being skewed by endovenous heat-induced thrombosis in older reports.[1,2,5,6] However, deep vein thrombosis and pulmonary embolism— although rare—are a reality of venous therapies, with deaths of relatively young patients being reported in the press.[7,8] Occurrence of these outcomes attests to a need for some form of targeted thromboprophylaxis in this patient group and, given the potential for litigation and the absence of good evidence and limited professional consensus, should be of significant concern for practising specialists. The recent precedent set by the judgement in Montgomery vs. Lanarkshire Health Board signals the importance of addressing such potentially serious complications.[9]

## Strategies for managing deep vein thrombosis prophylaxis

The risk of deep venous thrombosis and pulmonary embolism is well recognised by vascular specialists. Phlebologists have extended the practice of graduated compression stockings and anticoagulant thromboprophylaxis from their typical use in managing the risk of perioperative venous thromboembolism in patients undergoing general surgery or open varicose veins surgery to managing this risk in patients undergoing endovenous interventions. Low molecular weight heparin has long been the mainstay of pharmacological thromboprophylaxis in general surgery, where it is associated with significant reductions in postoperative deep vein thrombosis.[10] Caprini's summary of the relative efficacy of thromboprophylaxis methods showed that compared with placebo, the incidence of total deep vein thrombosis was reduced by approximately 44% with graduated compression stockings and by 76% with low molecular weight heparin.[10] However, the extent to which graduated compression stockings and low molecular weight heparin confer additional benefit over aggressive mobilisation following ambulatory endovenous treatment is not known.[11] Relevant evidence is virtually non-existent because of the difficulties of conducting high quality research in this area. The relatively rare incidence of venous thromboembolism in this patient group and the very large numbers that would be required makes randomised controlled trials impractical.

This absence of trial evidence (and limited guidelines recommendations) for thromboprophylaxis in patients undergoing ambulatory endovenous treatment has resulted in variable thromboprophylaxis management in UK (and probably international as well) endovenous practice. Venous thromboembolism guidelines from England's National Institute for Health and Care Excellence (NICE) and the American College of Chest Physicians (ACCP) focus on in-patients undergoing major surgery rather than those undergoing venous interventions.[12–14] Only the Scottish Intercollegiate Guideline Network (SIGN) make specific recommendation for both venous surgery and endovenous procedures. They advocate graduated compression stockings use only for patients undergoing endovenous procedures unless a patient has additional thromboembolic risk factors—in which case, heparin thromboprophylaxis is added.[15] However, SIGN concede that evidence for these recommendations is only based on non-analytic studies and expert opinion. This limited direct guidance, the relatively minor trauma of endovenous treatments and patients' almost immediate return to preoperative levels of mobility has led some phlebologists to question the need for ever administering pharmacological thromboprophylaxis to this cohort.

## The need for a targeted venous thromboembolism risk protocol for endovenous patients

Management of deep vein thrombosis risk in surgical practice should be based on objective risk stratification, with higher risk individuals receiving appropriate mechanical and low molecular weight heparin thromboprophylaxis.[12,16,17] Procedure- and patient-based risk assessment protocols are typically used. Procedure-based protocols depend on operation type (site and level of surgical trauma) and duration with major procedures, extended duration and prolonged immobilisation signalling elevated risk and mandating thromboprophylaxis. Such protocols are of limited usefulness for patients undergoing local anaesthetic endovenous interventions that usually last significantly less than 60-minutes and are invariably followed by immediate mobilisation. Likewise, patient-based risk assessment protocols such as Caprini scores and the UK Department of Health venous thromboembolism tool are best suited to patients undergoing inpatient care as many of the formative risk factors are not applicable to endovenous patients.[17–19]

## A suggested new scoring system

Because of this existing background of uncertainty and variable practice, we have worked towards developing a risk assessment protocol that focuses upon factors directly applicable to patients undergoing endovenous intervention with the aim of providing more meaningful and targeted deep vein thrombosis risk stratification. While developing our proposed "Worcester score", we performed a questionnaire survey of vein specialists; therefore, the survey was conducted on members of the Vascular Society for Great Britain and Ireland and delegates attending the 2016 Charing Cross International Symposium and the 2016 joint meeting of the Venous Forum and the European Venous Forum (Questionnaire).

Unfortunately, the response rate was poor in all three instances and no attempt was made to collate the data for presentation. However, six factors most frequently cited as being significant by respondents were selected and the authors agreed a simple weighting of one or two for each score to produce the Worcester protocol and scoring system. The six weighted factors are as follows: patients score one point each for obesity (defined as a body mass index of >30), contraceptive medication or

## Current Perceptions of DVT risk factors in endovenous Varicose Vein surgery

### Endovenous practice

1. Do you perform endovenous procedures for varicose veins / chronic venous insufficiency?

○ Yes

○ No

2. How significant would you consider the following risk factors for VTE following endovenous surgery? *(indicate on the visual analogue scale)*:

| | Very low risk | | | | | | | | | Very high risk |
|---|---|---|---|---|---|---|---|---|---|---|
| Age ≥75 | ○ | ○ | ○ | ○ | ○ | ○ | ○ | ○ | ○ | ○ |
| Age 61 - 74 | ○ | ○ | ○ | ○ | ○ | ○ | ○ | ○ | ○ | ○ |
| Age 41 - 60 | ○ | ○ | ○ | ○ | ○ | ○ | ○ | ○ | ○ | ○ |
| BMI >30 | ○ | ○ | ○ | ○ | ○ | ○ | ○ | ○ | ○ | ○ |
| Procedure duration >1 hour | ○ | ○ | ○ | ○ | ○ | ○ | ○ | ○ | ○ | ○ |
| Reduced mobility/Impaired calf-pump function | ○ | ○ | ○ | ○ | ○ | ○ | ○ | ○ | ○ | ○ |
| Smoking | ○ | ○ | ○ | ○ | ○ | ○ | ○ | ○ | ○ | ○ |
| Use of HRT | ○ | ○ | ○ | ○ | ○ | ○ | ○ | ○ | ○ | ○ |
| Use of hormonal contraception | ○ | ○ | ○ | ○ | ○ | ○ | ○ | ○ | ○ | ○ |
| Long haul flight (>3 hours); 4 weeks pre- or post- procedure | ○ | ○ | ○ | ○ | ○ | ○ | ○ | ○ | ○ | ○ |
| Personal history of VTE | ○ | ○ | ○ | ○ | ○ | ○ | ○ | ○ | ○ | ○ |
| Family History of VTE | ○ | ○ | ○ | ○ | ○ | ○ | ○ | ○ | ○ | ○ |
| Past history of malignancy | ○ | ○ | ○ | ○ | ○ | ○ | ○ | ○ | ○ | ○ |
| Inherited thrombophilia | ○ | ○ | ○ | ○ | ○ | ○ | ○ | ○ | ○ | ○ |
| Moderate/Major surgery within 12 weeks | ○ | ○ | ○ | ○ | ○ | ○ | ○ | ○ | ○ | ○ |

3. Would you prescribe conventional pharmacological VTE prophylaxis (low molecular weight heparin) in the presence of the following risk factors?

| | YES | NO |
|---|---|---|
| Age ≥75 | ○ | ○ |
| Age 61 - 74 | ○ | ○ |
| Age 41 - 60 | ○ | ○ |
| BMI > 30 | ○ | ○ |
| Procedure duration >1 hour | ○ | ○ |
| Reduced mobility/Impaired calf-pump function | ○ | ○ |
| Smoking | ○ | ○ |
| Use of HRT | ○ | ○ |
| Use of hormonal contraception | ○ | ○ |
| Personal history of VTE | ○ | ○ |
| Family history of VTE | ○ | ○ |
| Past history of malignancy | ○ | ○ |
| Inherited thrombophilia | ○ | ○ |
| Moderate/Major surgery within 12 weeks | ○ | ○ |

| Targeted factors | Score |
|---|---|
| Obesity (BMI >30) | 1 |
| Hormonal medication | 1 |
| Thrombophlebitis | 1 |
| 1$^{ary}$ /1$^{st}$ degree VTE | 2 |
| Limb immobility | 2 |
| Thrombophilia* | 2 |

| Total score | Risk |
|---|---|
| 0 Points | Low |
| 1 Points | Moderate |
| 2 Points | High |

**Table 1:** The Worcester venous thromboembolism risk score for endovenous procedures. Patients with a history of cancer or inflammatory conditions such as inflammatory bowel disease or rheumatoid arthritis are automatically classified as high risk

hormone replacement therapies (HRT) that increase venous thromboembolism risk, and symptomatic (active) superficial vein thrombosis. They score two points each for history of proven venous thromboembolism, any compromise of calf "muscle-pump" function, defined as inability to walk to/from the intervention room, and known thrombophilia. Patients' total score then stratifies their risk as low (score 0), moderate (score 1) or high (score ≥2).

As previously indicated, the rarity of venous thromboembolism events following endovenous treatment has made it impractical to test this score in any type of randomised study. We have compared this unvalidated Worcester protocol with the UK Department of Health protocol in a retrospective study. The two scores were then compared to our original clinical decision to give low molecular weight heparin (used as a surrogate for clinician determined increased venous thromboembolism risk) on a historical cohort of patients on a local database.

Overall, 276 patients treated during an 18-month period (from November 2014) were assessed with the score. Their average age was 55 years and just over half (55%) of them were women. Twenty-one patients were clinically assessed as being at increased risk of venous thromboembolism and were treated prophylactically with extended low molecular weight heparin. Indications for treatment included: active thrombophlebitis, use of hormonal therapy, history of venous thromboembolism and raised body mass index. No venous thromboembolism occurred in this cohort.

Of 36 patients (13%) classified as moderate or high risk according to the Department of Health risk score, 47% had been given prophylactic treatment. However, four patients who were scored as low risk had also been clinically assessed as being at increased risk. The Worcester risk score deemed 60 patients (22%) to be at moderate or high risk—capturing all patients who had been clinically assessed as being at increased risk (Figure 1). The score, therefore, appears to be more discriminating than the Department of Health protocol in predicting the clinical decision to give low molecular weight heparin in this patient cohort. This provides—albeit weak—evidence that the Worcester score may be a more effective risk assessment tool than the existing protocol in this patient group.

## Duration of deep vein thrombosis prophylaxis

After thromboprophylaxis has been assessed, as indicated, duration of low molecular weight heparin thromboprophylaxis is a second area of controversy and variability in endovenous practice. In a poll at the 2014 UK-Venous Forum meeting, a clear majority of specialists favoured single-dose low molecular weight heparin as their choice for thromboprophylaxis despite conflicting evidence from haematologists. Haematologists' argument against this practice is based on epidemiological evidence from the Million Women Study (Sweetland *et al*) relating to post-procedural venous thromboembolism incidence and time since surgery.[20] This study assessed time since surgery and the relative risk of venous thromboembolism after inpatient surgery and day surgery. By demonstrating that both types of surgery are associated with a significantly elevated risk of postoperative deep vein thrombosis, it shows that the risk period is extended—commencing on the day of surgery and remaining elevated for weeks into the postoperative period. This extended risk period indicates that any prescribed thromboprophylaxis should be continued into the postoperative period to be protective during the patient's "at risk" phase.[20] Thus, clinicians who administer single dose low molecular weight heparin to patients assessed as being high risk for deep vein thrombosis may be failing to provide effective thromboprophylaxis.[11] If low molecular weight heparin prophylaxis, when indicated, is to be extended into the postoperative period, the actual duration of this treatment extension after endovenous treatment is not currently defined.

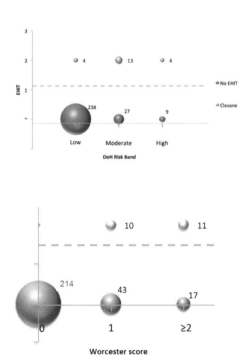

**Figure 1:** Charts showing predictive value of the Department of Health and Worcester scores *vs.* use of clinician-determined selective low molecular weight heparin (LWMH). Bubbles charts for the Department of Health and Worcester scores. Risk groups for each protocol are shown as blue bubbles, and green bubbles represent patients from each category who were clinically assessed to be at increased risk of venous thromboembolism (and given extended prophylactic LMWH). The bubble size reflects the number of patients in each category.

# Conclusion

Ambulatory endovenous treatments, like all invasive procedures, have the potential to induce venous thromboembolism with occasional devastating sequelae. All patients should be risk assessed and those at increased risk given appropriate thromboprophylaxis. However, applicable evidence and guidance remains sparse, and the validity and usefulness of existing risk-stratification models has been questioned. This has led to highly variable practice and controversy, potentially impacting venous thromboembolism outcomes after endovenous treatment. The proposed Worcester protocol is our response, until better evidence becomes available, to the need for a tailored risk assessment protocol aimed at standardising safe thromboprophylaxis and generating an evidence base for patients undergoing endovenous treatment.

In practice, all suitably mobile patients are immediately mobilised and appropriate graduated compression stockings are prescribed for those without peripheral vascular disease. We add low molecular weight heparin thromboprophylaxis for patients with moderate or high Worcester scores ($\geq 1$). Our practice is to extend low molecular weight heparin treatment for one week in moderate risk (Worcester score 1) and four weeks in high risk (Worcester Score $\geq 2$) patients.

Our future direction will focus on further questionnaire data to improve the Worcester protocol and on inviting validation of the present score against any existing endovenous databases. We also hope to conduct a prospective multicentre cohort study comparing use of the Worcester protocol with current practice.

## Summary

- Venous thromboembolism is a recognised but relatively rare complication of ambulatory endovenous procedures.

- There is need for targeted thromboprophylaxis in this patient group.

- Patients should be risk assessed and those at increased risk given appropriate thromboprophylaxis.

- Scarcity of evidence and guidance and limited usefulness of existing risk-stratification models has led to highly variable practice and controversy endovenous practice.

- A simple six-factor "Worcester protocol" is presented and may be more discriminating than existing protocols.

- Single shot low molecular weight heparin thromboprophylaxis (for preventing deep vein thrombosis), popular in the UK, is ineffective because the postoperative risk period is prolonged.

- Prescribed thromboprophylaxis should be continued postoperatively for effective protection, however, the actual duration of treatment extension is not currently defined.

- Independent validation of the Worcester score using any existing endovenous or in a prospective cohort study is invited.

# References

1. Marsh P, Price BA, Holdstock J, *et al.* Deep vein thrombosis (DVT) after venous thermoablation techniques: rates of endovenous heat-induced thrombosis (EHIT) and classical DVT after radiofrequency and endovenous laser ablation in a single centre. *Eur J Vasc Endovasc Surg* 2010; **40** (4): 521–27

2. Kulkarni S, Messenger DE, Slim FJA, *et al.* The incidence and characterization of deep vein thrombosis following ultrasound-guided foam sclerotherapy in 1000 legs with superficial venous reflux. *Journal of Vascular Surgery* 2013; **1** (3): 231–38.

3. Hingorani AP, Ascher E, Markevich N, *et al.* Deep venous thrombosis after radiofrequency ablation of greater saphenous vein: a word of caution. *J Vasc Surg* 2004; **40** (3): 500–04.

4. Carradice D, Leung C, Chetter I. Laser; best practice techniques and evidence. *Phlebology* 2015; **30** (2 Suppl): 36-41

5. Kabnick LS, Ombrellino M, Agis H, *et al.* Endovenous heat induced thrombus (EHIT) at the superficial-deep venous junction: a new post-treatment clinical entity, classification and potential treatment strategies. 18th Annual Meeting of the American Venous Forum, Miami, Florida; 2006.

6. Sutton PA, El-Dhuwaib Y, Dyer J, Guy AJ. The incidence of post-operative venous thromboembolism in patients undergoing varicose vein surgery recorded in Hospital Episode Statistics. *Ann R Coll Surg Eng* 2012; **9 4**(7): 481–83.

7. The Daily Mail. Mother-of-two's death after varicose vein surgery 'could have been prevented', her husband claims. http://www.dailymail.co.uk/health/article-2980924/Mother-two-s-death-varicose-vein-surgery-prevented-husband-claims.html (date accessed 08.02.17).

8. RTE News. Inquest into the death of Karen McCabe adjourned until May. http://www.rte.ie/news/2016/0218/769058-inquest-varicose-veins-surgery-death (date accessed 08.02.17).

9. United Kingdom Supreme Court. Judgement: Montgomery Vs Lanarkshire Health Board (2015). https://www.supremecourt.uk/decided-cases/docs/UKSC_2013_0136_Judgment.pdf (date accessed 08.02.17).

10. Caprini JJ. Chapter 41: Thrombotic Risk Assessment: A Hybrid Approach. The Vein Book (ed. Bergan JJ). 2007 Elselvier inc.

11. Goodyear SJ, Nyamekye I. Rational anti-DVT prophylaxis for ambulatory varicose veins procedures. In: Greenhalge R. M. (Ed.) Vascular and Endovascular Challenges Update. London: BIBA Publishing, 2016, pp. 541-549

12. National Clinical Guideline Centre. Acute and Chronic Conditions (UK). Venous Thromboembolism: Reducing the Risk of Venous Thromboembolism (Deep Vein Thrombosis and Pulmonary Embolism) in Patients Admitted to Hospital. National Institute for Clinical and Health Excellence: Guidance. http://bit.ly/2kH7B6N (date accessed 08.02.17)

13. Kahn SR, Lim W, Dunn AS, *et al.* Prevention of VTE in Nonsurgical PatientsPrevention of VTE in Nonsurgical Patients: Antithrombotic Therapy and Prevention of Thrombosis, 9th ed: American College of Chest Physicians Evidence-Based Clinical Practice Guidelines. *Chest* 2012; **141** (2_suppl): e195S-–e226S

14. Gloviczki P, Comerota AJ, Dalsing MC, *et al.* The care of patients with varicose veins and associated chronic venous diseases: Clinical practice guidelines of the Society for Vascular Surgery and the American Venous Forum. *J Vasc Surg* 2011; **53**: 2S-48S (May 2011 Supplement).

15. Scottish Intercollegiate Guideline Network. Guideline 122: Prevention and management of venous thromboembolism: http://www.sign.ac.uk/pdf/sign122.pdf (date accessed 08.02.17).

16. National Institute for Health and Care Excellence. Venous thromboembolism in adults: reducing their risk in hospital (Quality Standard 3). http://bit.ly/2kNctd2 (date accessed 08.02.17)

17. Department of Health. Risk assessment for venous thromboembolism (VTE).

18. Caprini JJ. Chapter 41: Thrombotic Risk Assessment: A Hybrid Approach. The Vein Book (ed. Bergan JJ). 2007 Elselvier inc.

19. Rogers SO Jr, Kilaru RK, Hosokawa P, *et al.* Multivariable predictors of postoperative venous thromboembolic events after general and vascular surgery: results from the patient safety in surgery study. *J Am Coll Surg* 2007; **204** (6):1211–21

20. Sweetland S, Green J, Liu B, *et al.* Million Women Study collaborators.Duration and magnitude of the postoperative risk of venous thromboembolism in middle aged women: prospective cohort study. *BMJ* 2009; **339**: b4583.

# Leg ulceration

# Biological strategies for wound healing

M Kanapathy, J Hunckler, A Mosahebi and T Richards

## Introduction

Wound management represents a significant financial and resource burden to the healthcare system with the prevalence of patients with wounds in the UK alone estimated to be approximately 2.2 million, requiring over 40 million healthcare visits and consuming about 340 million dressings annually.[1,2] Between £2.3 billion and £3.1 billion is spent in caring for patients with chronic wounds in the UK alone.[3] Chronic wounds account for a burdening problem with over 100,000 new ulcers anticipated every year, with an ageing population and rising prevalence of obesity and diabetes.[4] On average, 61% of chronic wounds take up to a year to heal.[2] Hence, measures to enhance wound healing are beneficial to patients, also crucial to reduce cost and burden of wound management.

The wound healing process is still an unclear, highly orchestrated series of mechanisms, involving different and interlinked sets of cellular events and biological cascades. This complexity makes the creation and validation of an efficient new treatment a challenge, despite being highly necessary to reduce the healthcare burden and improve the patient's quality of life. This chapter outlines three strategies for wound healing that are currently being studied at our centre: epidermal graft, platelet-rich plasma with autologous adipose derived stem cell, and electrical stimulation therapy.

## Epidermal grafting for wound healing

Epidermal grafts for wound healing involves the transfer of the epidermal layer from an area of healthy skin to the wound bed. The epidermal grafts are harvested by applying continuous negative pressure on the donor site to promote blister formation (Figure 1). The roof of the blister, which is the epidermis, is then excised and transferred to the wound. The superficial nature of the graft enables this autologous skin grafting to be performed in a relatively pain free manner in an outpatient setting with minimal or no donor site morbidity.

The epidermal graft has been reported to behave more like a tissue engineered skin graft or a cultured keratinocyte sheet, which stimulates the wound to regenerate by itself rather than to provide instant wound coverage as seen with full-thickness skin graft and split thickness skin graft. Cultured keratinocytes have been used for resurfacing burn wounds and in the treatment of skin ulcers since the 1970s. However, the clinical application of the cultured keratinocytes has been limited by the short-term and long-term results: variable graft take rate, limited mechanical

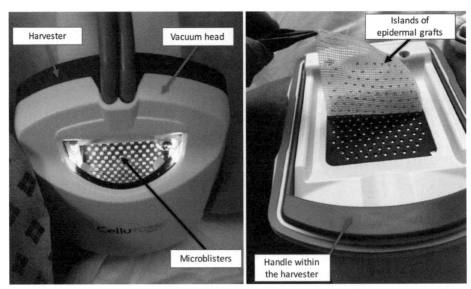

**Figure 1:** The harvest technique. The microblisters, visible through the window of the vacuum head, were raised within half an hour by combining negative pressure of 400–500mmHg and temperature of 40 degrees Celcius. The vacuum head was then detached, leaving behind the harvester. The handle within the harvester, attached to an in-built blade, was then pulled up to excise the roof of the blister. The epidermal grafts were then transferred using a silicon dressing to the wound.

resistance, hyperkeratosis, scar contracture, ulceration and blister formation due to reaction towards foreign fibroblasts in feeder media. These results, accompanied by the long culture time (typically requiring three to four weeks), the fragility of the sheets, and the high cost, has limited the use of this technique to only specialised facilities.

Epidermal grafts are advantageous as they do not require a carrier system, additional culture time, or a specialised facility. The epidermal graft harvesting systems separate the epidermis from the dermis at the dermal-epidermal junction while preserving the histological architecture of the epidermis, constituents of which contributes to its unique wound healing mechanism. The healing by epidermal graft is influenced by the interplay of three main mechanisms: keratinocyte activation, growth factor secretion and re-epithelialisation from the wound edge. *In vitro* studies showed that the migrating keratinocytes from the transplanted grafts synthesise several growth factors, namely the vascular endothelial growth factor, hepatocyte growth factor, granulocyte colony-stimulating factor, platelet-derived growth factor, and transforming growth factor α. The migrating keratinocytes also deposit a variety of extracellular matrix components, such as laminin, fibronectin, and type IV collagen.

In a pilot study done in our centre at the Royal Free Hospital London involving 35 patients, seven out of 10 patients achieved complete healing within six weeks, a healing rate which is comparable to split skin graft. None of the patients had donor site scarring. In another study that we conducted to evaluate and compare the patient-reported outcome measure between epidermal and split-skin grafts revealed that complete satisfaction with donor site appearance was observed in 100% of the epidermal graft cases (and 50% of split skin cases). Noticeability, adverse problems and overall satisfaction were significantly better in epidermal graft cases. Furthermore, our cost evaluation study revealed that the cost per patient for epidermal graft was £431 and £1,489 for split skin graft, with an annual saving of £126,960 based on 10 grafts per month.

Several clinical trials are currently underway to investigate the efficacy of epidermal graft in the clinical setting using the cellutome epidermal harvesting system. We are currently undertaking a randomised controlled trial to evaluate the efficacy of epidermal graft against split skin graft (EPIGRAAFT Trial).[5] This trial will also include mechanistic analysis to further understand the difference in the mechanism of wound healing between the two techniques. Another large randomised multicentre controlled trial is comparing the safety and effectiveness of epidermal graft combined with multi-layered compression therapy for the healing of venous leg ulcers.[6] The findings from these high-quality trials will define the efficacy of this technique and further improve our understanding of the mechanism of healing by epidermal graft.

## Platelet-rich plasma and autologous adipose derived stem cells for wound healing

Platelet-rich plasma is an autologous blood-derived product enriched in platelets, growth factors, chemokines and cytokines. It is a reservoir of essential growth factors, including platelet-derived growth factor, vascular endothelial growth factor, transforming growth factor-beta 1, and insulin-like growth factor which facilitate repair and healing. Platelet-derived biologic mediators have two primary effects on wound healing: recruiting and activating cells that effect wound healing, and regulation of angiogenesis.[7] Platelets may also have antimicrobial and immune modulation properties which help to reduce wound infection and facilitate healing. Several authors have found improved wound healing in a variety of wounds including burns, chronic ulcers and traumatic wounds when platelet-rich plasma is applied to non-healing wounds or when combined with split skin grafts. However, the evidence is limited with two systematic reviews illustrating no clear benefit of platelet-rich plasma on wound healing, owing to the poor-quality evidence available.

The use of fat graft for wound healing is becoming more common. Adipose-derived stem cells or mesenchymal stem cells found in fat are believed to facilitate healing through differentiation into cells that effect wound healing, e.g. fibroblasts, keratinocytes. They also release pro-healing growth factors and anti-inflammatory cytokines as well as healing-related peptides such as leptin and adiponectin which together may enhance wound healing. Several studies have shown significant improvement in wound healing with fat grafting including use in chronic wounds, burns, skin fibrosis, traumatic wounds, diabetic ulcers and osteoarthritis.

When used in combination, platelet-rich plasma may increase the survival of the fat grafts. This is believed to be due to the pro-angiogenic effects of platelet-rich plasma, which allows early vascularisation of the fat therefore reversing the early ischaemic phase of the graft. Another pro-survival effect may be the release of anti-inflammatory chemokines, which help reduce inflammation and swelling which encourage degeneration of the graft. Hypotheses also exist that suggest platelet-rich plasma may provide nutrient support to the fat cells through its plasma component and that the fibrin component allows formation of a scaffold for fat cells. A few small studies have demonstrated a significant improvement in retention of fat grafts when combined with platelet-rich plasma in both facial and breast grafting. Cervelli *et al* also demonstrated excellent re-epithelialisation of chronic lower limb wounds when platelet-rich plasma and fat grafting were combined.

However, current evidence is limited to phase 1 clinical trials evaluating the safety and efficacy of fat grafting and platelet-rich plasma in wound healing as well as pre-clinical study. We are currently evaluating the efficacy of fat grafting for wound healing, and to further investigate the outcome of platelet-rich plasma and fat graft in combination. We hypothesise that the combination of platelet-rich plasma and fat graft would speed and improve healing further. We wish to compare the wound healing outcome between the groups, and whether an improved healing is achieved with combination of autologous fat graft with platelet-rich plasma.

## Electrical stimulation therapy

Across the tissues of the human body, asymmetric ionic flows generate endogenous electrical potentials. A transepithelial electrical potential, named skin battery, is naturally generated by the movement of ions through Na+/K+ ATPase pumps of the epidermis.[8] The current of injury, which is essential for normal wound healing, is generated during skin injury and creates an electrical potential across the wound.[8,9] Healing is arrested when the flow of current is disturbed or stopped by prolonged opening, such as in the case of chronic wound. We hypothesise that, by applying an exogenous electrical stimulation on the chronic wound, the current of injury would be simulated and reactivated, leading to healing of the wound.

The effect of electrical stimulation has already been tested *in vitro* on different cell types involved in wound healing, such as macrophages, fibroblasts, epidermal cells, bacteria, and endothelial cells, and have reported changes in cell migration, proliferation and orientation, and increase in proteins and DNA synthesis. The mechanisms by which cells sense and respond to electrical stimulation remain relatively unclear, making *in vitro* studies essential. This is why we want to highlight the importance of the polarity of the applied current on the collective cell behaviour during a scratch-wounded healing assay *in vitro*.

When applied on *in vivo* models and clinical studies, electrical stimulation therapy has shown interesting positive effects on wound closure and healing rate. An *in vivo* study of acute wounds has shown that electrical stimulation accelerate wound healing in a diabetic rat model where the wound closure is usually delayed.[10] Moreover, the reduced expression of Collagen-I, α-Smooth muscle actin and transforming growth factor-β1 of the diabetic model were restored back to normal with electrical stimulation, suggesting that the electrical stimulation treatment might enhance the healing of acute diabetic wounds. Several clinical studies have been conducted in the last few years on chronic[11] and acute wounds,[12] reporting faster healing and upregulation of vascular endothelial growth factor and platelet growth factor when electrical stimulation therapy is applied. In electrical stimulation therapy, there are mainly four type of current used in wound healing: direct current, alternative current, pulsed current and transcutaneous electrical nerve stimulation. However, there is a considerable variation in study design, outcome measures, electrical stimulation parameters, and treatment duration, and dose, thus exploring further evidence on the optimal approach of electrical stimulation for the treatment of cutaneous wound healing is crucial.

# Conclusion

These biological strategies for wound healing hold promise as a potential alternative to the conventional therapies as it stimulates endogenous wound healing, relatively inexpensive, and ultimately improves the quality of life of patients. The increased number of publications in the last couple of years testifies to the growing clinical popularity of these techniques. However, more work needs to be done to better understand the mechanism of healing at the cellular level in order to propose an evidence-based clinical pathway.

## Summary

- Newer strategies are required to overcome current strategies of managing chronic wounds.

- Epidermal grafting is an option for autologous skin grafting which can be performed in the outpatient setting without anaesthesia and results in no donor site morbidity.

- Platelet-rich plasma and autologous adipose derived stem cell can enhance healing of chronic wounds by secreting pro-healing cytokines and growth factors.

- Electrical stimulation therapy may be able to restore the electrical potential across wounds to reactivate endogenous healing.

# References

1. Brigham PA, McLoughlin E. Burn incidence and medical care use in the United States: estimates, trends, and data sources. *The Journal of Burn Care & Rehabilitation* 1996; **17** (2): 95–107.
2. Guest JF, Ayoub N, McIlwraith T, *et al*. Health economic burden that different wound types impose on the UK's National Health Service. *Int Wound J* 2017; **14** (2): 322–33.
3. Phillips CJ, Humphreys I, Fletcher J, *et al*. Estimating the costs associated with the management of patients with chronic wounds using linked routine data. *Int Wound J* 2016; **13** (6): 1193–97.
4. Sen CK, Gordillo GM, Roy S, *et al*. Human skin wounds: A major and snowballing threat to public health and the economy. *Wound Repair and Regeneration* 2009; **17** (6): 763–71.
5. Kanapathy M, Hachach-Haram N, Bystrzonowski N, *et al*. Epidermal grafting *versus* split-thickness skin grafting for wound healing (EPIGRAAFT): study protocol for a randomised controlled trial. *Trials* 2016; **17** (1): 245.
6. SerenaGroup I. Clinical Trial to Evaluate Blister Graft Utilizing a Novel Harvesting Device for Treatment of Venous Leg Ulcers (Cellutome). In: ClinicalTrials.gov [Internet]. Bethesda (MD): National Library of Medicine (US). http://bit.ly/2l7pQ3y (date accessed 24 February 2017).
7. Frechette JP, Martineau I, Gagnon G. Platelet-rich plasmas: growth factor content and roles in wound healing. *Journal of Dental Research* 2005; **84** (5): 434–49.
8. Zhao M, Song B, Pu J, *et al*. Electrical signals control wound healing through phosphatidylinositol-3-OH kinase-|[gamma]| and PTEN. *Nature* 2006; **442**: 457–60.
9. Reid B, Song B, McCaig CD, Zhao M. Wound healing in rat cornea: the role of electric currents. *FASEB Journal* 2005; **19** (3): 379–86.
10. Kim TH, Cho H-Y, Lee SM. High-voltage pulsed current stimulation enhances wound healing in diabetic rats by restoring the expression of collagen, α-smooth muscle actin, and TGF-β1. *The Tohoku journal of Experimental Medicine* 2014; **234** (1): 1–6.
11. Magnoni C, Rossi E, Fiorentini C, *et al*. Electrical stimulation as adjuvant treatment for chronic leg ulcers of different aetiology: an RCT. *Journal of Wound Care* 2013; **22** (10): 525–26
12. Ud-Din S, Sebastian A, Giddings P, Colthurst J, *et al*. Angiogenesis is induced and wound size is reduced by electrical stimulation in an acute wound healing model in human skin. *PloS One* 2015; **10** (4): e0124502